CURRICULUM DEVELOPMENT FOR MEDICAL EDUCATION

CURRICULUM DEVELOPMENT FOR MEDICAL EDUCATION

A SIX-STEP APPROACH

Fourth Edition

Edited by

Patricia A. Thomas, MD

David E. Kern, MD, MPH

Mark T. Hughes, MD, MA

Sean A. Tackett, MD, MPH

Belinda Y. Chen, MD

JOHNS HOPKINS UNIVERSITY PRESS | BALTIMORE

© 2022 Johns Hopkins University Press
All rights reserved. Published 2022
Printed in the United States of America on acid-free paper
2 4 6 8 9 7 5 3 1

Johns Hopkins University Press
2715 North Charles Street
Baltimore, Maryland 21218-4363
www.press.jhu.edu

Library of Congress Cataloging-in-Publication Data

Names: Thomas, Patricia A. (Patricia Ann), 1950– editor. | Kern, David E., editor. |
Hughes, Mark T., editor. | Tackett, Sean, 1982– editor. | Chen, Belinda Y., 1966– editor.
Title: Curriculum development for medical education : a six-step approach / edited by
Patricia A. Thomas, MD, David E. Kern, MD, MPH, Mark T. Hughes, MD, MA,
Sean A. Tackett, MD, MPH, Belinda Y. Chen, MD.
Description: Fourth edition. | Baltimore : Johns Hopkins University Press, [2022] |
Includes bibliographical references and index.
Identifiers: LCCN 2021048343 | ISBN 9781421444093 (hardcover ; alk. paper) | ISBN 9781421444109
(paperback ; alk. paper) | ISBN 9781421444116 (ebook)
Subjects: MESH: Curriculum | Education, Medical
Classification: LCC R737 | NLM W 18 | DDC 610.71/1—dc23/eng/20211101
LC record available at https://lccn.loc.gov/2021048343

A catalog record for this book is available from the British Library.

*Special discounts are available for bulk purchases of this book. For more information,
please contact Special Sales at specialsales@jh.edu.*

To the many faculty members
who strive to improve medical education
by developing, implementing, and evaluating
curricula in the health sciences

Contents

Preface

Embedded in a contemporary building awash in natural light sits a windowless class-room in quiet darkness. The carpeted floor has a geometric design, but there is no seating. When not in use, multiple wall-mounted LED screens stare blankly into space. As students file into the room, they receive and adjust their HoloLens headsets and see, suspended in space, a room-size image of the human spine. Students walk around, peering from above and below, locating and highlighting structures with finger gestures. The faculty member directs the teaching session with a tablet noting the relationships of the circulatory system, the sensory and motor tracks, and the bony structures. This 40-minute augmented reality session replaces hours of cadaveric dissection in the human anatomy curriculum.

Not far away, a group of medical, nursing, physician assistant, and social work students, who comprise the board of the student-run clinic, meet with a community leader to plan an outreach effort to increase high blood pressure screening and referral in a local neighborhood. Dual-degree students and their advisor discuss their thesis work—identifying potential gene-editing targets in human disease. A longitudinal clerkship student meets with his faculty advisor to discuss his Urban Health Pathway learning portfolio.

These are just a few examples of the transformational changes in health professions educational programs that have occurred over the past decade. Tectonic shifts in the life sciences, the nature of knowledge, and social structures have intersected and, in many cases, redirected health professions education. New technologies for learning, new models of collaborative care, and increasing attention to the needs of communities have called for curricula to be developed, updated, and in some cases, transformed. Learners are more diverse, more facile in the world of digital and social media, and hungry for the skills that will help them make a difference with their chosen careers.

Curriculum Development for Medical Education: A Six-Step Approach has been in use by health educators across the professions and around the world for more than 20 years. Designed as a practical, generic, and timeless approach to curriculum development, it has proven to be an agile, stalwart resource in this era of rapid educational change. Widely cited, it has an international reputation; it has been translated into Chinese, Japanese, and Spanish. Its home program has undergone its own modifications and evolution, from an in-person longitudinal faculty development workshop to a program that also includes online, shorter, interprofessional, and student-oriented workshops.

As the editors began discussions for the fourth edition in 2019, we reflected that the themes of the third edition—competency-based education, interprofessional education, and educational technology—were broadly adopted and developed, now with a robust literature of successful implementation and enhancements. Our experience working with international colleagues taught us that the book could better acknowledge international curricular exemplars. We had also been told by readers that more attention to health equity as a curricular focus was needed. Having worked with a national consortium of medical schools addressing health systems sciences, we recognized the health of populations and communities as a complex domain in particular need of a structured approach to its introduction into an educational program.

The year 2020 was its own tectonic shift. The coronavirus pandemic exposed stark realities of wealth and health inequity, both locally and internationally, that led to appalling COVID-19 mortality. Sophisticated health systems were woefully inadequate to the task of population surges of illness. Calls for social justice came from street marchers as well as international leaders. Educational programs, abruptly limited by the loss of in-person teaching and student access to clinical sites, quickly implemented technology to fill in the gaps. As educators, we experienced our own "HoloLens" moment of viewing our work through new lenses. Seeing the incomplete nature of our curricular structures, we committed to addressing these shortcomings.

The fourth edition uses these contemporary themes through updated examples and references throughout the book. Given the complexity of a health systems science topic such as health equity, we added a new chapter. We continue to emphasize the themes of "Interprofessionalism and Collaborative Practice" and "Technology" from the previous edition and added new themes of "Internationalism" and "Health Systems Sciences" in this edition.

Each chapter underwent extensive review by the editorial group. Each integrates text and examples that reflect the interprofessional and international audience for this book. We have also increased emphasis on the care of populations, equity, interprofessional collaboration, and the use of technology. In addition, several chapters have noteworthy updates. Chapter 2, Problem Identification and General Needs Assessment, which has always grounded curriculum development in improving health outcomes, has new emphasis on the interplay between roles of health care professionals, patients, educators, and society, and it presents qualitative as well as quantitative methods in understanding the current and ideal approaches to a health problem. Chapter 3, Targeted Needs Assessment, expands the discussion of learning environment to include the virtual and workplace environments, and it acknowledges that some curricula have vastly expanded targeted learners with the use of massive open online courses (MOOCs) and other online platforms. Chapter 4, Goals and Objectives, has an enhanced discussion of competencies and entrustable professional activities (EPAs) and their relationship to goals and objectives. Chapter 5, Educational Strategies, integrates an expanded discussion of learning theory and research related to the choice of educational methods. Chapter 6, Implementation, acknowledges the breadth of expertise and people needed to implement a modern curriculum, offers more detail in understanding costs, and introduces design thinking and change agency. Chapter 7, Evaluation and Feedback, has a new section that addresses theory and general considerations underlying evaluation, integrates qualitative and mixed-method approaches throughout, and discusses the issue of implicit bias in evaluation. Chapter 9, Dissemination, addresses the protection of participants, intellectual property, open access journals, and social media in greater detail than previous editions. Chapter 10, Curriculum Development for Larger Programs, includes well-being as a core value in a large program; it also includes a discussion of disability and accommodations and addresses the tools for programmatic assessment in a competency-based curriculum.

Appendix A for this edition once again presents a summary of the six steps for three curricula representing the continuum in medical education. In addition, these three examples show the progressive use of the six-step model, including a short three-day course, a two-year residency training program, an interprofessional postgraduate training program, and ongoing continuous professional development.

We welcome as a new editor to this edition Sean A. Tackett, a faculty member with expertise in international medical education and medical education research. Our new authors are Mamta K. Singh and Heidi L. Gullett, for the new Chapter 11, and Appendix A authors Amit K. Pahwa, Deanna Saylor, and Mary L. O'Connor Leppert, all of whom have participated in the longitudinal Curriculum Development Program at Johns Hopkins.

Eric B. Bass has stepped away as author, with our thanks for his foundational contribution as previous editor and author of Chapter 2 and co-author for Chapter 9. We also acknowledge our external reviewers for Chapter 7, Ken Kolodner and Joseph Carrese, for their statistical and qualitative research expertise, respectively.

We extend our sincerest thanks to contributions not only of our peer educators and colleagues but also of the many participants in workshops and programs whose input has improved the six-step model over many years. As with each previous edition, many of the participants in the Johns Hopkins Faculty Development Program in Curriculum Development have generously contributed their projects as examples in this edition.

Contributors

Chadia N. Abras, PhD, Vice Provost and Director of Institutional Assessment, Johns Hopkins University Office of the Provost, Johns Hopkins University, and Associate Professor, Johns Hopkins University School of Education, Baltimore, Maryland

Belinda Y. Chen, MD, Assistant Professor, Department of Medicine, Division of General Internal Medicine, Johns Hopkins University School of Medicine, and Director, Programs in Curriculum Development, Johns Hopkins Faculty Development Program, Baltimore, Maryland

Heidi L. Gullett, MD, MPH, Charles Kent Smith, MD, and Patricia Hughes Moore, MD, Professorship in Medical Student Education in Family Medicine, Associate Professor of Family Medicine, and Fellow, the Institute for Integrative Health, Center for Community Health Integration, Case Western Reserve University School of Medicine, Cleveland, Ohio

Mark T. Hughes, MD, MA, Assistant Professor, Department of Medicine, Division of General Internal Medicine and Palliative Medicine, and Core Faculty, Johns Hopkins Berman Institute of Bioethics, Johns Hopkins University School of Medicine, Baltimore, Maryland

David E. Kern, MD, MPH, Emeritus Professor of Medicine, Johns Hopkins University School of Medicine, Past Director, Division of General Internal Medicine, Johns Hopkins Bayview Medical Center, and Past Director, Programs in Curriculum Development, Johns Hopkins Faculty Development Program, Baltimore, Maryland

Brenessa M. Lindeman, MD, MEHP, Associate Professor, Department of Surgery, Section Chief and Fellowship Director for Endocrine Surgery, and Assistant Dean for Graduate Medical Education, University of Alabama at Birmingham, Birmingham, Alabama

Pamela A. Lipsett, MD, MHPE, Warfield M. Firor Endowed Professorship, Professor, Departments of Surgery, Anesthesiology, and Critical Care Medicine, and School of Nursing; Assistant Dean for Assessment and Evaluation, School of Medicine; Program Director, General Surgery Residency Program and Surgical Critical Care Fellowship Program; and Co-director, Surgical Intensive Care Units, Johns Hopkins University School of Medicine, Baltimore, Maryland

Mary L. O'Connor Leppert, MB BCh, Associate Professor of Pediatrics, Kennedy Krieger Institute, Johns Hopkins University School of Medicine, Baltimore, Maryland

Amit K. Pahwa, MD, Associate Professor of Medicine and Pediatrics, Health System Science Core Theme Director, Associate Director of Pediatrics Core Clerkship, and Director of Advanced Clerkship in Internal Medicine, Johns Hopkins University School of Medicine

Deanna Saylor, MD, MHS, Assistant Professor of Neurology, Johns Hopkins University School of Medicine, Baltimore, Maryland, and Program Director, Neurology Post-Graduate Training Program, University of Zambia School of Medicine, Lusaka, Zambia

Mamta K. Singh, MD, MS, Jerome Kowal, MD, Professor in Geriatric Health Education, Professor of Medicine, Case Western Reserve University School of Medicine, Cleveland, Ohio, and Director, Health Professions Education, Evaluation, and Research Advanced Fellowship and VA Quality Scholars, VA Northeast Ohio Health Care System, Cleveland, Ohio

Sean A. Tackett, MD, MPH, Associate Professor of Medicine, Johns Hopkins University School of Medicine, and International Medical Education Director, Division of General Internal Medicine, Johns Hopkins Bayview Medical Center, Baltimore, Maryland

Patricia A. Thomas, MD, Professor of Medicine Emerita, Johns Hopkins University School of Medicine, Baltimore, Maryland

CURRICULUM DEVELOPMENT FOR MEDICAL EDUCATION

Introduction

Patricia A. Thomas, MD, and David E. Kern, MD, MPH

PURPOSE

The purpose of this book is to provide a practical, theoretically sound, evidence-informed approach to developing, implementing, evaluating, and continually improving educational experiences in the health professions.

TARGET AUDIENCE

This book is designed for use by curriculum developers and others who are responsible for the educational experiences of health professional students, residents, fellows, faculty, and clinical practitioners. Although this book was originally written from the perspective of physician education, the approach has been used effectively in other health professions education. It should be particularly helpful to those who are developing or planning to develop a curriculum.

DEFINITION OF CURRICULUM

In this book, a curriculum is defined as *a planned educational experience.* This definition encompasses a breadth of educational experiences, from one or more sessions on a specific subject to a year-long course (face-to-face or online), from a clinical rotation or clerkship to an entire training program.

RATIONALE FOR THE BOOK

Health professionals often have responsibility for planning educational experiences, frequently without having received training or acquired experience in such endeavors, and usually in the presence of limited resources and significant institutional constraints. Accreditation bodies, however, require *written* curricula with fully developed educational objectives, educational methods, and evaluation.[1-8]

Ideally, health professional education should change as our knowledge base changes and as the needs, or the perceived needs, of patients, clinical practitioners, and society change. Some contemporary demands for change and curriculum development are listed in Table I.1. This book assumes that health professional educators will benefit from learning a practical, generic, and timeless approach to curriculum development that can address current as well as future needs.

Table I.1.   Some Contemporary Demands for Curriculum Development in Health Professional Education

---

Outcomes (See Chapter 2, Step 1)
Health professions educational programs and institutions should do the following:
- Respond to current and future health care needs of society[9–21]
- Mitigate costs of education and training[21–23]
- Facilitate entry and support advancement of people from diverse backgrounds into the professions[21,23–26]
- Aim to improve the health of the local community, including underserved populations[15,19,25,27–32]
- Train the number of primary care physicians and specialty physicians required to meet societal needs[17,18,22,24,25,29]

Goals and Objectives (See Chapter 4, Step 3)
Educational programs should graduate health professionals who can do the following:
- Practice patient-centered care[9–12,15,18,33–35]
- Work collaboratively in interprofessional teams[9,11–21,24,36–38]
- Promote patient safety and health systems continuous quality improvement[10–13,15,18,20,21,33,35,37,38–40]
- Improve health of populations by using population- and community-centered approaches to providing health care[15,16,20,23–25,27,37,41]
- Use effective communication, patient and family education, and behavioral change strategies[1,2,8,15,16,24,35,36]
- Access, assess, and apply the best scientific evidence to clinical practice (evidence-based medicine, or EBM)[1–11,15,38,40]
- Use technology and information effectively to assist in accomplishing all the above[2,10,11,16–20,24,25,37]

Content Areas (See Chapter 5, Step 4)
Educational programs should improve instruction and learning in the following areas:
- Professional identity formation[42,43]
- Professionalism, values, and ethics[9,12,15,18,20, 36–38,44]
- Leadership, management, teamwork, and self-awareness[12,15–21,23,35]
- Health systems sciences[9,12,15,20,24,33]
- Social and structural determinants of health in populations and communities[10,12,15,16,19,23,24,27,37,45,46]
- Adaptive expertise to maximize problem-solving in changing environments[20,45,47]

Methods (See Chapter 5, Step 4)
Educational programs should modify current methods to accomplish the following:
- Construct educational interventions based on the best evidence available[40,48,49]
- Address the informal and hidden curricula of an institution that can promote or extinguish what is taught in the formal curricula[15,50,51]
- Enhance interprofessional education[18,21,34,36,37]
- Increase the quantity and quality of clinical training in community-based ambulatory, subacute, and chronic care settings, while reducing the amount of training on inpatient services of acute hospitals, as necessary, to meet training needs[22,29–32,37]
- Effectively integrate advancing technologies into health professional curricula, such as simulation, virtual reality, and interactive electronic interfaces[9,18,19,24,37,39–41]
- Develop faculty to meet contemporary demands[15,19,24,37,52]

Assessment (See Chapter 7, Step 6)
Educational programs across the continuum should do the following:
- Move to outcomes-defined, rather than time-defined, criteria for promotion and graduation (i.e., competency-based education)[2,9,15,19,24,37,52]
- Certify competence in the domains of patient care, knowledge for practice, practice-based learning and improvement, systems-based practice, interprofessional collaboration, and personal and professional development[2,9,39,40,53]
- Evaluate the efficacy of educational interventions[9,39,48]

BACKGROUND INFORMATION

The approach described in this book has evolved over the past 34 years, during which time the authors have taught curriculum development and evaluation skills to over 1,000 participants in continuing education courses and the Johns Hopkins Faculty Development Program (JHFDP). The more than 300 participants in the JHFDP's 10-month Longitudinal Program in Curriculum Development have developed and implemented more than 130 curricula in topics as diverse as skills building prior to training in clinical settings, clinical reasoning and shared decision-making, high-value care, chronic illness and disability, surgical skills assessment, laparoscopic surgical skills, transitions of patient care, cultural competence, social determinants of health, professionalism and social media, and international residency curricula (see Appendix A). The authors have also developed and facilitated the development of numerous curricula in their educational and administrative roles.

AN OVERVIEW OF THE BOOK

Chapter 1 presents an overview of a six-step approach to curriculum development. *Chapters 2 through 7* describe each step in detail. *Chapter 8* discusses how to maintain and improve curricula over time. *Chapter 9* discusses how to disseminate curricula and curricular products within and beyond institutions. *Chapter 10* discusses additional issues related to larger, longer, and integrated curricula.

A new chapter, *Chapter 11*, has been added to this edition to illustrate how the six-step approach can be applied to the new competency of health systems science, with a particular focus on addressing health equity and community needs—an area of burgeoning interest in health professions education.

Throughout the book, *examples* are provided to illustrate major points, especially in the contexts of the themes for the fourth edition: interprofessional education (defined as the presence of students from more than one health or social care profession) and collaborative practice, applications in international settings, use of technology, and health systems science (including health care delivery, population/community health, and health equity). Examples frequently come from the real-life curricular experiences of the authors or their colleagues, although they may have been adapted for the sake of brevity or clarity. The authors have purposefully included, as much as possible, published examples to emphasize how curriculum development contributes to educational scholarship.

Chapters 2 through 11 end with *questions* that encourage the reader to review the principles discussed in each chapter and apply them to a desired, intended, or existing curriculum. In addition to lists of *references cited* in the text, these chapters include annotated lists of *general references* that can guide the reader who is interested in pursuing a particular topic in greater depth.

Appendix A provides examples of curricula that have progressed through all six steps and that range from newly developed curricula to curricula that have matured through repetitive cycles of implementation. The three curricula in Appendix A include examples from undergraduate (medical student), postgraduate (resident), and continuing professional development. *Appendix B* provides the reader with a selected list of published and unpublished resources for curricular development, faculty development, and funding of curricular work.

REFERENCES CITED

1. Liaison Committee on Medical Education, *Functions and Structure of a Medical School: Standards for Accreditation of Medical Education Programs Leading to the MD Degree*, March 2021, accessed October 7, 2021, https://lcme.org/publications/.
2. "Common Program Requirements (Residency)," Accreditation Council for Graduate Medical Education, 2020, accessed October 6, 2021, https://www.acgme.org/what-we-do/accreditation/common-program-requirements/.
3. "Accreditation Criteria," Accreditation Council for Continuing Medical Education, 2020, accessed May 26, 2021, https://www.accme.org/accreditation-rules/accreditation-criteria.
4. World Federation of Medical Education, *Basic Medical Education WFME Global Standards for Quality Improvement* (Copenhagen, Denmark: WFME, 2015).
5. "Standards for Accreditation of Baccalaureate and Graduate Nursing Programs," American Association of Colleges of Nursing, 2018, accessed May 26, 2021, https://www.aacnnursing.org/CCNE-Accreditation/Accreditation-Resources/Standards-Procedures-Guidelines.
6. American Nurses Credentialing Center, *2015 ANCC Primary Accreditation Provider Application Manual* (Silver Spring, MD: American Nurses Credentialing Center, 2015).
7. "Accreditation Standards for Physician Assistant Education," 5th ed., Accreditation Review Commission on Education for the Physician Assistant, Inc., 2019, accessed May 26, 2021, http://www.arc-pa.org/accreditation/standards-of-accreditation/.
8. "Accreditation Standards and Key Elements for the Professional Program in Pharmacy Leading to the Doctor of Pharmacy Degree: 'Standards 2016,'" Accreditation Council for Pharmacy Education (Chicago: ACPE, 2015), accessed May 26, 2021, https://www.acpe-accredit.org/pdf/Standards2016FINAL.pdf.
9. Susan R. Swing, "The ACGME Outcome Project: Retrospective and Prospective," *Medical Teacher* 29, no. 7 (2007): 648–54, https://doi.org/10.1080/01421590701392903.
10. Institute of Medicine (IOM), *Crossing the Quality Chasm: A New Health System for the 21st Century* (Washington, DC: National Academies Press, 2001).
11. Institute of Medicine, "The Core Competencies Need for Health Care Professionals," in *Health Professions Education: A Bridge to Quality*, ed. Ann C. Greiner and Elisa Knebel (Washington, DC: National Academies Press, 2003), https://doi.org/10.17226/10681.
12. Donald M. Berwick and Jonathan A. Finkelstein, "Preparing Medical Students for the Continual Improvement of Health and Health Care: Abraham Flexner and the New 'Public Interest,'" *Academic Medicine* 85, no. 9 Suppl. (2010): S56–65, https://doi.org/10.1097/ACM.0b013e3181ead779.
13. Donald M. Berwick, Thomas W. Nolan, and John Whittington, "The Triple Aim: Care, Health, and Cost," *Health Affairs* 27, no. 3 (2008): 759–69, NLM, https://doi.org/10.1377/hlthaff.27.3.759.

14. Institute of Medicine Committee on Planning a Continuing Health Professional Education, *Redesigning Continuing Education in the Health Professions* (Washington, DC: National Academies Press, 2010), https://doi.org/10.17226/12704.

15. Susan E. Skochelak, Maya Hammoud, and Kimberly D. Lomis, *Health Systems Science: AMA Education Consortium,* 2nd ed. (St. Louis: Elsevier, 2020).

16. Stephanie R. Starr et al., "Science of Health Care Delivery as a First Step to Advance Undergraduate Medical Education: A Multi-institutional Collaboration," *Healthcare (Amst)* 5, no. 3 (2017): 98–104, https://www.sciencedirect.com/science/article/pii/S2213076416301415.

17. Kenneth M. Ludmerer, "The History of Calls for Reform in Graduate Medical Education and Why We Are Still Waiting for the Right Kind of Change," *Academic Medicine* 87, no. 1 (2012): 34–40, https://doi.org/10.1097/ACM.0b013e318238f229.

18. Catherine R. Lucey, "Medical Education: Part of the Problem and Part of the Solution," *JAMA Internal Medicine* 173, no. 17 (2013): 1639–43, https://doi.org/10.1001/jamainternmed.2013.9074.

19. Association of Faculties of Medicine of Canada, *The Future of Medical Education in Canada* (Ottawa: AFMC, 2010).

20. "Outcomes for Graduates 2018," General Medical Council, 2018, accessed May 26, 2021, https://www.gmc-uk.org/education/standards-guidance-and-curricula/standards-and-outcomes/outcomes-for-graduates.

21. National Academies of Sciences, Engineering, and Medicine, *The Future of Nursing 2020–2030: Charting a Path to Achieve Health Equity* (Washington, DC: National Academies Press, 2021), https://doi.org/10.17226/25982.

22. Institute of Medicine, *Graduate Medical Education That Meets the Nation's Health Needs* (Washington, DC: National Academies Press, 2014), https://doi.org/10.17226/18754.

23. Melanie Raffoul, Gillian Bartlett-Esquilant, and Robert L. Phillips Jr. "Recruiting and Training a Health Professions Workforce to Meet the Needs of Tomorrow's Health Care System," *Academic Medicine* 94, no. 5 (2019): 651–55, https://doi.org/10.1097/acm.0000000000002606.

24. Julio Frenk et al., "Health Professionals for a New Century: Transforming Education to Strengthen Health Systems in an Interdependent World," *The Lancet* 376, no. 9756 (2010): 1923–58, https://doi.org/10.1016/s0140-6736(10)61854-5.

25. "Global Consensus for Social Accountability of Medical Schools, Consensus Document," World Federation for Medical Education, 2010, accessed May 28, 2021, https://wfme.org/home/projects/social-accountability/.

26. Alda Maria R. Gonzaga et al., "A Framework for Inclusive Graduate Medical Education Recruitment Strategies," *Academic Medicine* 95, no. 5 (2020): 710–16, https://doi.org/10.1097/acm.0000000000003073.

27. Charles Boelen et al., "Accrediting Excellence for a Medical School's Impact on Population Health," *Education for Health (Abingdon)* 32, no. 1 (2019): 41–48, https://doi.org/10.4103/efh.EfH_204_19.

28. James Rourke, "Social Accountability: A Framework for Medical Schools to Improve the Health of the Populations They Serve," *Academic Medicine* 93, no. 8 (2018): 1120–24, https://doi.org/10.1097/acm.0000000000002239.

29. Brian M. Ross, Kim Daynard, and David Greenwood, "Medicine for Somewhere: The Emergence of Place in Medical Education," *Educational Research and Review* 9, no. 22 (2014): 1250–65.

30. Mora Claramita et al., "Community-Based Educational Design for Undergraduate Medical Education: A Grounded Theory Study," *BMC Medical Education* 19, no. 1 (2019): 258, https://doi.org/10.1186/s12909-019-1643-6.

31. "Closing the Gap in a Generation: Health Equity through Action on the Social Determinants of Health," Commission on Social Determinants of Health (Geneva: World Health Organization, 2008), accessed May 26, 2021, https://www.who.int/social_determinants/thecommission/finalreport/en/.

32. Wagdy Talaat and Zahra Ladhani, "Community Based Education in Health Professions: Global Perspectives" (Cairo: WHO Regional Office for the Eastern Mediterranean, 2014), accessed May 26, 2021, https://www.hrhresourcecenter.org/node/5568.html.

33. Paul A. Hemmer et al., "AMEE 2010 Symposium: Medical Student Education in the Twenty-First Century—a New Flexnerian Era?," *Medical Teacher* 33, no. 7 (2011): 541–46, https://doi.org/10.3109/0142159x.2011.578178.

34. Kevin B. Weiss, James P. Bagian, and Thomas J. Nasca, "The Clinical Learning Environment: The Foundation of Graduate Medical Education," *JAMA* 309, no. 16 (2013): 1687–88, https://doi.org/10.1001/jama.2013.1931.

35. Jason Russell Frank, Linda Snell, and Jonathan Sherbino, *CanMEDS 2015 Physician Competency Framework* (Ottawa: Royal College of Physicians and Surgeons of Canada, 2015).

36. Interprofessional Education Collaborative, *Core Competencies for Interprofessional Collaborative Practice: 2016 Update* (Washington, DC: Interprofessional Education Collaborative, 2016), accessed October 8, 2021, https://www.ipecollaborative.org/ipec-core-competencies.

37. George E. Thibault, "Reforming Health Professions Education Will Require Culture Change and Closer Ties between Classroom and Practice," *Health Affairs* 32 no. 11 (2013): 1928–32, https://doi.org/10.1377/hlthaff.2013.0827.

38. "CLER Pathways to Excellence: Expectations for an Optimal Clinical Learning Environment to Achieve Safe and High-Quality Patient Care," Version 2.0, CLER Evaluation Committee (Chicago: Accreditation Council for Graduate Medical Education, 2019), https://doi.org/10.35425/ACGME.0003.

39. Robert T. Englander et al., "Toward Defining the Foundation of the MD Degree: Core Entrustable Professional Activities for Entering Residency," *Academic Medicine* 91, no. 10 (2016): 1352–58, https://doi.org/10.1097/acm.0000000000001204.

40. Ronald M. Cervero and Julie K. Gaines, "The Impact of CME on Physician Performance and Patient Health Outcomes: An Updated Synthesis of Systematic Reviews," *Journal of Continuing Education in the Health Professions* 35, no. 2 (2015): 131–38, https://doi.org/10.1002/chp.21290.

41. Hayley Croft et al., "Current Trends and Opportunities for Competency Assessment in Pharmacy Education—a Literature Review." *Pharmacy (Basel)* 7, no. 2 (2019), https://doi.org/10.3390/pharmacy7020067.

42. Molly Cooke, David M. Irby, and Bridget C. O'Brien, *Educating Physicians: A Call for Reform of Medical School and Residency* (Stanford, CA: Jossey-Bass, 2010).

43. John Goldie, "The Formation of Professional Identity in Medical Students: Considerations for Educators," *Medical Teacher* 34, no. 9 (2012): e641–48, https://doi.org/10.3109/0142159x.2012.687476.

44. Richard A. Cooper and Alfred I. Tauber, "Values and Ethics: A Collection of Curricular Reforms for a New Generation of Physicians," *Academic Medicine* 82, no. 4 (2007): 321–23, https://doi.org/10.1097/01.Acm.0000259373.44699.90.

45. Maria Mylopoulos et al., "Preparation for Future Learning: A Missing Competency in Health Professions Education?," *Medical Education* 50, no.1 (2015): 115–23, https://doi.org/10.1111/medu.12893.

46. Patricia A. Cuff and Neal A. Vanselow, eds., *Improving Medical Education: Enhancing the Behavioral and Social Science Content of Medical School Curricula* (Washington, DC: National Academies Press, 2004), https://doi.org/10.17226/10956.

47. William B. Cutrer et al., "Fostering the Development of Master Adaptive Learners: A Conceptual Model to Guide Skill Acquisition in Medical Education," *Academic Medicine* 92, no. 1 (2017): 70–75, https://doi.org/10.1097/acm.0000000000001323.

48. R. M. Harden et al., "Best Evidence Medical Education," *Advances in Health Science Education Theory and Practice* 5, no. 1 (2000): 71–90, https://doi.org/10.1023/a:1009896431203.

49. "The BEME Collaboration," Best Evidence Medical and Health Professional Education, accessed May 26, 2021, www.bemecollaboration.org.

50. Melanie Neumann et al., "Empathy Decline and Its Reasons: A Systematic Review of Studies with Medical Students and Residents," *Academic Medicine* 86, no. 8 (2011): 996–1009, https://doi.org/10.1097/ACM.0b013e318221e615.

51. Frederick Hafferty and Joseph O'Donnell, eds., *The Hidden Curriculum in Health Professional Education* (Hanover, NH: Dartmouth College Press, 2014).

52. Ligia Cordovani, Anne Wong, and Sandra Monteiro, "Maintenance of Certification for Practicing Physicians: A Review of Current Challenges and Considerations," *Canadian Medical Journal* 11, no. 1 (2020): e70–e80, https://doi.org/10.36834/cmej.53065.

53. Robert T. Englander et al., "Toward a Common Taxonomy of Competency Domains for the Health Professions and Competencies for Physicians," *Academic Medicine* 88, no. 8 (2013): 1088–94, https://doi.org/10.1097/ACM.0b013e31829a3b2b.

CHAPTER ONE

Overview
A Six-Step Approach to Curriculum Development

David E. Kern, MD, MPH

ORIGINS AND ASSUMPTIONS

The six-step approach described in this monograph derives from the generic approaches to curriculum development set forth by Taba,[1] Tyler,[2] Yura and Torres,[3] and others,[4] and from the work of McGaghie et al.[5] and Golden,[6] who advocated the linking of curricula to health care needs. It is similar to models for clinical, health promotion, and social services program development, with Step 4, Educational Strategies, replacing program intervention.[7–10]

Underlying assumptions are fourfold. First, educational programs have aims or goals, whether or not they are clearly articulated. Second, health professional educators have a professional and ethical obligation to meet the needs of their learners, patients, and society. Third, health professional educators should be held accountable for the outcomes of their interventions. And fourth, a logical, systematic approach to curriculum development will help achieve these ends.

RELATIONSHIP TO ACCREDITATION

Accrediting bodies for undergraduate, graduate, and continuing health professions education in the United States and internationally usually require formal curricula that include goals, objectives, and explicitly articulated educational and evaluation strategies based on needs.[11–19] Some degree programs must also meet governmental standards for licensing. Undergraduate and postgraduate medical curricula must address core clinical competencies.[11,12] The achievement of milestones for each competency is required for residency training.[20] Current trends in translating competencies into clinical practice, such as entrustable professional activities (EPAs)[21,22] (see Chapter 4), provide additional direction and requirements for Step 3 (Goals and Objectives), Step 4 (Educational Strategies), and Step 6 (Evaluation and Feedback), while grounding curricula in societal needs (Step 1, Problem Identification and General Needs Assessment).

A SIX-STEP APPROACH (FIGURE 1.1)

Step 1: Problem Identification and General Needs Assessment

This step begins with the *identification and critical analysis of a health need or other problem.* The need may relate to a specific health problem, such as the provision of care to patients infected with an emerging infectious disease, or to a group of problems, such as the provision of routine gynecologic care by primary care providers. It may relate to qualities of health care providers, such as the need for them to develop

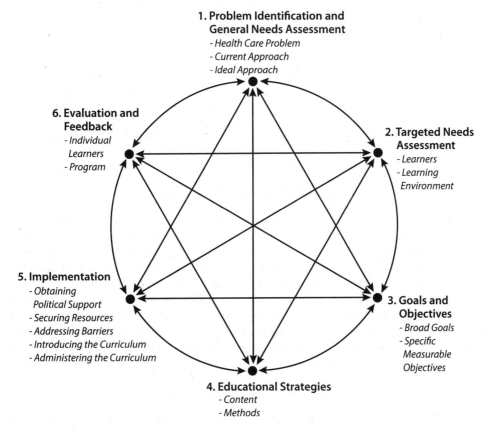

Figure 1.1.   A Six-Step Approach to Curriculum Development

as self-directed, lifelong learners who can provide effective care as medical knowledge and practice evolve. Or it may relate to the health needs of society in general, such as whether the quantity and type of health care workers being produced are appropriate. A complete problem identification requires an analysis of the *current approach* of patients, health professionals, the health care education system, and society, in general, to addressing the identified need. This is followed by identification of an *ideal approach* that describes how patients, health professionals, the health care education system, and society should be addressing the need. The difference between the ideal approach and the current approach represents a *general needs assessment*.

Step 2: Targeted Needs Assessment

This step involves assessing the needs of one's targeted group of learners and their learning environment(s), which may be different from the needs of learners in general. It enables desired integration of a specific curriculum into an overall curriculum or educational program. It also develops communication with and support from stakeholders, and it aligns one's curriculum development strategy with potential resources.

> **EXAMPLE:** *Problem Identification, General and Targeted Needs Assessment.* The problem identification and general needs assessment for a curriculum designed to improve the provision of cost-effective/high-value care (HVC) revealed that, while the United States had the highest per capita spending on health care, it ranked twenty-fourth out of 188 nations in health outcomes and behind many less developed countries. Costs were becoming unsustainable. The major driver of unnecessary expenses was physician ordering of tests and procedures. There was consensus regarding the importance of HVC training and some guidelines for such training. While curricula were emerging in HVC at the residency and medical school level, none existed at all levels of medical school training. Most physicians identified a lack of any formal education in this area. In addition, the hidden and informal curricula in many institutions did not reinforce HVC practice. Ideally, training in HVC would address the knowledge, attitudes, skills, and behaviors related to cost-effective ordering. It would be ongoing and incremental throughout training. At the curriculum developers' medical school, curricular mapping revealed that HVC was not being formally taught. A targeted needs assessment of third-year medical students revealed that a minority were able to define or provide an example of HVC. The opportunity existed to integrate a HVC curriculum into an existing four-year curriculum in health systems science.[23]

Step 3: Goals and Objectives

Once the needs of targeted learners have been identified, goals and objectives for the curriculum can be written, starting with *broad or general goals* and then moving to *specific, measurable objectives.* Objectives may include cognitive (knowledge), affective (attitudinal), psychomotor (skill), and behavioral (real-life performance) objectives for the learner; process objectives related to the conduct of the curriculum; or even health, health care, or patient outcome objectives. The development of goals and objectives is critical because they help to determine curricular content and learning methods and help to focus the learner. They enable communication of what the curriculum is about to others and provide a basis for its evaluation. When resources are limited, prioritization of objectives can facilitate the rational allocation of those resources.

Step 4: Educational Strategies

Once objectives have been clarified, *curriculum content is chosen and educational methods are selected that will most likely achieve the educational objectives.*

EXAMPLE: *Educational Strategies.* Based on the above example of Steps 1 and 2, training-level-appropriate objectives were developed for knowledge, attitudes, and skills of first- through fourth-year medical students. Educational content related to understanding: the components of HVC; the impact of systems and individual behaviors on HVC practice; the impact of systems issues, such as reimbursement and insurance, on the practice of HVC; how to apply this knowledge to clinical decision-making both at the provider level and in provider-patient shared decision-making; and how to behave as an effective change agent at the clinical and systems levels. Topics were covered in three stages: (1) preclinical (basic understanding, systems issues, cognitive skills related to clinical decision-making, change agency), (2) an interval one-week block between clinical clerkships (applications to clinical decision-making, change agency), and (3) a final-year bootcamp preparing students for residency (applications to clinical decision-making). Educational methods focused on team-based learning (see Chapter 5) with didactics, session pretests, and application exercises. Application exercises included discussion for Stage 1, didactics and case discussion for Stage 2, and simulated patient exercises with feedback and discussion for Stage 3.[23]

EXAMPLE: *Congruent Educational Methods.*

Lower-level knowledge can be acquired from reading, in-person lectures, or online learning opportunities.

Case-based, problem-solving exercises that actively involve learners are methods that are more likely to improve clinical reasoning skills than attendance at lectures.

The development of physicians as effective team members is more likely to be promoted through their participation in and reflection on interprofessional cooperative learning and work experiences than through reading and discussing a book on the subject.

Interviewing, physical examination, and procedural skills will be best learned in simulation and practice environments that supplement practice with self-observation, observation by others, feedback, and reflection.

Step 5: Implementation

Implementation involves the implementation of both the educational intervention and its evaluation. It has *several components*: obtaining political support, identifying and procuring resources, identifying and addressing barriers to implementation, introducing the curriculum (e.g., piloting the curriculum on a friendly audience before presenting it to all targeted learners, phasing in the curriculum one part at a time), administering the curriculum, and refining the curriculum over successive cycles. Implementation is critical to the success of a curriculum. It is *the step that converts a mental exercise to reality.*

Step 6: Evaluation and Feedback

This step has several components. It usually is desirable to assess the performance of both *individuals* (individual assessment) and the *curriculum* (called "program evaluation"). The purpose of evaluation may be *formative* (to provide ongoing feedback so that the learners or curriculum can improve) or *summative* (to provide a final "grade" or evaluation of the performance of the learner or curriculum).

Evaluation can be used not only to drive the ongoing learning of participants and the improvement of a curriculum but also to gain support and resources for a curriculum and, in research situations, to answer questions about the effectiveness of a specific curriculum or the relative merits of different approaches.

EXAMPLE: *Evaluation.* The initial evaluation plan for the HVC curriculum described in the above examples was resource-limited but included several elements. Stage 1 knowledge acquisition was assessed using a knowledge exam pre- and post-intervention, with a comparison group who had not been exposed to the curriculum. Letters to a politician were used to assess application of serving as a change agent. Behaviors related to the practice of HVC and to serving as a change agent were assessed via end-of-clerkship evaluation forms completed by housestaff and attendings (Stage 2). Skills related to practicing HVC were assessed in simulation encounters during boot camp (Stage 3). Students ratings of the curriculum and its various components were collected via post-intervention surveys (Stages 1–3).[23]

THE INTERACTIVE AND CONTINUOUS NATURE OF THE SIX-STEP APPROACH

In practice, curriculum development does not usually proceed in sequence, one step at a time. Rather, it is a dynamic, interactive process. Progress is often made on two or more steps simultaneously. Progress on one step influences progress on another (as illustrated by the bidirectional arrows in Figure 1.1). As noted in the discussion and examples above, implementation (Step 5) actually began during the targeted needs assessment (Step 2). Limited resources (Step 5) may limit the number and nature of objectives (Step 3), as well as the extent of evaluation (Step 6) that is possible. Evaluation strategies (Step 6) may result in a refinement of objectives (Step 3). Evaluation (Step 6)—for example, pretests—may also provide information that serves as a needs assessment of targeted learners (Step 2). Time pressures, or the presence of an existing curriculum, may result in the development of goals, educational methods, and implementation strategies (Steps 3, 4, and 5) before a formal problem identification and needs assessment (Steps 1 and 2), so that Steps 1 and 2 are used to refine and improve an existing curriculum rather than develop a new one.

For a successful curriculum, curriculum development never really ends, as illustrated by the circle in Figure 1.1. Rather, the curriculum evolves, based on evaluation results (Step 6), changes in resources (Step 5), changes in targeted learners (Step 2), and changes in the material requiring mastery (Step 1). It undergoes a process of continous quality improvement (see Chapters 6, 8, and 10).

REFERENCES CITED

1. Hilda Taba, *Curriculum Development: Theory and Practice* (New York: Harcourt, Brace, & World, 1962), 1–515.
2. Ralph W. Tyler, *Basic Principles of Curriculum and Instruction* (Chicago: University of Chicago Press, 1949), 1–83.
3. Helen Yura and Gertrude J. Torres, eds., *Faculty-Curriculum Development: Curriculum Design by Nursing Faculty*, Publication No. 15-2164 (New York: National League for Nursing, 1986), 1–371.
4. Kent J. Sheets, William A. Anderson, and Patrick C. Alguire, "Curriculum Development and Evaluation in Medical Education," *Journal of General Internal Medicine* 7, no. 5 (1992): 538–43, https://doi.org/10.1007/bf02599461.
5. William McGaghie et al., *Competency-Based Curriculum Development in Medical Education* (Geneva: World Health Organization, 1978), 1–99.
6. Archie S. Golden, "A Model for Curriculum Development Linking Curriculum with Health Needs," in *The Art of Teaching Primary Care*, ed. Archie S. Golden, Dennis G. Carlsen, and Jan L. Hagen (New York: Springer Publishing Co.,1982), 9–25.

7. Nancy G. Calley, *Program Development for the 21st Century: An Evidence-Based Approach to Design, Implementation, and Evaluation* (Thousand Oaks, CA: Sage Publications, 2011).

8. James F. McKenzie, Brad L. Neiger, and Rosemary Thackeray, *Planning, Implementing, and Evaluating Health Promotion Programs: A Primer*, 6th ed. (San Francisco, CA: Benjamin Cummings Publishing, 2012).

9. Thomas C. Timmreck, *Planning, Program Development and Evaluation: A Handbook for Health Promotion, Aging and Health Services* (Boston: Jones and Bartlett Publishers, 2003).

10. Bernard J. Healey and Robert S. Zimmerman Jr., *The New World of Health Promotion: New Program Development, Implementation, and Evaluation* (Burlington, MA: Jones and Bartlett Learning, 2010), 3–106.

11. Liaison Committee on Medical Education, *Functions and Structure of a Medical School: Standards for Accreditation of Medical Education Programs Leading to the MD Degree*, March 2021, accessed September 15, 2021, https://www.lcme.org/publications/.

12. "Common Program Requirements (Residency)," Accreditation Council for Graduate Medical Education, 2020, accessed September 15, 2021, https://www.acgme.org/what-we-do/accreditation/common-program-requirements/.

13. "Accreditation Criteria," Accreditation Council for Continuing Medical Education, 2020, accessed September 15, 2021, https://www.accme.org/accreditation-rules/accreditation-criteria.

14. "Standards," World Federation for Medical Education, accessed September 15, 2021, https://wfme.org/standards/.

15. Accreditation Council for Graduate Medical Education–International (ACGME-I), accessed September 15, 2021, https://www.acgme-i.org/.

16. "Standards for Accreditation of Baccalaureate and Graduate Nursing Programs," American Association of Colleges of Nursing, accessed September 15, 2021, https://www.aacnnursing.org/CCNE-Accreditation/Accreditation-Resources/Standards-Procedures-Guidelines.

17. "Credentialing for Continuing Nursing Education," ANNC Accreditation/American Nurses Credentialing Center, accessed September 15, 2021, https://www.nursingworld.org/organizational-programs/accreditation/.

18. "Accreditation Standards for Physician Assistant Education," 5th ed., Accreditation Review Commission on Education for the Physician Assistant, accessed September 15, 2021, http://www.arc-pa.org/accreditation/standards-of-accreditation/.

19. "Accreditation Standards and Key Elements for the Professional Program in Pharmacy Leading to the Doctor of Pharmacy Degree: Standards 2016," Accreditation Council for Pharmacy Education, accessed September 15, 2021, https://www.acpe-accredit.org/pdf/Standards2016FINAL.pdf.

20. Thomas J. Nasca et al., "The Next GME Accreditation System—Rationale and Benefits," *New England Journal of Medicine* 366, no.11 (2012): 1051–56, https://doi.org/10.1056/nejmsr1200117.

21. Ara Tekian et al., "Entrustment Decisions: Implications for Curriculum Development and Assessment," *Medical Teacher* 42, no. 6 (2020): 698–704, https://doi.org/10.1080/0142159x.2020.1733506.

22. "Core Entrustable Professional Activities for Entering Residency," Association of American Medical Colleges, accessed September 15, 2021, https://www.aamc.org/what-we-do/mission-areas/medical-education/cbme/core-epas.

23. Example adapted with permission from the curricular project of Christopher Steele, MD, MPH, MS, in the Johns Hopkins Longitudinal Program in Faculty Development, cohort 32, 2018–19.

CHAPTER TWO

Step 1
Problem Identification and General Needs Assessment

. . . building the foundation for meaningful objectives

Belinda Y. Chen, MD

Medical instruction does not exist to provide individuals with an
opportunity of learning how to make a living, but in order to make
possible the protection of the health of the public.
—Rudolf Virchow

Many reasons may prompt someone to begin work on a health care curriculum. Indeed, continuing developments in medical science and technology call for efforts to keep health professions education up to date, whether it be new knowledge to be disseminated (e.g., new information about an emerging virus like Ebola or SARS-CoV-2) or a new skill to be mastered (e.g., point-of-care ultrasound). Sometimes, educational leaders issue a mandate to improve performance in selected areas based on feedback from learners, suboptimal scores on standardized examinations, or recommendations from educational accrediting bodies (e.g., national standards for competency-based training or patient safety and quality). Other times, educators want to take advantage of new learning technology (e.g., simulation/virtual reality) or need to respond to changes in the learning environment (e.g., virtual conferences that allow for distance learning to overcome geographic separation). Regardless of where one enters the curriculum development paradigm, it is critical to take a step back and consider the responsibilities of an educator. Why is a new or revised curriculum worth the time and effort needed to plan and implement it well? Since the ultimate purpose of health professions education is to improve the health of the public, what is the health problem or outcome that needs to be addressed? What is the ideal role of a planned educational experience in improving such health outcomes? This chapter offers guidance on how to define the problem, determine the current and ideal approaches to the problem, and synthesize all of the information in a general needs assessment that clarifies the gap the curriculum will fill.

DEFINITIONS

The first step in designing a curriculum is to identify and characterize the health care problem that will be addressed by the curriculum, how the problem is currently being addressed, and how it ideally should be addressed. The description of the current and ideal approaches to the problem is called a *general needs assessment*. Because the difference between the current and ideal approaches can be considered part of the problem that the curriculum will address, Step 1 can also simply be called *problem identification*.

IMPORTANCE

The better a problem is defined, the easier it will be to design appropriate curricula to address the problem. All of the other steps in the curriculum development process depend on having a clear understanding of the problem (see Figure 1.1). Problem identification (Step 1), along with targeted needs assessment (Step 2), is particularly helpful in focusing a curriculum's goals and objectives (Step 3), which in turn help to focus the curriculum's educational strategies and evaluation (Steps 4 and 6). Step 1 is especially important in justifying dissemination of a successful curriculum because it supports its generalizability. Steps 1 and 2 also provide a strong rationale that can help the curriculum developer obtain support for curriculum implementation (Step 5).

DEFINING THE HEALTH CARE PROBLEM

The ultimate purpose of a curriculum in health professions education is to equip learners to address a problem that affects the health of the public or a given population. Frequently, the problem of interest is complex (see Chapter 11). However, even the simplest health issue may be refractory to an educational intervention, if the problem has not been defined well. A comprehensive definition of the problem should consider the epidemiology of the problem, as well as the impact of the problem on patients, health professionals, medical educators, and society (Table 2.1).

In defining the problem of interest, it is important to explicitly identify *whom* the problem affects. Does the problem affect people with a particular disease (e.g., frequent disease exacerbations requiring hospitalization of patients with asthma), or does the problem affect society at large (e.g., inadequate understanding of behaviors associated with acquiring an emerging infectious disease)? Does the problem directly or indirectly affect health professionals and their trainees (e.g., physicians inadequately prepared to participate effectively as part of interprofessional teams)? Does the problem affect health care organizations (e.g., a need to foster the practice of patient-centered care or to meet the needs of the populations it serves)? The problem of interest may involve different groups. The degree of impact has implications for curriculum development because a problem that is perceived to affect many people may be granted more attention and resources. Educators will be able to choose the most appropriate target audience for a curriculum, formulate learning objectives, and develop curricular content when they know the characteristics and behaviors of those affected by the health problem of interest.

Once those who are affected by the problem have been identified, it is important to elaborate on *how* they are affected. What is the effect of the problem on clinical outcomes, quality of life, quality of health care, use of health care services, medical and nonmedical costs, patient and clinician satisfaction, work and productivity, and the functioning of society? How common and how serious are these effects?

EXAMPLE: *Problem Identification.* A trauma-informed physical exam curriculum published on MedEd-PORTAL included a succinct, referenced problem identification in the introductory paragraph. Their problem identification includes definition of "trauma" with examples of categories of trauma, notes a prevalence of a history of trauma in over 89% of people living in the United States based on a national survey, cites an association between trauma and chronic health conditions (such as depression, diabetes, cardiovascular disease, and substance use), and references evidence that trauma can negatively affect health outcomes through altering patients' sense of safety, autonomy, and trust, their relationships with health professionals, and their utilization of health care services.[1]

Table 2.1. Identification and Characterization of the Health Care Problem

Whom does it affect?
   Patients
   Health professionals
   Medical educators
   Society

What does it affect?
   Clinical outcomes
   Quality of life
   Quality of health care
   Use of health care and other resources
   Medical and nonmedical costs
   Patient and provider satisfaction
   Work and productivity
   Societal function

What is the *quantitative and qualitative importance* of the effects?

GENERAL NEEDS ASSESSMENT (TABLE 2.2)

Current Approach

Having defined the nature of the health care problem, the next task is to assess current efforts to address the problem. The process of determining the current approach to a problem is sometimes referred to as a "job analysis" because it is an assessment of the "job" that is currently being done to deal with a problem.[2] To determine the current approach, the curriculum developer should ask what is being done by each of the following:

   a. Patients (including their families, significant others, and caregivers)
   b. Health professionals (including the systems within which they practice)
   c. Health professions educators (including the environments in which they teach)
   d. Society (including community networks, health care payers, policymakers)

Knowing what *patients* are doing and not doing regarding a problem may influence decisions about curricular content. For example, are patients using noneffective treatments or engaging in activities that exacerbate a problem, behaviors that need to be reversed? Or are patients predisposed to engage in activities that could alleviate the problem, behaviors that need to be encouraged?

Knowing how *health professionals* are currently addressing the problem is especially relevant because they are frequently the target audience for curricula. In the general needs assessment, one of the challenges is to determine how health professionals vary in their approaches to a problem. Many studies of clinical practice between and within countries have demonstrated substantial variations in both adherence to recommended practices and use of either ineffective or harmful practices.[3-5]

EXAMPLE: *Current Approach by Health Professionals.* The ABIM (American Board of Internal Medicine) Foundation reported that three out of four physicians surveyed agreed that the frequency with which

Table 2.2.   The General Needs Assessment

What is *currently* being done by each of the following?
   Patients
   Health professionals
   Medical educators
   Society

What personal and environmental factors affect the problem?
   Predisposing
   Enabling
   Reinforcing

What *ideally* should be done by each of the following?
   Patients
   Health professionals
   Medical educators
   Society

What are the key *differences* between the current and ideal approaches?

---

doctors order unnecessary tests was a serious problem for America's health care system. The majority of American physicians surveyed estimated that the average physician ordered unnecessary medical tests and procedures at least once a week. The Choosing Wisely campaign encouraged specialty societies to identify interventions in which there was a discrepancy between recommended and actual use. Having identified specific health care problems of unnecessary variations in practice, this campaign then highlighted opportunities for patients and health professionals to work together to reduce waste and low-value care. Educational efforts on a variety of levels were then directed toward reducing low-value care and promoting high-value care.[6,7]

Most problems important enough to warrant a focused curriculum are encountered in many different places, so it is wise to explore what other *educators* are currently doing to help patients and health professionals address the problem. Much can be learned from the previous work of educators who have tried to tackle the problem of interest. For example, curricular materials may exist already and be of great value in developing a curriculum for one's own target audience. A plethora of existing curricula may highlight the need for evaluation tools to help educators determine which methods are most effective in achieving desired outcomes. This is particularly important because time and resources available for education are usually limited. A dearth of relevant curricula will reinforce the need for innovative curricular work.

EXAMPLE: *Interprofessional Education.* Reports from the World Health Organization and the National Academy of Medicine called for greater interprofessional education (IPE) to improve health outcomes through fostering the development of coordinated interprofessional teams that work together to promote quality, safety, and systems improvement.[8,9] Those developing curricula in interprofessional education should be familiar with the guidelines and competencies established by the Interprofessional Education Collaborative.[10,11] However, even within the guidelines, there is substantial room for variation. New curriculum developers could learn from a scoping review of published nursing curricula that includes a table of teaching and learning methods used and evaluation instruments and outcomes.[12] Subsequent articles build on this experience and share additional lessons learned from implementation in specific settings, such as primary care within the Veterans Administration.[13] The peer-reviewed website MedEdPORTAL groups IPE curricula in its Interprofessional Education Collection for easier searching.[14]

Curriculum developers should also consider what *society* is doing to address the problem. This will help to improve understanding of the societal context of current efforts to address the problem, taking into consideration potential barriers and facilitators that influence those efforts.

EXAMPLE: *Impact of Societal Approach to Opioid Overdose on Curricular Planning.* In 2017, the opioid crisis was declared a public health emergency in the United States. In designing a curriculum to help health professionals learn to address drug overdoses, it is helpful to know how society handles the distribution and administration of naloxone. Medical and pharmacy educators at one institution noted that their institution was in one of the 30 states with expanded naloxone access for at-risk patients, relatives, and first responders. Therefore, their curriculum included instructions on not only how to prescribe naloxone but also how to administer it and teach others to do so. They were also able to obtain naloxone kits to distribute to the trained first responders.[15]

To understand fully the current approach to addressing a health care problem, curriculum developers need to be familiar with perspectives on human behavior. The ecological perspective emphasizes multiple influences on behavior, including at the individual, interpersonal, institutional, community, and public policy levels.[16] Interventions are more likely to be successful if they address multiple levels of influence on behavior. Most educational interventions will focus primarily on individual and/or interpersonal factors, but some may be part of larger interventions that also target environmental and policy-level factors to support healthful behaviors (e.g., teaching not just nutritional principles but also how to inquire about and address food insecurity in partnership with others).[17]

When focusing on the individual and interpersonal levels of influence on behavior, curriculum developers should consider the fundamental principles of modern theories of human behavior change.[18] While it is beyond the scope of this book to discuss specific theories in detail, three concepts seem particularly important: (1) human behavior is mediated by what people know and think; (2) knowledge is necessary, but not sufficient, to cause a change in behavior; and (3) behavior is influenced by the environment as well as by individual beliefs, motivations, and skills.

In the light of these key concepts, curriculum developers need to consider *multiple types of factors* that may aggravate or alleviate the problem of interest. Factors that can influence the problem can be classified as predisposing factors, enabling factors, or reinforcing factors.[19] *Predisposing factors* are the knowledge, attitudes, and beliefs that influence a person's motivation to change (or not to change) behaviors related to a problem. *Enabling factors* are generally personal skills and societal or environmental forces that make a behavioral or environmental change possible. *Reinforcing factors* are the rewards and punishments that encourage continuation or discontinuation of a behavior.

> **EXAMPLE:** *Predisposing, Enabling, and Reinforcing Factors.* Correct use of personal protective equipment (PPE) is important in health care settings to reduce the transmission of infectious disease. However, workers have been shown to have variable usage patterns. In designing curricula for health professionals related to improving infection control, it would be helpful for a curriculum developer to be aware of a paper that systematically reviewed qualitative studies of factors that impact a worker's ability to safely don and doff PPE.[20] Predisposing factors may include motivations for adhering to recommendations for PPE use, such as self-preservation and perception of risk of transmission. Enabling factors could include availability of PPE resources, location of specific donning/doffing stations, presence of environmental cues such as cards, and social influences. Reinforcing factors could include social influences, independent observers, and rewards for compliance.

By considering all aspects of how a health care problem is addressed, one can determine the most appropriate role for an educational intervention in addressing the problem, keeping in mind that an educational intervention by itself usually cannot solve all aspects of a complex health care problem.

Ideal Approach

After examination of the current approach to the problem, the next task is to determine the ideal approach to the problem. Determination of the ideal approach will require careful consideration of the multiple levels of influence on behavior, as well as the same fundamental concepts of human behavior change described in the preceding section. The process of determining the ideal approach to a problem is sometimes referred to as a "task analysis," which can be viewed as an assessment of the specific "tasks" that need to be performed to appropriately deal with the problem.[2,21] To determine the ideal approach to a problem, the curriculum developer should ask what patients, health professionals, health professions educators, and society should each do to deal most effectively with the problem.

To what extent should *patients* be involved in handling the problem themselves? In many cases, the ideal approach will require education of patients and families affected by, or at risk of having, the problem.

EXAMPLE: *Role of Patients/Families.* Parents of children discharged from a neonatal intensive care unit (NICU) generally have not received any instruction about the developmental milestones that should be expected of their children. Neonatology care teams need to address the role that parents play in observing a child's development.[22,23]

Which *health professionals* should deal with the problem, and what should they be doing? Answering these questions can help the curriculum developer to target learners and define the content of a curriculum appropriately. If more than one type of health professional typically encounters the problem, the curriculum developer must decide what is most appropriate for each type of clinician and whether the curriculum will be modified to meet the needs of each type of clinician or will target just one group of health professionals.

EXAMPLE: *Role of Health Professionals.* Curriculum developers aiming to improve attention to hospitalized patients' spiritual needs recognized the roles of both physicians and chaplains. They subsequently developed an interprofessional curriculum in which chaplain trainees were embedded in the medical team. Chaplain trainees learned about the hospital environment, the culture of rounds, and the medical team's thinking about the plan of care. Medical trainees learned from the chaplain trainees about how to use a spirituality assessment tool to elicit needs and the value of involving chaplains in various patient care situations.[24]

What role should *health professions educators* have in addressing the problem? Determining the ideal approach for medical educators involves identifying the appropriate target audiences, the appropriate content, the best educational strategies, and the best evaluation methods to ensure effectiveness. Reviewing previously published curricula that address similar health care problems often uncovers elements of best practices that can be used in new curricular efforts.

EXAMPLE: *Identifying Appropriate Audiences, Content, and Methods.* Interns and residents have traditionally been trained to be on "code teams," but students can also be in clinical situations where improved competence in basic resuscitation can make a difference in patient outcomes. Basic life support (BLS) and advanced cardiovascular life support (ACLS) training can increase familiarity with cardiac protocols but have been shown to be inadequate in achieving competency as defined by adherence to protocols. Deliberate practice through simulation is an educational method that could potentially improve students' achievement of competency in these critical skills. A curriculum was created, implemented, and evaluated with these outcomes in mind.[25]

EXAMPLE: *Identifying Best Practices.* Since the Institute of Medicine's *Unequal Treatment* report, there have been numerous attempts to address health care disparities in undergraduate medical education.[26] Curriculum developers tasked with developing approaches to health disparities within their local environment could search PubMed and find a validated cultural competence assessment instrument, the Tool for Assessing Cultural Competency Training (TACCT), that could be used in a needs assessment or evaluation of a curriculum.[27] They could also learn how others have developed and described frameworks for the scope of related domains, such as cultural competence.[28] Reading about a consortium of 18 medical schools funded to address health disparities through medical education back in 2004 could lead not only to shareable curricular resources but also to potential colleagues with experience in teaching this topic.[29] Reviewing lessons learned by other educators can prevent unnecessary duplication of effort and identify opportunities to advance the field.[30]

Keep in mind, however, that educators may not be able to solve the problem by themselves. When the objectives are to change the behavior of patients or health professionals, educators should define their role relative to other interventions that may be needed to stimulate and sustain behavioral change.

What role should *society* have in addressing the problem? While curriculum developers usually are not in the position to effect societal change, some of their targeted learners may be, now or in the future. A curriculum, therefore, may choose to address current societal factors that contribute to or alleviate a problem (such as advertisements, political forces, organizational factors, and government policies). Sometimes, curriculum developers may want to target or collaborate with policymakers as part of a comprehensive strategy for addressing a public health problem.

> **EXAMPLE:** *Curricula to Influence Social Action.* Canadian medical students recognized that homeless and vulnerably housed populations experienced higher rates of preventable all-cause mortality compared to the general public. The Canadian Federation of Medical Students established a task force to create a curricular framework for helping students develop knowledge, attitudes, and skills to care for such populations. The task force included not only students and educators but also public health officials and persons who had experienced homelessness. Among the core competencies they identified based on literature review and group consensus was "advocacy"—being able to advocate for system-level change within health care systems and in greater society. Educational strategies discussed included providing opportunities for community service learning and mentorship with collaborators outside the health care sector to facilitate social action.[31]

The ideal approach should serve as an important, but not rigid, guide to developing a curriculum. One needs to be flexible in accommodating others' views and the many practical realities related to curriculum development. For this reason, it is useful to be transparent about the basis for one's "ideal" approach: individual opinion, consensus, the logical application of established theory, or scientific evidence. Obviously, one should be more flexible in espousing an "ideal" approach based on individual opinion than an "ideal" approach based on strong scientific evidence.

Differences between Current and Ideal Approaches

Having determined the current and ideal approaches to a problem, the curriculum developer can identify the differences between the two approaches. The gap identified by this *general needs assessment* should be the main target of any plans for addressing the health care problem. As mentioned above, the differences between the current and ideal approaches can be considered part of the problem that the curriculum will address, which is why Step 1 is sometimes referred to, simply, as *problem identification*.

OBTAINING INFORMATION ABOUT NEEDS

Each curriculum has unique needs for information about the problem of interest. In some cases, substantial information already exists and simply must be identified. In other cases, much information is available, but it needs to be systematically reviewed and synthesized. Frequently, the information available is insufficient to guide a new curriculum, in which case new information must be collected. Depending on the availability of relevant information, different methods can be used to identify and characterize a health care problem and to determine the current and ideal approaches to that problem. The most commonly used methods are listed in Table 2.3.

By carefully obtaining information about the need for a curriculum, educators will demonstrate that they are using a scholarly approach to curriculum development. This is an important component of educational scholarship, as defined by a consensus

Table 2.3.   Methods for Obtaining the Necessary Information

Review of Available Information
    Evidence-based reviews of educational and clinical topics
    Published original studies
    Clinical practice guidelines
    Published recommendations on expected competencies
    Reports by professional organizations or government agencies
    Documents submitted to educational clearinghouses
    Curriculum documents from other institutions
    Patient education materials prepared by foundations or professional organizations
    Patient support organizations
    Public health statistics
    Clinical registry data
    Administrative claims data

Use of Consultants/Experts
    Informal consultation
    Formal consultation
    Meetings of experts

Collection of New Information
    Surveys of patients, practitioners, or experts
    Focus group(s)
    Nominal group technique
    Group judgment methods (Delphi method)
    Liberating structures
    Daily diaries by patients and practitioners
    Observation of tasks performed by practitioners
    Time and motion studies
    Critical incident reviews
    Study of ideal performance cases or role-model practitioners (appreciative inquiry)

---

conference on educational scholarship that was sponsored by the Association of American Medical Colleges (AAMC).[32] A scholarly approach is valuable because it will help to convince learners and other educators that the curriculum is based on up-to-date knowledge of the published literature and existing best practices.

Finding and Synthesizing Available Information

The curriculum developer should start with a *well-focused review of information that is already available*. A *literature review*, including journal articles and textbooks, is generally the most efficient method for gathering information about a health care problem, what is currently being done to deal with it, and what ideally should be done. An informationist (health services librarian) can be extremely helpful in accessing the health and education literature, as well as databases that contain pertinent information. However, the curriculum developer should formulate specific questions to guide the review and the search for relevant information. Without focused questions, the review will be inefficient and less useful.

The curriculum developer should look for published *reviews* as well as any *original studies* about the topic. If a published review is available, it may be possible to rely on it, with just a quick look for new studies performed since the review was completed. The Best Evidence in Medical Education (BEME) Collaboration is a good source of high-quality evidence-based reviews of topics in medical education.[33] Depending on the topic, other evidence-based medicine resources may also contain valuable information, especially the Cochrane Collaboration, which produces evidence-based reviews on a wide variety of clinical topics.[34] If a formal review of the topic has not yet been done, it will be necessary to search systematically for relevant original studies. In such cases, the curriculum developer has an opportunity to make a scholarly contribution to the field by performing and publishing a review of that health professions education topic. It should include a carefully documented and comprehensive search for relevant studies, with explicitly defined criteria for inclusion in the review, as well as a verifiable methodology for extracting and synthesizing information from eligible studies.[35–39] By examining historical and social trends, the review may yield insights into future needs, in addition to current needs.

For many clinical topics, it is wise to look for pertinent *clinical practice guidelines*, because the guidelines may clearly delineate the ideal approach to a problem. In some countries, practice guidelines can be accessed through a government health agency, such as the National Institute for Health and Care Excellence (NICE) in the United Kingdom.[40] Other organizations also publish clinical guidelines. For example, the American Diabetes Association publishes its standards for medical care in diabetes annually as a journal supplement.[41] One way to find guidelines is to search PubMed and apply the "guideline" filter to search results. When different guidelines conflict, the curriculum developer can critically appraise the methods used to develop the guidelines to determine which recommendations should be included in the ideal approach.[42]

When designing a curriculum, educators need to be aware of any recommendations or statements by accreditation agencies or professional organizations about the *competencies* expected of practitioners. For example, any curriculum for internal medicine residents in the United States should take into consideration the core competencies set by the Accreditation Council for Graduate Medical Education (ACGME), specific milestones for internal medicine, and the certification requirements of the ABIM.[43–45] Similarly, any curriculum for medical students in the United States or Canada should take into consideration the accreditation standards of the Liaison Committee on Medical Education (LCME) and the core entrustable professional activities (EPAs) that medical school graduates should be able to perform when starting residency training, as defined by the graduate medical education accreditation authorities.[46,47] Within any clinical discipline, a corresponding professional society may issue a consensus statement about core competencies that should guide training in that discipline. A good example is the Society of Hospital Medicine, a national professional organization of hospitalists, which commissioned a task force to prepare a framework for curriculum development based on the core competencies in hospital medicine.[48] Often, the ideal approach to a problem will be based on this sort of authoritative statement about expected competencies. It is also important to check for updates to such statement. For example, as point-of-care ultrasound (POCUS) became possible, leaders needed to consider whether POCUS-training should be a core competency for hospital medicine.[49]

Educational clearinghouses can be particularly helpful to the curriculum developer because they may provide specific examples of what is being done by other medical educators to address a problem. The most useful educational clearinghouses tend to be those that have sufficient support and infrastructure to have some level of peer review, as well as some process for keeping them up to date. One particularly noteworthy clearinghouse for medical education is the MedEdPORTAL launched in 2005 by the AAMC.[50] This database includes a variety of peer-reviewed curriculum documents that have been prepared by medical and dental educators from many institutions. Clearinghouses are also maintained by some specialty and topic-oriented professional organizations. For example, the Society for Academic Emergency Medicine maintains a list of online academic resources that includes websites, online modules, curricular examples, podcasts, and free open access medical education (FOAMed) reusable learning objects, such as graphics, diagrams, cases, images, and videos.[51]

Other sources of available information also should be considered, especially when the published literature is sparse (see "Curricular Resources" in Appendix B). Data sources such as government publications, preprint curricula, data collected for other organizations, patents, and informal symposia proceedings are termed the "gray literature." For example, the AAMC maintains a database of medical school curricular data collected from curriculum management systems in use at many US and Canadian medical schools.[52] The database includes information about the content, structure, delivery, and assessment of medical school curricula and aggregated reports. Data related to specific topics of interest may be accessible through its website. Other sources of information include *reports by professional societies or government agencies*, which can highlight deficiencies in the current approach to a problem or make recommendations for a new approach to a problem. In some cases, it may be worthwhile to contact *colleagues at other institutions* who are performing related work and who may be willing to share information that they have developed or collected. For some health care problems, foundations or professional organizations have prepared *patient education materials*, and these can provide information about the problem from the patient perspective, as well as material to use in one's curriculum. Areas in which patient education materials suggest to patients "consult your physician" represent areas that physicians should be prepared to address with patients. Consultation with an informationist can be very helpful in identifying relevant data sources from both the standard peer-reviewed journals and the educational and gray literature.

Public health statistics, *clinical registry data*, and *administrative claims data* can be used for obtaining information about the incidence or prevalence of a problem. Libraries often have reports on the vital statistics of the population, which are published by the government. Clinical registry data may be difficult to access directly, but a search of the literature on a particular clinical topic can often identify reports from clinical registries. In the United States, the federal government and many states maintain administrative claims databases that provide data on the use of inpatient and outpatient medical services. Such data can help to define the magnitude of a clinical problem. Because of the enormous size of these databases, special e•pertise is needed to perform analyses of such data. Though these types of databases rarely have the depth of information that is needed to guide curriculum planning, they do have potential value in defining the extent of the health care problem.

Even though the curriculum developer may be an expert in the area to be addressed by the curriculum, it is wise to ask other experts how they interpret the information about a problem, particularly when the literature gives conflicting information or when there is uncertainty about the future direction of work in that area. In such cases, *expert opinions* can be obtained by consultation or by organizing a meeting of experts to discuss the issues. For most curricula, this can be done on a relatively informal basis with local experts. Occasionally, the problem is so controversial or important that the curriculum developer may wish to spend the additional time and effort necessary to obtain formal input from outside experts.

Collecting New Information

When the available information about a problem is so inadequate that curriculum developers cannot draw reasonable conclusions, it is desirable to *collect new information* about the problem. Information gathering can take numerous forms involving both quantitative and qualitative methodologies. The key feature that differentiates Step 1 from Step 2 is that, in Step 1, the curriculum developer seeks information that is broadly generalizable, not targeted.

In-person interviews with a small sample of patients, students, practitioners, medical educators, or experts can yield information relatively quickly, but for a general needs assessment, the sample must be chosen carefully to be broadly representative. Such interviews may be conducted individually or in the format of a *focus group* of 8–12 people, where the purpose is to obtain in-depth views regarding the topic of concern.[53] Obtaining consensus of the group is not the goal; rather, the goal is to elicit a range of perspectives. Another small-group method occasionally used in needs assessment is the *nominal group technique*, which employs a structured, sometimes iterative approach to identifying issues, solutions, and priorities.[54] The outcome of this technique is an extensive list of brainstormed and rank-ordered ideas. When the objective is not only to generate ideas or answers to a question but also to move a group toward agreement, an iterative process called the *Delphi method* can be used with participants who either meet repeatedly or respond to a series of questions over time. Participant responses are fed back to the group on each successive cycle to promote consensus. It is important to use such processes accurately to obtain true consensus.[55,56] When seeking information from a diverse group of stakeholders, use of *liberating structures*—simple rules to guide interaction and innovative thinking about a shared issue—may help to organize and facilitate the experience.[57]

When quantitative and representative data are desired, it is customary to perform a systematic *questionnaire or interview survey*.[58,59] For the general needs assessment, it is particularly important to ensure that questionnaires are distributed to an appropriate sample so that the results will be generalizable. Surveys can be now be done via text and social media in addition to mail, phone, and email. (See the General References at the end of this chapter and references in Chapter 3 for more information on survey methodology.)

EXAMPLE: *Gathering New Information for a General Needs Assessment.* A national needs assessment of competencies for general and expert practice of POCUS was done for Canadian emergency medicine (EM) physicians. A response rate of over 80% was obtained from experts, practicing physicians, and trainees. The results were published in the *Canadian Journal of Emergency Medicine* so that educators across Canada could use these results to guide curricular development.[60]

EXAMPLE: *Choosing Appropriate Sample for a General Needs Assessment.* A different algorithmic approach for EM POCUS curricula in less-resourced countries in Africa was described by a group of emergency medicine leaders from eight different African countries. While core competency documents by the International Federation of Emergency Medicine were reviewed as a starting place, this group of educators also pointed out that simply adopting priorities of programs from resource-rich countries would not prepare learners to meet the needs of their patients. For example, they mentioned that aortic procedures and central-line placement are rarely done in their ERs. Rather, use of POCUS for determining whether precious IV fluids should be administered or to aid in differential diagnosis of abdominal pain in the absence of other commonly used imaging modalities would make a greater impact in their settings.[61]

Sometimes, more intensive methods of data collection are necessary. When little is known about the current approach to a clinical problem, educators may ask practitioners or patients to complete *daily diaries or records of activities*. Alternatively, they may utilize *work sampling* (direct observation of a sample of patients, practitioners, or medical educators in their work setting), *time and motion studies* (which involve observation and detailed analysis of how patients and/or practitioners spend their time), *critical incident reviews* (in which cases having desired and undesired outcomes are reviewed to determine how the process of care relates to the outcomes), or *review of ideal performance cases* (using appreciative inquiry to discover what has enabled achievement in the past as a way to help to improve future performance).[62–66] These methods require considerable time and resources but may be valuable when detailed information is needed about a particular aspect of clinical practice. Electronic medical record systems can sometimes provide helpful data, though one should take measures to ensure confidentiality and relevance (data collected for billing or patient care purposes may or may not be applicable to the educational research questions at hand).[67,68]

What is most important is identifying accurate and relevant data to guide understanding of the health problem for the purpose of curriculum development. Therefore, regardless of what methods are used to obtain information about a problem, it is necessary to synthesize that information in an efficient manner. A logical, well-organized report, with tables that summarize the collected information, is one of the most common methods for accomplishing the synthesis. A well-organized report has the advantages of efficiently communicating this information to others and being available for quick reference in the future. Collected reference materials and resources can be filed for future access.

TIME AND EFFORT

Some problems are complex enough to require a great deal of time to understand them adequately. However, when original data needs to be collected, less complex problems that have not been studied may require more time and effort than more complex problems that have been well studied. Those involved in the development of a curriculum must decide how much they are willing to spend, in terms of time, effort, and other resources, for problem identification and general needs assessment. An inadequate commitment to Step 1 could lead to a curriculum that is poorly focused and unlikely to address the problem effectively, or to a subsequent waste of effort expended in "reinventing the wheel" when adoption or adaptation of an existing curriculum could have addressed the gap. Investing too much time and effort in Step 1 runs the risk of leaving insufficient resources for the other steps in the curriculum development process. Careful consideration of the nature of the problem is necessary to achieve an appropriate balance.

One of the goals of this step is for the curriculum developer to become enough of an expert in the area to make decisions about curricular objectives and content. The curriculum developers' prior knowledge of the problem area, therefore, will also determine the amount of time and effort needed for this step.

The time and effort spent on defining the problem of interest in a scholarly manner may yield new information or new perspectives that warrant publication in the medical literature (see Chapter 9, Dissemination). However, the methods employed in the problem identification and general needs assessment should be rigorously applied and described if the results are to be published in a peer-reviewed journal. The curriculum developer must decide whether the academic value of a scholarly publication related to Step 1 is worth the additional time and effort. A sound, if less methodologically rigorous, problem identification and needs assessment that is used for planning the curriculum could also be used for the introduction and discussion of a scholarly publication about evaluation results or novel educational strategies.

Sharing a previously well-articulated Step 1 can serve as a foundation that allows other curriculum developers to focus more time and energy on other steps. Otherwise, time pressures, or the inheritance of an existing curriculum, may result in a situation in which the curriculum is developed before an adequate problem identification and general needs assessment has been written. In such situations, a return to this step may be helpful in explaining or improving an existing curriculum.

CONCLUSION

To address a health care problem effectively and efficiently, a curriculum developer must define the problem carefully and determine the current and ideal approaches to the problem. A curriculum by itself may not solve all aspects of the problem, particularly if the problem is a complex one. However, the difference between the ideal and current approaches will often highlight deficiencies in the knowledge, attitudes, skills, or behavior of practitioners. Educational efforts can be directed toward closing those gaps. Thus, this step is essential in focusing a curriculum so that it can make a meaningful contribution to solving the problem.

The conclusions drawn from the general needs assessment may or may not apply to the particular group of learners or institution(s) targeted by a curriculum developer. For this reason, it is necessary to assess the specific needs of one's targeted learners and institution(s) (see Chapter 3) before proceeding with further development of a curriculum.

QUESTIONS

For the curriculum you are coordinating or planning, please answer the following questions:

1. What is the *health care problem* that will be addressed by this curriculum?

2. *Whom* does the problem affect?

3. *What* effects does the problem have on these people?

4. How important is the problem, *quantitatively and qualitatively*?

5. Based on your current knowledge, what are patients/families, health professionals, educators, and policymakers doing *currently* to address the problem?

	Patients	Health Professionals	Educators	Society
Current Approach				
Ideal Approach				

6. Based on your current knowledge, what should patients, health professionals, educators, and policymakers *ideally* be doing to address the problem?

7. To complete a *general needs assessment*, what are the differences between the current and ideal approaches?

8. What are the key areas in which your knowledge has been deficient in answering these questions? Given your available resources, what *methods* would you use to correct these deficiencies? (See Table 2.3.)

GENERAL REFERENCES

Altschuld, James W., and Ryan Watkins, eds. *Needs Assessment: Trends and a View toward the Future*. Hoboken, NJ: Jossey-Bass, 2014.
    A concise overview guide to theories and trends by experienced authors in the field of needs assessment. This volume of the journal includes articles on asset-based needs assessment and contextual assessments, considerations for international work, and tools for data collection including web-based, crowd-sourcing, photovoice, and big data. It also references a website (www.needsassessment.org) that contains links to free books and actual assessment tool templates. 128 pages.

Glanz, Karen, Barbara K. Rimer, and K. Viswanath, eds. *Health Behavior: Theory, Research, and Practice*. 5th ed. San Francisco: Jossey-Bass, 2015.
    The classic public health textbook that covers the past, present, and future of health behavioral interventions. Helpful for considering the big picture of a health problem and options for influencing behaviors on the levels of patients, professionals, educators, and society.

O'Brien, Bridget C., Kirsty Forrest, Marjo Wijenn-Meijer, and Olle ten Cate. "A Global View of Structures and Trends in Medical Education." In *Understanding Medical Education: Evidence, Theory, and Practice*, edited by Tim Swanwick, Kirsty Forrest, and Bridget C. O'Brien, 7–22. Hoboken, NJ: John Wiley & Sons, 2019.
    This is the lead chapter of a book that attempts to provide a global perspective on medical education. The authors review the structure of medical education in different countries and the interplay between medical education and health systems, cultural and societal factors, globalization, and technology. A helpful read to understand factors that can affect the current and ideal approaches to medical education.

Sklar, David P. "What Would Excellence in Health Professions Education Mean If It Addressed Our Most Pressing Health Problems?," *Academic Medicine* 94, no. 1 (January 2019): 1–3. https://doi.org/10.1097/ACM.0000000000002474.

> One of many excellent editorial/commentaries written by Dr. David Sklar, editor of *Academic Medicine*, to promote thinking about the ways the education of health professionals should and could be more closely tied to health care problems and outcomes.

REFERENCES CITED

1. Sadie Elisseou et al., "A Novel, Trauma-Informed Physical Examination Curriculum for First-Year Medical Students," *MedEdPORTAL* 15 (2019), https://doi.org/10.15766/mep_2374-8265.10799.
2. Archie S. Golden, "A Model for Curriculum Development Linking Curriculum with Health Needs," in *The Art of Teaching Primary Care*, ed. Archie S. Golden, Dennis G. Carlson, and Jan L. Hagen (New York: Springer Publishing Co., 1982), 9–25.
3. John E. Wennberg, "Practice Variations and Health Care Reform: Connecting the Dots," *Health Affairs* Suppl Variation (2004), VAR140-4, https://doi.org/10.1377/hlthaff.var.140.
4. Paul Glasziou et al., "Evidence for Underuse of Effective Medical Services around the World," *The Lancet* 390, no. 10090 (2017): 169–77, https://doi.org/10.1016/S0140-6736(16)30946-1.
5. Shannon Brownlee et al., "Evidence for Overuse of Medical Services around the World," *The Lancet* 390, no. 10090 (2017), 156–68, https://doi.org/10.1016/S0140-6736(16)32585-5.
6. "Choosing Wisely: A Special Report on the First Five Years," ABIM and Consumer Reports Foundation, accessed May 28, 2021, https://www.choosingwisely.org/wp-content/uploads/2017/10/Choosing-Wisely-at-Five.pdf.
7. Michelle P. Lin et al., "Emergency Physician Knowledge, Attitudes, and Behavior regarding ACEP's Choosing Wisely Recommendations: A Survey Study," *Academic Emergency Medicine* 24, no. 6 (2017): 668–75, https://doi.org/10.1111/acem.13167.
8. WHO Study Group on Interprofessional Education and Collaborative Practice, *Framework for Action on Interprofessional Education and Collaborative Practice* (Geneva, Switzerland: World Health Organization, 2010).
9. Institute of Medicine (US) Committee on the Health Professions Education Summit, *Health Professions Education: A Bridge to Quality*, ed. Ann Greiner and Elisa Knebel (Washington DC: National Academies Press, 2003).
10. Interprofessional Education Collaborative Expert Panel, *Core Competencies for Interprofessional Collaborative Practice: Report of an Expert Panel* (Washington, DC: Interprofessional Education Collaborative, 2011).
11. Interprofessional Education Collaborative, *Core Competencies for Interprofessional Collaborative Practice: 2016 Update* (Washington, DC: Interprofessional Education Collaborative, 2016), accessed October 8, 2021, https://www.ipecollaborative.org/ipec-core-competencies.
12. Natalie L. Murdoch, Sheila Epp, and Jeanette Vinek, "Teaching and Learning Activities to Educate Nursing Students for Interprofessional Collaboration: A Scoping Review," *Journal of Interprofessional Care* 31, no. 6 (2017): 744–53, https://doi.org/10.1080/13561820.2017.1356807.
13. Nancy D. Harada et al., "Interprofessional Transformation of Clinical Education: The First Six Years of the Veterans Affairs Centers of Excellence in Primary Care Education," *Journal of Interprofessional Care* online (2018), https://doi.org/10.1080/13561820.2018.1433642.
14. "MedEdPORTAL Interprofessional Education Collection," Association of American Medical Colleges, accessed October 1, 2021, https://www.mededportal.org/interprofessional-education.
15. Raagini Jawa et al., "Rapid Naloxone Administration Workshop for Health Care Providers at an Academic Medical Center," *MedEdPORTAL* 16 (2020), https://doi.org/10.15766/mep_2374-8265.10892.

16. James F. Sallis and Neville Owen, "Ecological Models of Health Behaviors," in *Health Behavior: Theory, Research, and Practice,* ed. Karen Glanz, Barbara K. Rimer, and Kasisomayajula Viswanath (San Francisco: Jossey-Bass, 2015), 48.

17. "Food Insecurity and Health: A Toolkit for Physicians and Health Care Organizations," Feeding America, accessed October 1, 2021, https://hungerandhealth.feedingamerica.org/wp-content/uploads/2017/11/Food-Insecurity-Toolkit.pdf.

18. Karen Glanz, Barbara K. Rimer, and Kasisomayajula Viswanath, *Health Behavior: Theory, Research, and Practice*, 5th ed. (San Francisco: Jossey-Bass, 2015), 512.

19. Lawrence W. Green and Marshall W. Kreuter, *Health Program Planning: An Educational and Ecological Approach* (New York: McGraw-Hill, 2005).

20. Jos H. Verbeek et al., "Personal Protective Equipment for Preventing Highly Infectious Diseases Due to Exposure to Contaminated Body Fluids in Healthcare Staff," *Cochrane Database of Systematic Reviews*, no. 5 (2020), https://doi.org//10.1002/14651858.CD011621.pub5.

21. Gary M. Arsham, August Colenbrander, and Bruce E. Spivey, "A Prototype for Curriculum Development in Medical Education," *Journal of Medical Education* 48, no. 1 (1973): 78–84, https://doi.org/10.1097/00001888-197301000-00011.

22. Loren Berman et al., "Parent Perspectives on Readiness for Discharge Home after Neonatal Intensive Care Unit Admission," *Journal of Pediatrics* 205 (2019): 98–104.e4, https://doi.org/10.1016/j.jpeds.2018.08.086.

23. Ayuko Komoriyama et al., "A Journey through Follow-Up for Neurodevelopmentally At-Risk Infants—a Qualitative Study on Views of Parents and Professionals in Liverpool," *Child: Care, Health & Development* 45, no. 6 (2019): 808–14, https://doi.org/10.1111/cch.12713.

24. Patrick Hemming et al., "Demystifying Spiritual Care: An Interprofessional Approach for Teaching Residents and Hospital Chaplains to Work Together," *Journal of Graduate Medical Education* 8, no. 3 (2016): 454–55, https://doi.org/10.4300/JGME-D-15-00637.1.

25. Julianna Jung and Nicole A. Shilkofski, "Appendix A: Essential Resuscitation Skills for Medical Students," in *Curriculum Development for Medical Education: A Six-Step Approach*, 3rd ed., ed. Patricia A. Thomas et al. (Baltimore: Johns Hopkins University Press, 2015), 236–45.

26. Institute of Medicine, *Unequal Treatment: Confronting Racial and Ethnic Disparities in Health Care*, ed. Brian D. Smedley, Adrienne Y. Stith, and Alan R. Nelson (Washington, DC: National Academies Press, 2003), 780.

27. Désirée Lie, "Revising the Tool for Assessing Cultural Competence Training (TACCT) for Curriculum Evaluation: Findings Derived from Seven US Schools and Expert Consensus," *Medical Education Online* 13, no. 11 (2008): 1–11, https://doi.org/10.3885/meo.2008.Res00272.

28. Katie Crenshaw et al., "What Should We Include in a Cultural Competence Curriculum? An Emerging Formative Evaluation Process to Foster Curriculum Development," *Academic Medicine* 86, no. 3 (2011): 333–41, https://doi.org/10.1097/ACM.0b013e3182087314.

29. Olivia Carter-Pokras et al., "Surmounting the Unique Challenges in Health Disparities Education: A Multi-Institution Qualitative Study," *Journal of General Internal Medicine* 25, no. S2 (2010): S108–14, https://doi.org/10.1007/s11606-010-1269-1.

30. Cristina Gonzalez, Aaron Fox, and Paul Marantz, "The Evolution of an Elective in Health Disparities and Advocacy: Description of Instructional Strategies and Program Evaluation," *Academic Medicine* 90, no. 12 (2015): 1636–40, https://doi.org/10.1097/ACM.0000000000000850.

31. Syeda Shanza Hashmi et al., "A Student-Led Curriculum Framework for Homeless and Vulnerably Housed Populations," *BMC Medical Education* 20, no. 1 (2020): 232, https://doi.org/10.1186/s12909-020-02143-z.

32. Deborah Simpson et al., "Advancing Educators and Education by Defining the Components and Evidence Associated with Educational Scholarship," *Medical Education* 41, no. 10 (2007): 1002–9, https://doi.org/10.1111/j.1365-2923.2007.02844.x.

33. "The BEME Collaboration," Best Evidence Medical and Health Professional Education, accessed October 1, 2021, https://www.bemecollaboration.org.
34. Cochrane Library, accessed October 1, 2021, https://www.cochranelibrary.com.
35. Darcy Reed et al., "Challenges in Systematic Reviews of Educational Intervention Studies," *Annals of Internal Medicine* 142, no. 12 (2005): 1080–89, https://doi.org/10.7326/0003-4819 -142-12_part_2-200506211-00008.
36. William C. McGaghie et al., "Varieties of Integrative Scholarship," *Academic Medicine* 90, no. 3 (2015): 294–302, https://doi.org/10.1097/ACM.0000000000000585.
37. David Moher et al., "Preferred Reporting Items for Systematic Reviews and Meta-Analyses: The Prisma Statement," *PLOS Medicine* 6, no. 7 (2009): e1000097, https://doi.org/10.1371 /journal.pmed.1000097.
38. Morris Gordon and Trevor Gibbs, "STORIES Statement: Publication Standards for Healthcare Education Evidence Synthesis," *BMC Medicine* 12 (2014): 143, https://doi.org/10.1186 /s12916-014-0143-0.
39. Risha Sharma et al., "Systematic Reviews in Medical Education: A Practical Approach: AMEE Guide 94," *Medical Teacher* 37, no. 2 (2015): 108–24, https://doi.org/10.3109/0142159x.2014 .970996.
40. "NICE Guidance," National Institute for Health and Care Excellence, accessed October 1, 2021, https://www.nice.org.uk/guidance.
41. "Introduction: Standards of Medical Care in Diabetes—2021," *Diabetes Care* 44, no. Suppl 1 (2021): S1–S2, https://doi.org/10.2337/dc21-Sint.
42. "The AGREE II Instrument," AGREE Next Steps Consortium (2017), accessed October 1, 2021, http://www.agreetrust.org/resource-centre/agree-ii.
43. "Common Program Requirements (Residency)," Accreditation Council for Graduate Medical Education, accessed October 1, 2021, https://www.acgme.org/what-we-do/accreditation /common-program-requirements/.
44. "The Internal Medicine Milestone Project," ACGME and American Board of Internal Medicine, July 2015, accessed October 1, 2021, https://www.acgme.org/Portals/0/PDFs/Milestones /InternalMedicineMilestones.pdf.
45. "Becoming Certified: Policies," American Board of Internal Medicine, accessed May 31, 2021, https://www.abim.org/certification/policies/.
46. Liaison Committee on Medical Education, *Functions and Structure of a Medical School: Standards for Accreditation of Medical Education Programs Leading to the MD Degree*, March 2021, accessed October 1, 2021, https://lcme.org/publications/.
47. "Core Entrustable Professional Activities for Entering Residency: Curriculum Developer's Guide," 2014, Association of American Medical Colleges, accessed October 6, 2021, https:// www.aamc.org/what-we-do/mission-areas/medical-education/cbme/core-epas/publications.
48. Sylvia C. W. McKean et al., "How to Use the Core Competencies in Hospital Medicine: A Framework for Curriculum Development," *Journal of Hospital Medicine* 1 (2006): 57–67, https://doi.org/10.1002/jhm.86.
49. Nilam J. Soni et al., "Point-of-Care Ultrasound for Hospitalists: A Position Statement of the Society of Hospital Medicine," 2019, https://doi.org/10.12788/jhm.3079.
50. MedEdPORTAL: The Journal of Teaching and Learning Resources, accessed October 6, 2021, https://www.mededportal.org.
51. "SAEM Online Academic Resources (SOAR)," Society for Academic Emergency Medicine, accessed October 6, 2021, https://www.saem.org/education/saem-online-academic-resources.
52. "Curriculum Inventory," Association of American Medical Colleges, accessed October 6, 2021, https://www.aamc.org/what-we-do/mission-areas/medical-education/curriculum -inventory.
53. Renée E. Stalmeijer, Nancy McNaughton, and Walther N. K. A. Van Mook, "Using Focus Groups in Medical Education Research: AMEE Guide No. 9," *Medical Teacher* 36, no. 11 (2014): 923–39, https://doi.org/10.3109/0142159X.2014.917165.

54. Susan Humphrey-Murto et al., "Using Consensus Group Methods Such as Delphi and Nominal Group in Medical Education Research," *Medical Teacher* 39, no. 1 (2017): 14–19, https://doi.org/10.1080/0142159X.2017.1245856.

55. Susan Humphrey-Murto et al., "The Use of the Delphi and Other Consensus Group Methods in Medical Education Research: A Review," *Academic Medicine* 92, no. 10 (2017): 1491–98, https://doi.org/10.1097/ACM.0000000000001812.

56. Thomas Foth et al., "The Use of Delphi and Nominal Group Technique in Nursing Education: A Review," *International Journal of Nursing Studies* 60, (2016): 112–20, https://doi.org/10.1016/j.ijnurstu.2016.04.015.

57. Liberating Structures, accessed October 6, 2021, https://www.liberatingstructures.com.

58. Karen A. Burns et al., "A Guide for the Design and Conduct of Self-Administered Surveys of Clinicians," *Canadian Medical Association Journal* 79, no. 3 (2008): 245–52, https://doi.org/10.1503/cmaj.080372.

59. Hunter Gehlbach, Anthony R. Artino, and Steven J. Durning, "AM Last Page: Survey Development Guidance for Medical Education Researchers," *Academic Medicine* 85, no. 5 (2010): 925, https://doi.org/10.1097/ACM.0b013e3181dd3e88.

60. Lisa M. Fischer et al., "Emergency Medicine Point-of-Care Ultrasonography: A National Needs Assessment of Competencies for General and Expert Practice," *Canadian Journal of Emergency Medicine* 17, no. 1 (2015): 74–88, https://doi.org/10.2310/8000.2013.131205.

61. Margaret Salmon et al., "Getting It Right the First Time: Defining Regionally Relevant Training Curricula and Provider Core Competencies for Point-of-Care Ultrasound Education on the African Continent," *Annals of Emergency Medicine* 69, no. 2 (2017): 218–26, https://doi.org/10.1016/j.annemergmed.2016.07.030.

62. Lena Mamykina, David K. Vawdrey, and George Hripcsak, "How Do Residents Spend Their Shift Time? A Time and Motion Study with a Particular Focus on the Use of Computers," *Academic Medicine* 91, no. 6 (2016): 827–32, https://doi.org/10.1097/ACM.0000000000001148.

63. Daniel Wong et al., "How Hospital Pharmacists Spend Their Time: A Work-Sampling Study," *Canadian Journal of Hospital Pharmacy* 73, no. 4 (2020): 272–78, https://doi.org/10.4212/cjhp.v73i4.3026.

64. Alison Steven et al., "Critical Incident Techniques and Reflection in Nursing and Health Professions Education," *Nurse Educator* 45, no. 6 (2020): E57–E61, https://doi.org/10.1097/NNE.0000000000000796.

65. William T. Branch, "Use of Critical Incident Reports in Medical Education: A Perspective," *Journal of General Internal Medicine* 20, no. 11 (2005): 1063–67, https://doi.org/10.1111/j.1525-1497.2005.00231.x.

66. John Sandars and Deborah Murdoch-Eaton, "Appreciative Inquiry in Medical Education," *Medical Teacher* 39, no. 2 (2017): 123–27, https://doi.org/10.1080/0142159X.2017.1245852.

67. Amanda L. Terry et al., "A Basic Model for Assessing Primary Health Care Electronic Medical Record Data Quality," *BMC Medical Informatics and Decision Making* 19, no. 1 (2019): 30, https://doi.org/10.1186/s12911-019-0740-0.

68. Vineet Arora, "Harnessing the Power of Big Data to Improve Graduate Medical Education: Big Idea or Bust?," *Academic Medicine* 93, no. 6 (2018): 833–834, https://doi.org/10.1097/ACM.0000000000002209.

Step 2
Targeted Needs Assessment

. . . refining the foundation

Mark T. Hughes, MD, MA

DEFINITION

A targeted needs assessment is a process by which curriculum developers apply the knowledge learned from the general needs assessment to their particular learners and learning environment. Curriculum developers must understand their learners and their learning environment to develop a curriculum that best suits their needs and addresses the health problem characterized in Step 1. In Step 2, curriculum developers identify specific needs by assessing *the differences between ideal and actual characteristics of the targeted learner group and the differences between ideal and actual characteristics of their learning environment.*

IMPORTANCE

The targeted needs assessment serves many functions. It allows the health problem to be framed properly for the intended curriculum. It clarifies the challenges and opportunities for subsequent curriculum development steps. It involves stakeholders in the process of making curricular decisions. It is one of the first steps in engaging and motivating learners in their own education. By involving those who are investing in the curriculum in the targeted needs assessment process, curriculum developers cultivate relationships and build trust, which will be important for implementation of the curriculum (see Chapter 6). A well-done targeted needs assessment can ensure that resources are being used effectively. Done appropriately, the targeted needs assessment prevents duplication of what is already being done, teaching what is already known, or teaching above the level of the targeted learners. It helps to shape the educational plan and design assessments that confirm preparedness for future learning or work. Stated simply, the targeted needs assessment provides the data to justify curricular decisions.[1]

Step 2 encourages the curriculum developer to move the focus from the health problem to the targeted learners. The general needs assessment from Step 1 serves as a guide for developing the targeted needs assessment (see Chapter 2). The general needs assessment can provide the rationale for a curricular approach, but that approach must still consider the characteristics of the curriculum developer's intended learners. The published literature used to support the general needs assessment may be dated, and curriculum developers will need to update the curriculum design based on current practice. A model curriculum from another institution, found in the literature search for Step 1, may require modification to fit one's own learners. A published curriculum may have been delivered to another type of learner with a different knowledge base or a different learning preference.

The needs of a curriculum's targeted learners are likely to be somewhat different from the needs of learners identified in the general needs assessment. A curriculum's targeted learners may already be proficient in one area of general need but have particular learning needs in another area. Some objectives may already be taught in other parts of the overall teaching program but need to be further developed in the new curricular segment. Stakeholders, such as clerkship or program directors, may want specific learner objectives, competencies, or milestones to interact with and reinforce topics addressed in other curricula.

The targeted needs assessment should occur at two levels: (1) the targeted learners (their current and past experiences; their strengths and weaknesses in knowledge, attitudes, skills, and behaviors), and (2) the targeted learning environment (the existing curriculum; other characteristics of the learners' environment that influence whether/how learning occurs and is reinforced; the needs of key stakeholders).

IDENTIFICATION OF TARGETED LEARNERS

Before curriculum developers can proceed with the targeted needs assessment, they must first identify their targeted learners. Targeted learners can be patients, practitioners, practitioners-in-training, or students. Often curriculum developers are assigned the targeted learners, such as health professional students or resident physicians-in-training.

Ideally, however, the choice of targeted learners would flow from the problem identification and general needs assessment (see Chapter 2). The targeted learners would be the group most likely, with further learning, to contribute to the solution of the problem.

> **EXAMPLE:** *Selecting Targeted Learners.* In an effort to address health inequities in rural communities in Canada due to an undersupply of physicians, educators at the Northern Ontario School of Medicine used a demographic scoring system at the time of admission to select learners who were raised and had family in the region or in other rural locations. This resulted in targeted learners who had an established place-identity and who, it was hoped, would be more invested in a "place-based" educational program aiming to keep graduates in the region to practice rural medicine.[2,3]

When curriculum developers have already been assigned their targeted learners, it is worth considering how an educational intervention directed at the targeted learners could contribute to solving the health problem of concern. For instance, understanding the targeted learners' developmental stage can help in determining what aspects of the problem are addressed by delivery of the curriculum. The targeted learner group should not be just a convenience sample of available learners.

Depending on the curriculum, targeted learners may be a small group, as with a lecture or seminar, or number in the thousands, as with a massive open online course (MOOC).[4] Targeted learners may be based at one institution or across multiple institutions. While curriculum developers may intend a target audience, they should also appreciate that other learners may be exposed to the curriculum (e.g., an online curriculum intended for internal medicine residents is used by family nurse practitioner students). It is also important to understand how the targeted learners will interact with other learners within the health professions and how their learning can influence others. Defining the characteristics of the targeted learners in the targeted needs assessment can help other educators determine how representative they are to other learners. Thus, if resources permit, curriculum developers should create a targeted needs assessment with an eye on its generalizability to other learners.

DESCRIPTION OF THE TARGETED LEARNING ENVIRONMENT

Curriculum developers must also assess their targeted learners' environment(s). If the curriculum devotes unnecessary resources to areas already addressed and mastered in the targeted learning environment, it will be inefficient. If the curriculum devotes insufficient resources or attention to areas of concern within the targeted environment, then it will not be fully effective. If a topic is not taught in the curriculum, learners may consciously or unconsciously view those issues as unimportant to their professional formation.[5] In addition to the planned or formal curriculum, curriculum developers must be attentive to the other experiences within the learning environment that shape learners' values. The unplanned interactions among student peers and between students and teachers create a culture of the learning environment that will influence learners' current and future thoughts and behaviors.[6,7] The informal, collateral, or hidden curricula can motivate learners and reinforce knowledge or skills taught in the formal curriculum, or they can counter the attitudes and behaviors that educators wish to promote. Since clinical training involves professional acculturation, it is important to understand the sociocultural underpinning of the clinical learning environment.[8,9] Priming students to attune themselves to the hidden curriculum within their environment can be one strategy within the formal curriculum to mitigate its influence.[10]

CONTENT

Content about Targeted Learners

Once targeted learners have been identified, the next step in the targeted needs assessment is to decide on the information about the targeted learners that is most needed. Such information might include expectations regarding the extent of knowledge and skills needed (which will differ, for instance, between a medical student and a senior resident); previous and already planned training and experiences; scope of current responsibilities (for instance, service obligations of resident physicians); existing proficiencies (cognitive, affective, psychomotor behaviors); perceived deficiencies and needs (from evaluators' and/or learners' perspectives); measured deficiencies in knowledge or skills; reasons for past poor performance; learners' capacities and motivations to improve performance; tolerance for ambiguity[11,12] and readiness to change; attitudes about the curricular topic; preferred learning methods; and targeted learners' experiences with different learning strategies (Table 3.1).

For learners in a work environment, it is important to learn the scope of their work responsibilities, the competencies necessary to fulfill those responsibilities, and the training and non-training requirements necessary for the learner to become competent.[13] Non-training requirements include character or personality traits conducive to fulfilling tasks in a particular work environment (e.g., ability to work in a fast-paced environment). Different kinds of learners in a work environment may have different learning needs in light of their work responsibilities.

EXAMPLE: *Expectations Regarding Scope of Knowledge and Skills Needed.* The nursing education council in a large health system developed an innovative approach to learners' needs assessments. After a literature review, draft assessment surveys for clinical nurses, nurse managers/directors, advanced practice registered nurses, and nurse executives were developed and finalized through an iterative process and consultant feedback. Surveys were administered electronically across the health system. Nurses preferred online education, citing lack of time as a barrier to continuing education. An education action plan was developed, targeting the most preferred topics identified in the needs assessment: clinical nurses favored education on workplace culture, nurse managers desired education on motivating and influencing others, and advanced practice nurses wanted more training in dealing with difficult people.[14]

EXAMPLE: *Learners and Prior Experience.* Curriculum developers planning education programs for point-of-care ultrasound in resource-limited settings need to understand their trainees' prior experience with ultrasonography. For example, have they referred a patient for ultrasonography at a health facility? Have they ever personally used an ultrasound machine before? Have they had formal instruction in ultrasonography? If so, was it lecture-based or hands-on skills training? Curriculum developers can include objective measures of the targeted learners' capabilities in diagnostic imaging to determine whether ultrasound training would aid the learners' diagnostic capacity. For learners with prior experience in the use of ultrasound, curriculum developers can design developmentally appropriate training to enhance their capacity. In addition, educators need to understand how the targeted learners anticipate applying ultrasound in their clinical practice and the barriers that can affect continuing education about, and sustained use of, ultrasonography.[15]

EXAMPLE: *Learners' Knowledge, Attitudes, and Barriers.* Because internal medicine trainees at the main health system in Qatar come from diverse geographic backgrounds in the Middle East, North Africa, and Asia, curriculum developers sought to determine their knowledge of and attitudes toward evidence-based medicine (EBM). EBM aptitude was measured by the Assessing Competency in Evidence Based Medicine (ACE) tool. Education background and demographic information was collected via survey, and attitudes about EBM, self-rated aptitude, and barriers to institutional EBM implementation were assessed

Table 3.1.   Content Potentially Relevant to a Targeted Needs Assessment

Content about Targeted Learners
Expectations regarding extent of knowledge and skills needed
Previous training and experiences relevant to the curriculum
Already planned training and experiences relevant to the curriculum
Scope of current responsibilities and requirements necessary to become competent
Existing characteristics/proficiencies/practices
    Cognitive: knowledge, problem-solving abilities
    Affective: attitudes, values, beliefs, role expectations
    Psychomotor: skills/capabilities (e.g., history, physical examination, procedures,
        counseling)
    Current behaviors/practices
Perceived and measured deficiencies and learning needs
Attitudes and motivations of learners to improve performance
Tolerance for ambiguity and readiness to change
Preferences and experiences regarding different learning strategies
    Synchronous (educator sets time, such as with noon lecture)
    Asynchronous (learner decides on learning time, such as with e-learning)
    Duration (amount of time learner thinks is needed to learn or that they can devote to learning)
    Methods (e.g., readings, lectures, online learning resources, large- and small-group
        discussions, problem-based learning, team-based learning, peer teaching,
        demonstrations, role-plays/simulations, supervised experience)

Content about Targeted Learning Environment
Related existing curricula and need for enhancement or modification
Needs of stakeholders other than the learners (course directors, clerkship directors, program
    directors, faculty, accrediting bodies, and others)
Barriers, enablers, and reinforcing factors that affect learning by the targeted learners
    Barriers (e.g., time, unavailability, or competition for resources)
    Enablers (e.g., learning portfolios, electronic medical record reminders)
    Reinforcing factors (e.g., incentives such as grades, awards, recognition)
Resources (e.g., patients and clinical experiences, faculty, role models and mentors,
    information resources, access to hardware and software technology, audiovisual
    equipment, simulation center)
Informal and collateral curriculum

by Likert scale questions. The needs assessment found knowledge gaps, and most learners rated themselves as having beginner or intermediate abilities in EBM. Trainees had favorable views toward implementing EBM in their clinical practice, but barriers included lack of knowledge, resources, and time.[16]

EXAMPLE: *Learners' Experience and Perceived Deficiencies.* To assess management skills of consultation-liaison psychiatry directors, a new forum of the Academy of Consultation-Liaison Psychiatry performed a needs assessment of its members through a voluntary, anonymous online survey. In addition to learning about the directors' experience level, the survey asked respondents to rate the importance of 14 managerial tasks and their level of confidence as a leader in those tasks. Lower confidence in managerial skills was seen with newer directors, prompting the study authors to advocate for institutions and department chairs to invest in health management training.[17]

EXAMPLE: *Measuring Learners' Deficiencies in the Clinical Setting.* Recognizing a need for clinician training in caring for older adults with multimorbidity, educators took audio recordings of 30 clinic visits between internal medicine residents and their primary care patients aged 65 and older with two or more chronic conditions. The curriculum developers wished to ascertain current practice and opportunities for improvement in the five guiding principles for the care of older adults with multimorbidity: patient preferences, interpreting the evidence, prognosis, clinical feasibility, and optimizing therapies and the care plan. Audio recordings were transcribed and then qualitatively analyzed to determine themes. Most discussions between residents and patients related to at least one of the guiding principles. Residents missed many opportunities to apply the guiding principles, especially with regard to eliciting patient preferences and talking about prognosis. The educational gaps identified in the targeted needs assessment guided curriculum developers to incorporate prognosis into the internal medicine residency training.[18]

With knowledge about the targeted learners' needs, characteristics, and preferences, curriculum developers will be better equipped to design a curriculum given available resources.

Content about the Targeted Learning Environment

Concomitant with acquiring information about the learners, curriculum developers must also understand the environment in which their curriculum is to be delivered. For instance, does a curriculum addressing the problem already exist, and if so, what has been its track record (in terms of both learner satisfaction and achievement of learning objectives)? Curriculum developers may discover that the existing or planned curriculum is adequate to meet learners' knowledge and skill needs but that programmatic or system changes are needed to facilitate subsequent application of the knowledge and skills in clinical settings.

> **EXAMPLE:** *Programmatic Change for Training in Telemedicine.* In 2017, the Veterans Health Administration's Office of Rural Health initiated a program to increase telerehabilitation services. Clinical rehabilitation providers in the rural sites had the knowledge and skills to provide "hands-on" rehabilitation services, but they needed training in how to deliver rehabilitation through telecommunications technology. Centrally located "Hub" sites with expertise in delivering telerehabilitation provided mentorship and training to "Spoke" sites in rural areas. Mentors from the Hubs were interviewed and identified barriers needing attention at the Spokes, including personnel, space, equipment, and broadband availability.[19]

In assessing the learning environment, curriculum developers may find that the trainees' clinical training experiences do not match their learning needs.

> **EXAMPLE:** *Learners in the Clinical Learning Environment.* Curriculum developers designing a curriculum on minimally invasive gynecologic surgery found that learners rotating at four different hospitals received little objective assessment of their surgical skills. Although case logs indicated involvement in laparoscopic and robotic hysterectomies, upper-level residents felt less prepared to perform them relative to abdominal hysterectomies. Consequently, curriculum developers augmented mastery skill development in the operating room with simulation and centralized faculty evaluation of procedural videos to provide better objective measurement of surgical performance.[20]

Sometimes changes in the learning environment, such as evolving needs of stakeholders, create opportunities for delivering curricular content.

> **EXAMPLE:** *Learners, Their Environment, and Other Stakeholders.* In New York during the COVID-19 pandemic, when clinical rotations were limited for medical students, a service learning program was developed to address the pandemic's dramatic effect on chronic health disparities. Education about the social determinants of health (SDOH) went from passive learning to experiential learning. Medical students and faculty developed a screening tool to assess SDOH. Students called patients and used the screening tool to connect patients with necessary resources or referrals. The SDOH screening tool increased student competency in addressing social determinants of health and was subsequently incorporated into the women's health clerkship.[21]

Information about the targeted environment might include the needs of key stake-holders other than patients or learners (faculty, educational leaders, accrediting bodies). For instance, curriculum developers may find that faculty members are not prepared to teach what needs to be learned, and faculty development thus becomes an important factor in curricular planning.

EXAMPLE: *Needs of Stakeholders Other Than Learners.* Curriculum developers planning a quality improvement curriculum for residents in general preventive medicine needed to incorporate a clinical component in their training. To assess the learning environment of the preventive medicine residents, preceptors at the clinical sites were surveyed. Preceptors expressed interest in working with the preventive medicine residents and thought their presence would improve patient care, but the preceptors lacked training in quality improvement and teamwork strategies. Thus, curriculum developers needed to modify their curricular approach by making the preceptors secondary targeted learners in order to enhance the educational experience of the primary targeted learners—the preventive medicine residents.[22]

EXAMPLE: *An Evolving Learning Environment and Need for Faculty Development.* A new Master of Education in the Health Professions (MEHP) degree program was developed to prepare health professionals to teach effectively, for schools and training programs related to medicine, public health, nursing, and other health professions. Curriculum developers planned to deliver the first year of the curriculum during in-person sessions and then, eventually, to transition to an exclusively online curriculum. The targeted needs assessment discovered that prospective learners preferred the online option because they were geographically distant from the home institution and wanted to minimize commute time. Plus, more asynchronous learning fit better into the targeted learners' schedules. Curriculum developers recruited faculty from various health professional schools and schools of education and learned in the targeted needs assessment that faculty members required training in how to deliver their content in an online format. This faculty development and transition to online training enabled the program to become international in scope.[23]

It is also important to understand the barriers, enablers, and reinforcing factors (see Chapter 2) in the environment that affect learning by the targeted learners. For example, is a resident too busy with clinical responsibilities to devote time to other educational pursuits? Are there established, designated time slots for delivering the formal curriculum? Are there aspects of the medical culture that promote or inhibit the application of learning? Are there incentives for learning or improving performance? Are faculty members motivated and enthusiastic to teach, and are they sufficiently incentivized to deliver the curriculum?

EXAMPLE: *Inadequate Team Skills Training, Need for Faculty Development.* Curriculum developers for a multifaceted interprofessional curriculum wanted to offer students various opportunities to learn and practice interprofessional teamwork competencies. A framework for creating opportunities for collaborative care was developed that included curricular and extracurricular learning experiences for students, as well as faculty development for team skills training. The targeted needs assessment revealed that successful implementation of the curriculum would require continuing education for faculty so that they would have the knowledge, skills, and values to work collaboratively in interprofessional teams and to role-model these behaviors for students. In addition to being taught basic team skills, faculty members were rewarded for work that involved interprofessional collaboration. Over time, demonstration of faculty interprofessional collaboration was acknowledged as a criterion for faculty promotion and existing university faculty awards.[24]

Curriculum developers need to determine if sufficient resources are available for learning and applying what is learned in practice. Is there an ample supply of patients with whom learners can practice their clinical skills? Are appropriate technologies (e.g., computers, diagnostic equipment, simulation services) available? Are there opportunities to collaborate with other departments or disciplines to share resources?

Lastly, can the targeted needs assessment determine whether (or in what way) the informal or collateral curriculum will affect learning the new content? (See Table 3.1.)

METHODS

General Considerations

Curriculum developers may already have some of the information about their targeted learners and their environment; other information may have to be acquired. Data already in existence may provide information relevant to curriculum developers and obviate the need for independent data collection. Some examples are local results of national questionnaires (e.g., the matriculation and graduation questionnaires from the Association of American Medical Colleges, or AAMC), standardized examinations (e.g., in-service training and specialty board examinations), procedure and experience logs, related curricula in which the targeted learners participate, and audit results. Comparison of institutional data to a national dataset like the AAMC questionnaires might show either that one's learners deviate from that national sample in a specific way that enables tailoring of the curriculum or that one's learners are representative of national trends, setting the stage for generalizability of targeted needs assessment results later in the curriculum development process. Curriculum management software is another source of already collected data that can help curriculum developers determine what is happening in their institution with respect to a topic of interest. Such software is used to track and map information on a school's curricula, and it can help curriculum developers place and integrate curricular content appropriately.[25] This information is increasingly being required by accreditation bodies. The AAMC Curriculum Inventory collates information from US and Canadian MD and DO degree-granting accredited schools to create a publicly available benchmarking and reporting tool on the content, structure, delivery, and assessment of curricula.[26]

When the desired information about the targeted learners is not already available to or known by the curriculum developers, they must decide how to acquire it. As with problem identification and general needs assessment (see Chapter 2), curriculum developers must decide *how much time, effort, and resources should be devoted to this step*. A commitment of too little time and effort risks development of an inefficient or ineffective curriculum. A commitment of too much time and effort can diminish the resources available for other critical steps, such as the development of effective educational strategies, successful implementation of the curriculum, and evaluation. Because resources are almost always limited, curriculum developers will need to *prioritize* their information needs. Questions that can be helpful in determining prioritization include the following:

- Will the data obtained change or influence what curriculum developers propose to do?
- What are the long-term plans for using the information that is gathered?

Once the information that is required has been decided, curriculum developers should decide on the *best method to obtain this information, given available resources*. In making this decision, they should ask the following questions:

1. What standards of representativeness, validity, and accuracy will be required?
2. Will *subjective or objective* measures be used?
3. Will *quantitative or qualitative data* be preferable?

As with curriculum evaluation, a variety of measurement methods and analytic tools can be employed in the targeted needs assessment (see Chapter 7).

> **EXAMPLE:** *Assessing Education Needs with Simulation.* In developing a curriculum on team leadership skills, curriculum developers used unannounced in situ simulations of cardiac arrest to assess the behavior of first-year residents acting as code team leaders. Simulated cardiac arrests were video-recorded, and standardized checklists were used by observers to judge the quality of team leadership in the resuscitation. The simulations allowed course directors to find areas of opportunity for learning, which informed the subsequent curriculum.[27]

Conducting a literature review can clarify the construct for the targeted needs assessment and determine if validated instruments already exist.[28] The purpose and ultimate utility of the targeted needs assessment for aiding the curriculum development process can help in deciding which method to pursue (see Table 3.2). If there is strong disagreement within the group responsible for developing the curriculum about the knowledge, attitude, skill, or performance deficits of the targeted learners, a more rigorous, representative, objective, and quantitative assessment of learner needs may be required. If a curriculum developer is new to an institution or unfamiliar with the learners and the learning environment and needs to get a "big picture" sense of the targeted needs assessment, collection and analysis of in-depth qualitative data gathered from a sample of selected learners and faculty may be most useful. This can be accomplished by interviews or focus groups to learn how stakeholders conceptualize the issue at hand.[28] If the curriculum developers have limited or no experience in using a needs assessment method, it is wise to seek *advice or mentorship from those with expertise* in the method.

Before applying a method formally to the group of targeted learners, it is important to *pilot* the data collection instrument on a convenient, receptive audience. Piloting of a questionnaire on a few friendly learners and faculty can provide feedback on whether the questionnaire is too long or whether some of the questions are worded in a confusing manner. This kind of informal feedback can provide specific suggestions on improved wording and format, on what questions can be eliminated, and on whether any new questions need to be added before the questionnaire is sent to a larger pool of survey respondents. This ensures a better chance of acquiring valid information from the targeted learners or other stakeholders.

If publication or dissemination of the findings of one's targeted needs assessment is anticipated, the work is likely to be considered educational research. Often with publication of a targeted needs assessment, curriculum developers will need to address issues related to the protection of human subjects, including whether study subjects provided informed consent and whether they perceived participation as voluntary or coercive. Before collecting data, curriculum developers should consider consultation with their institutional review board (see Chapters 6, 7, and 9).

Specific Methods

Specific methods commonly used in the needs assessment of targeted learners, and the advantages and disadvantages of each method, are shown in Table 3.2. Strategic planning sessions with stakeholders can help later with implementation of the curriculum.[29–31]

Table 3.2.   Advantages/Disadvantages of Different Needs Assessment Methods

Method	Advantages	Disadvantages
Informal discussion (in-person, over phone, via online platform, through social media, or by email)	Convenient Inexpensive Rich in detail and qualitative information Method for identifying stakeholders	Lack of methodological rigor Variations in questions Interviewer biases
Formal interviews	Standardized approach to interviewee Methodological rigor possible Questions and answers can be clarified With good response rate, can obtain data representative of entire group of targeted learners Quantitative and/or qualitative information Means of gaining support from stakeholders	Methodological rigor requires trained interviewers and measures of reliability Costly in terms of time and effort, especially if methodological rigor is required Interviewer bias and influence on respondent
Focus group discussions	Efficient method of "interviewing" several at one time (especially those with common trait) Learn about group behavior that may affect job performance (especially helpful to understand team-based learning) Group interaction may enrich or deepen information obtained Qualitative information	Requires skilled facilitator to control group interaction and minimize facilitator influence on responses Needs note taker or other means of recording information (e.g., audio ± video recording) Views of quiet participants may not be expressed No quantitative information Information may not be representative of all targeted learners Time and financial costs involved in data collection and analysis
Questionnaires	Standardized questions Methodological rigor relatively easy With good response rate, can obtain representative data Quantitative and/or qualitative information Can assess affective traits (attitudes, beliefs, feelings) Respondents can be geographically dispersed (web-based questionnaires increase the ease of reaching geographically dispersed respondents)	Requires skill in writing clear, unambiguous questions Answers cannot be clarified without resurveying Requires time and effort to ensure methodological rigor in survey development, data collection, and data analysis Dependent on adequate response rate (and resources devoted to achieving this) Requires time, effort, and skill to construct valid measures of affective traits

Method	Advantages	Disadvantages
Direct observation	Best method for assessing skills Can be informal or methodologically rigorous Informal observations can sometimes be accomplished as part of one's teaching or supervisory role	Can be time-consuming, especially if methodological rigor is desired Guidelines must be developed for standardized observations Observer generally must be knowledgeable of behavior being observed Observer bias Impact of observer on observed Assesses ability, not real-life performance (unless observations are unobtrusive)
Tests	Efficient, objective means of assessing cognitive or psycho-motor abilities Tests of key knowledge items relatively easy to construct	Requires time, effort, and skill to construct valid tests of skills and higher-order cognitive abilities Test anxiety may affect performance Assesses ability, not real-life performance
Audits of current behaviors	Useful for medical record keeping and the provision of recorded care (e.g., tests ordered, provision of discrete preventive care measures, prescribed treatments) Potentially unobtrusive Assesses real-life performance Can be methodologically rigorous with standards, instructions, and assurance of inter- and intra-rater reliability	Requires development of standards Requires resources to pay and train auditors, time and effort to perform audit oneself May require permission from learner and/or institution to audit records Difficult to avoid or account for recording omissions Addresses only indirect, incomplete measures of care
Strategic planning sessions for the curriculum	Can involve targeted learners as well as key faculty Can involve brainstorming of learner needs and can gauge their readiness to change Can involve prioritization of needs and steps necessary to accomplish change Creates sense of involvement and responsibility in participants Assesses current program strengths and weaknesses Part of a larger organizational process that also identifies goals, objectives, and responsibilities	Requires skilled facilitator to ensure participation and lack of inhibition by all participants Requires considerable time and effort to plan and conduct successful strategic planning sessions and to develop the associated report

Surveys: Interviews, Focus Groups, and Questionnaires

Surveys are the most common type of targeted needs assessment used in educational scholarship. Surveys are collections and/or reviews of data that are usually systematically performed. Three types of survey frequently used in curriculum development are *interviews* (questions asked and recorded by an interviewer), *focus groups*, and *questionnaires* (usually self-administered). Curriculum developers can decide which method best suits their needs. In designing a survey, curriculum developers must decide on the sample population to be surveyed, whether the sample is randomly or purposefully selected, and the design of the survey (cross-sectional vs. longitudinal). Regardless of the type of survey administered, each question should have clearly delineated objectives and justification for its inclusion in the survey. The length of a survey and/or the sensitivity of its questions will influence the response rate by the sample population. Because response rates are critical for acquisition of representative data, curriculum developers should generally include only questions that can be acted on.[32] The sample population being surveyed should be notified about the survey, its purpose, what their responses will be used for, whether responses will be considered confidential, and the time needed to conduct the survey.

Interviews

Interviews can be conducted in person, by phone, or electronically (e.g., video conference, instant messaging). Interviews can be structured, unstructured, or semi-structured. Structured interviews allow for consistency of questions across respondents so that responses can be compared/contrasted, whereas unstructured or semi-structured interviews allow spontaneity and on-the-spot follow-up of interesting responses.

> **EXAMPLE:** *Interviews to Inform Curricular Reform.* Botswana revised its national Medical Internship Training Program in 2014. Medical interns at one district hospital voluntarily participated in one-on-one structured interviews that were transcribed and put into an electronic database. Interns provided information on their preferred learning activity format, timing of structured activities, ideal class size, impressions of current curriculum content (e.g., adequate exposure to HIV and tuberculosis but deficiencies in noncommunicable diseases and preventive medicine), opinions on the focus of the new curriculum (preference for skills development), desire for symptom-based curriculum over systems-based learning, and opinions on who should teach sessions.[33]

> **EXAMPLE:** *Qualitative Interviews to Define Competencies.* Psychiatry residents at the University of Toronto were interviewed by telephone or in person to learn about their experiences with telepsychiatry. Semi-structured interviews explored residents' perceptions of current and potential future telepsychiatry curricula, required competencies, barriers to gaining competencies, desired training opportunities, preferred learning methods, and attitudes toward technology in learning. Interview transcripts were thematically analyzed to characterize competencies. Competencies ranged from technical skills in using the telemedicine equipment to skills needed to conduct a psychiatric interview over technology. The needs assessment provided an evidence base for content and pedagogical methods, as well as evaluation criteria for achievement of the competencies.[34]

Several caveats should be kept in mind when developing, preparing for, and conducting an interview[35] (Table 3.3).

Table 3.3.   Tips for Developing, Preparing for, and Conducting an Interview

1.   Decide how information will be collected (notes by interviewer vs. recorded and transcribed) and the time needed to document responses.

2.   Develop an interview guide. This is especially important if multiple interviewers are used.

3.   Structure interview questions to facilitate conversation, with more general, open-ended questions up front, important questions toward the beginning, and sensitive questions at the end.

4.   Cluster questions with a common theme in a logical order.

5.   Clarify responses when necessary (use prompts such as the following: "Describe for me . . ."; "Tell me more . . ."; "Can you say more about that?"; "Can you give me an example?").

6.   Maintain a neutral attitude and avoid biasing interviewee responses (e.g., by discussing the responses of another interviewee).

7.   At the end of the interview, express gratitude and offer the interviewee an opportunity to express any additional questions or comments.

8.   Time permitting, summarize key points and ask permission to recontact interviewee for future follow-up questions.

Source: Sleezer et al.[35]

Focus Groups

Focus groups bring together people with a common attribute to share their collective experience with the help of a skilled facilitator. Focus groups are well suited to explore perceptions and feelings about particular issues. The groups should be of a manageable size (7 ± 2 is a good rule) and should engender an atmosphere of openness and respect-ful sharing. The facilitator should be familiar with the topic area and use language under-standable to the focus group participants (their typical jargon if a specialized group, lay-person language if a mixed group). Questions asked in a focus group often come in three forms: 1) developing an understanding of a topic (a "grand tour"); 2) brainstorming and pilot-testing ideas, with attention to their advantages/disadvantages; and 3) evaluating a program based on the experiences of the focus group participants. The facilitator should encourage participation, avoid closed-ended or leading questions, acknowledge re-sponses nonjudgmentally, manage those who are more willing or less willing to engage in the discussion, foster brainstorming in response to participants' answers, and keep track of time. Data are most often captured through digital audio recording devices and the recording is subsequently transcribed into text. After the focus group is completed, the facilitator should jot down notes about main themes discussed and any notable non-verbal interactions. Then the text should be analyzed, often with the use of software, and a report should be generated highlighting the key findings from the session.[36,37]

Questionnaires

Questionnaires, as opposed to interviews and focus groups, are completed by the in-dividual alone or with minimal assistance from another. They can be paper-based or electronic. Electronic resources can be survey-focused (e.g., www.surveymonkey.com, https://projectredcap.org/, or www.qualtrics.com) or part of learning management systems (e.g., www.blackboard.com). Software programs offer design flexibility. Good questionnaire design attends to ease of survey navigation, choice of response formats, and shared interpretation of visual cues.[38] Since online questionnaires can be accessed from a variety of platforms, including mobile devices, tablets, desktops, and laptops, curriculum developers need to be aware of the technological capabilities and preferences of the survey population.[39] It is important for response rates that questionnaires are viewable on a variety of web platforms.[40] In addition, online surveys may need additional privacy protections.[41] Often, websites for online questionnaires include software for data management and basic statistical analysis.

The just-in-time survey method is a strategy that can engage learners in the needs assessment process. Just-in-time can also be used to determine the knowledge content of upcoming lectures in a curriculum.

> **EXAMPLE:** *Targeted Needs Assessment in Preparation for Teaching Sessions.* In a surgery residency training program, residents were sent short readings on an upcoming topic and required to complete online study questions before their weekly teaching sessions. In addition to five open-ended questions that addressed key concepts of the reading, a standard question was always added to the list of weekly questions: "Please tell us briefly what single point of the reading you found most difficult or confusing. If you did not find any part of it difficult or confusing, please tell us what parts you found most interesting." Faculty members reviewed the survey responses to tailor the session content to residents' learning needs.[42]

Curriculum developers need to be mindful of several issues with regard to questionnaires. A questionnaire should contain instructions on how to answer questions. It is also generally advisable to include a cover letter or message with the questionnaire, explaining the rationale of the questionnaire and what is expected of the respondent. The cover letter or message can be the first step to develop respondents' buy-in for questionnaire completion, if it provides sufficient justification for the survey and makes the respondent feel vested in the outcome. If the questionnaire is sent electronically (by email, text message, chat message, etc.), the subject should be clearly stated. It is best if the message is personalized and from someone the prospective respondent knows.[40]

Questions should relate to the questionnaire objectives, and the respondent should be aware of the rationale for each question. Ask the more important questions early in the questionnaire to increase the odds they will be answered.[43] How questions are worded in a survey greatly affects the value of the information gleaned from them.[38,44,45] Pilot-testing to ensure clarity and understandability in both the format and the content of the questions is especially important, as no interviewer is present to explain the meaning of ambiguously worded questions.[28] Table 3.4 provides tips to keep in mind when writing questions.[28,32,39,43–46] Curriculum developers must be cognizant of the potential for nonresponse to particular items on the questionnaire and how this might affect the validity of the targeted needs assessment.[40,47,48]

Nonresponse to an entire survey is also possible and, when representative data are desired, *response rate* is critical. Nonresponse can result from nondelivery of the survey request, a prospective respondent's lack of awareness of the solicitation, or a respondent's conscious decision not to complete the questionnaire. Factors influencing a prospective respondent's cooperation include the amount of time, opportunity costs, or psychological cost involved in completing the questionnaire. Offering incentives,

Table 3.4.   Tips for Writing and Administering Questionnaire Questions

1. For paper-based questionnaires, make sure questions follow a logical order, key items are highlighted with textual elements (boldface, italics, or underline), the overall format is not visually complex or distracting, and the sequence of questions/pages is easy to follow.

2. For online questionnaires, develop a screen format that is appealing to respondents and displays easily across devices, highlight information that is essential to survey completion, provide error messages to help respondents troubleshoot issues, and use interactive and audiovisual capabilities sparingly to reduce respondent burden.

3. Ask for only one piece of information. Avoid a double-barreled item. The more precise and unambiguous the question is, the better.

4. Avoid biased, leading, vague, or negatively phrased questions.

5. Avoid abbreviations, colloquialisms, and phrases not easily understood by respondents.

6. Decide whether an open-ended or a closed-ended question will elicit the most fitting response. Open-ended answers (e.g., fill in the blank) will require more data analysis, so they should be used in a limited fashion when surveying a large sample. Closed-ended questions are used when the surveyor wants an answer from a prespecified set of response choices.

7. Make categorical responses (e.g., race) mutually exclusive and exhaust all categories (if necessary, using "other") in the offered list of options.

8. When more than one response is possible, offer the option of "check all that apply."

9. In using ordinal questions (where responses can be ordered on a scale by level of agreement, importance, confidence, usefulness, satisfaction, frequency, intensity, or comparison), make the scale meaningful to the topic area and easy to complete and understand based on the question thread and instructions. The response options should emphasize the construct of interest. Avoid absolute anchors like "always" and "never."

10. For ordinal questions (e.g., Likert scale), it is typical to have five response anchors. Reliability is reduced when there are too few anchors; too many may not provide meaningful data. Label each response option and have equal spacing between options.

11. For ordinal questions asking about potentially embarrassing or sensitive topics, it is generally best to put the negative end of the scale first.

12. For attitudinal questions, decide whether it is important to learn how respondents feel, how strongly they feel, or both.

13. Visually separate nonsubstantive response options (e.g., "not applicable") from substantive options

14. If demographic questions are asked, know how this information will influence the data analysis, what the range of answers will be in the target population, how specific the information needs to be, and whether it will be compared with existing datasets (in which case common terms should be used). Sometimes asking respondents to answer in their own words or numbers (e.g., date of birth, zip code, income) allows the surveyor to avoid questions with a burdensome number of response categories.

15. If demographic information is less critical to the needs assessment than other constructs, placing demographic questions at the end of the questionnaire may improve response rates on the key questions.

Sources: Adapted from Artino et al.;[28] Fink;[32] Dillman et al.;[39] Gehlbach and Artino;[43] Sullivan and Artino;[44] Artino et al.;[45] Sleezer et al.[46]

whether monetary or nonmonetary, can leverage completion of the questionnaire.[49] Incentives can range from nominal monetary amounts (even $1 can be an inducement) to a coffee shop gift card, or from group prizes to individual stakes in a lottery. Relevance of the questionnaire to the respondent also matters in their decision to participate, and salience may overcome any inclination toward nonresponse. Where and when the questionnaire will be administered may also affect response rates (e.g., at the end of a mandatory training session when time can be allotted for completing the questionnaire, or asynchronously so that respondents can complete the questionnaire at their own pace). Much of the literature on health professional response rates is based on mailed surveys, whereas most questionnaires now are administered electronically. If resources permit, mailed questionnaires may still have a role, however.[50,51] Letting the respondent self-select the mode of survey is an effective means of increasing response rates,[52] as learners may have preferred means of answering surveys. Curriculum developers need to ensure that questions asked by different methodologies are being interpreted in the same way by survey respondents. Other proven methods to improve response rates include making it easy for survey takers to respond (e.g., stamped return envelopes with handwritten addresses; easily navigable hyperlinks) and sending multiple reminders, preferably by mixed methods—regular mail, email, telephone.[39,40,52–54] Methods for following up with questionnaire nonrespondents may entail additional time and resources.

For questionnaires targeting physicians and health professional trainees, a general rule of thumb is to aim for response rates greater than 60%.[54,55] Response rates may differ depending on specialty.[56–58] Tips for increasing response rates on health professional surveys are presented in Table 3.5.[54,59–64]

Whatever survey method is used, the data need to be systematically collected and analyzed (see Chapter 7 for more detail on data analysis). If the needs assessment will be used for educational research, curriculum developers should adhere to guidelines for reporting survey-based educational research, including describing the rationale for using a survey, how the survey instrument was created and pretested, how it was administered, its response rate, and how its reliability and validity were assessed[28] (see Chapter 7). Curriculum developers should ask whether the targeted needs assessment collected useful information and what was learned in the process. Regardless of whether curriculum developers are analyzing quantitative data[65] or qualitative data,[66–68] they must always keep in mind that the targeted needs assessment is intended to focus the problem in the context of the targeted learners and their learning environment and to help shape the subsequent steps in curriculum development.

RELATION TO OTHER STEPS

The information one chooses to collect as part of the targeted needs assessment may be influenced by what one expects will be a *goal or objective* of the curriculum or by the *educational* and *implementation strategies* being considered for the curriculum. Subsequent steps—*Goals and Objectives*, *Educational Strategies*, *Implementation*, and *Evaluation and Feedback*—are likely to be affected by what is learned in the targeted needs assessment. The process of conducting a needs assessment can serve as advance publicity for a curriculum, engage stakeholders, and ease a curriculum's *implementation*. Information gathered as part of the targeted needs assessment can serve as *"pre-," or "before," data for evaluation* of the impact of a curriculum. For all of these

Table 3.5.   Tips for Increasing Questionnaire Response Rates

1. Consider reasons that professionals refuse to participate.
   a. Lack of time
   b. Unclear or low salience of the study (i.e., need to establish relevance)
   c. Concerns about confidentiality of results
   d. Some questions seem biased or do not allow a full range of choices on the subject
   e. Volume and length of survey
   f. Office staff who pose barrier to accessing the professional (especially in private practice)
2. Offer incentives to increase participation and convey respect for professional's time.
   a. Cash payment (even $1) > charitable inducement > donation to alma mater
   b. Not clear whether gift certificate has same motivating effect as cash
   c. Prepaid incentive > promised incentive (i.e., sent after survey returned)
   d. Small financial incentive > enrollment in lottery for higher amount
   e. For web survey, need to consider how liquid the monetary incentive is
   f. Token nonmonetary incentive has little to no impact on response rate
3. Design respondent-friendly questionnaire.
   a. Shorter survey (<1,000 words)
   b. Closed-ended questions get higher response rate than open-ended questions
   c. Attractive business format and standard paper size helps paper-based surveys
   d. Web surveys should be easy to navigate and monitor progress toward completion
   f. Mixed-methods reply approach helps (e.g., postal and/or electronic options)
4. Consider best means of contacting potential respondents and providing reminders
   a. Prenotification about survey (e.g., postal prenotification for web survey)
   b. Direct contact by professional peer helps
   c. Vary the type of appeal (i.e., value, utility, personal) made to motivate sample members in each contact
   d. For email notifications to web surveys, provide inviting subject line, avoid terms used by spammers, include URL to the survey, and ensure confidentiality
   e. Use several contacts (e.g., by email) and one additional contact (e.g., telephone call)
   f. Include replacement questionnaire (by mail or hyperlink) with follow-up contact
   g. For web surveys, send email reminders and postal mail for final reminder
5. Make it easy for sample member to respond
   a. For mail surveys, include return envelope with first class postage stamp
   b. For web surveys, make it easy to navigate to website hosting the survey
6. Personalize contact (cover letter, handwritten note, personalized envelope, phone call)
   a. Sample members with a close relationship to surveyor are more likely to respond
   b. Endorsement by opinion leader or professional association has mixed results

---

Sources: Adapted from Kellerman and Herold;[54] Field et al.;[59] VanGeest et al.;[60] Thorpe et al.;[61] Martins et al.;[62] Dykema et al.;[63] and Cho et al.[64]
Note: Most evidence comes from mailed surveys. Data on response rates for web surveys are limited.

reasons, it is wise to think through other steps, at least in a preliminary manner, before investing time and resources in the targeted needs assessment.

It is also worth realizing that one can learn a lot about a curriculum's targeted learners in the course of conducting the curriculum. This information can then be used as a targeted needs assessment for the next cycle of the curriculum (see Chapters 8 and 10).

EXAMPLE: *Step 6 Evaluation That Serves as Targeted Needs Assessment.* As part of their ambulatory medicine clinical experience, residents were evaluated by their preceptors through electronic medical record review of their patient panels. The evaluation found that, for the most part, residents were un-skilled in incorporating preventive care into office visits and in motivating patients to follow through with cancer screening recommendations. Focused training in these areas was developed for the next cycle of the ambulatory medicine clinical experience, and preceptors were prompted to ask about these issues during case presentations.

SCHOLARSHIP

A well-performed targeted needs assessment allows curriculum developers to disseminate information that may be relevant to other curriculum developers, especially to the extent that one's learners and learning environment(s) are similar to those elsewhere. This can be done in numerous formats (see Chapter 9) and is an important component of scholarship.

CONCLUSION

By clarifying the characteristics of one's targeted learners and their environment, the curriculum developer can help ensure that the curriculum being planned not only addresses important general needs but also is relevant and applicable to the specific needs of its learners and their learning institution. Performing the general needs assessment and the targeted needs assessment help make the curriculum developer an expert in the subject matter of a curriculum and its teaching. Steps 1 and 2 provide a sound basis for the next step, choosing the goals and objectives for the curriculum.

QUESTIONS

For the curriculum you are coordinating, planning, or would like to be planning, please answer or think about the following questions and prompts:

1. *Identify your targeted learners.* From the point of view of your problem identification and general needs assessment, will training this group as opposed to other groups of learners make the greatest contribution to solving the health care problem? If not, who would be a better group of targeted learners? Are these learners an option for you? Notwithstanding these considerations, is it nevertheless important to train your original group of targeted learners? Why?

2. To the extent of your current knowledge, *describe your targeted learners*. What are your targeted learners' previous training experiences, existing proficiencies, past and current performance, attitudes about the topic area and/or curriculum, learning style and needs, and familiarity with and preferences for different learning methods? What key characteristics do the learners share? What areas of heterogeneity should be highlighted?

3. To the extent of your current knowledge, *describe your targeted learning environment*. In the targeted learning environment, what other curricula exist or are being planned, what are the enabling and reinforcing factors and barriers to development and implementation of your curriculum, and what are the resources for learning? Who are the stakeholders (course directors, faculty, school administrators, clerkship and resi-

dency program directors, and accrediting bodies), and what are their needs with respect to your curriculum?

4. *What information* about your learners and their environment *is unknown* to you? *Prioritize* your information needs.

5. *Identify one or more methods* (e.g., informal and formal interviews, focus groups, questionnaires) by which you could obtain the most important information. For each method, *identify the resources* (time, personnel, supplies, space) required to develop the necessary data collection instruments and to collect and analyze the needed data. To what degree do you feel that each method is feasible?

6. Identify individuals on whom you could *pilot* your needs assessment instrument(s).

7. After conducting the targeted needs assessment, systematically ask whether useful information was collected and *what was learned in the process*.

8. Define how the targeted needs assessment *focuses the problem* in the context of your learners and their learning environment and *prepares you for the next steps*.

GENERAL REFERENCES

Learning Environment

Hafferty, Frederic W., and Joseph F. O'Donnell, eds. *The Hidden Curriculum in Health Professional Education*. Lebanon, NH: Dartmouth College Press / University Press of New England, 2014. Published 20 years after a landmark article in *Academic Medicine*, this book is a compilation of essays exploring the informal or hidden curriculum. It discusses the theoretical underpinnings of the concept and methodical approaches for assessing and addressing the informal or hidden curriculum. The curriculum developer in medical education will gain a better understanding of the social, cultural, and organizational contexts within which professional development occurs. 320 pages.

Needs Assessment

Morrison, Gary R., Steven M. Ross, Jennifer R. Morrison, and Howard K. Kalman. *Designing Effective Instruction*. 8th ed. Hoboken, NJ: John Wiley & Sons, 2019.
A general book on instructional design, including needs assessment, instructional objectives, instructional strategies, and evaluation. Chapters 2–4 deal with needs assessment. 512 pages.

Sleezer, Catherine M., Darlene F. Russ-Eft, and Kavita Gupta. *A Practical Guide to Needs Assessment*. 3rd ed. San Francisco: John Wiley & Sons (published by Wiley), 2014.
Practical how-to handbook on conducting a needs assessment, with case examples and toolkit. 402 pages.

Survey Design

Books

Dillman, Don A., Jolene D. Smyth, and Leah Melani Christian. *Internet, Phone, Mail, and Mixed-Mode Surveys: The Tailored Design Method*. 4th ed. Hoboken, NJ: John Wiley & Sons, 2014. Topics include writing questions, constructing questionnaires, survey implementation and delivery, mixed-mode surveys, and internet surveys. Presents a stepwise approach to survey implementation that incorporates strategies to improve rigor and response rates. Clearly written, with many examples. 509 pages.

Fink, Arlene. *How to Conduct Surveys: A Step-by-Step Guide*. 6th ed. Thousand Oaks, CA: SAGE Publications, 2017.
>   Short, basic text that covers question writing, questionnaire format, sampling, survey administration design, data analysis, creating code books, and presenting results. 224 pages.

Fowler, Floyd J. *Survey Research Methods (Applied Social Research Methods)*. 5th ed. Thousand Oaks, CA: SAGE Publications, 2014.
>   Short text on survey research methods, including chapters on sampling, nonresponse, data collection, designing questions, evaluating survey questions and instruments, interviewing, data analysis, and ethical issues. Focuses on reducing sources of error. 171 pages.

Krueger, Richard A., and Mary Anne Casey. *Focus Groups: A Practical Guide for Applied Research*. 5th ed. Thousand Oaks, CA: SAGE Publications, 2015.
>   Practical how-to book that covers uses of focus groups, planning, developing questions, determining focus group composition, moderating skills, data analysis, and reporting results. 252 pages.

Morgan, David L. *Basic and Advanced Focus Groups*. Thousand Oaks, CA: SAGE Publications, 2018.
>   Useful guide for designing, moderating, and analyzing focus groups. Compares and contrasts to interviews and includes a section on synchronous and asynchronous online focus groups. 216 pages.

Journal

VanGeest, Jonathan B., and Timothy P. Johnson, eds. "Special Issue: Surveying Clinicians." *Evaluation & the Health Professions* 36, no. 3 (2013): 275–407.
>   A theme issue reviewing methodologies for collecting information from physicians and other members of the interdisciplinary health care team. (1) "Facilitators and Barriers to Survey Participation by Physicians: A Call to Action for Researchers"; (2) "Sample Frame and Related Sample Design Issues for Surveys of Physicians and Physician Practices"; (3) "Estimating the Effect of Nonresponse Bias in a Survey of Hospital Organizations"; (4) "Surveying Clinicians by Web: Current Issues in Design and Administration"; and (5) "Enhancing Surveys of Health Care Professionals: A Meta-Analysis of Techniques to Improve Response."

Internet Resources

American Association for Public Opinion Research, accessed May 23, 2021, www.aapor.org.
>   The American Association for Public Opinion Research is a US professional organization of public opinion and survey research professionals, with members from academia, media, government, the nonprofit sector, and private industry. It sets standards for conducting surveys, offers educational opportunities in survey research, provides resources for researchers on a range of survey and polling issues, and publishes the print journal *Public Opinion Quarterly* and the e-journal *Survey Practice*.

Survey Research Methods Section, American Statistical Association, accessed May 23, 2021, https://community.amstat.org/surveyresearchmethodssection/home.
>   Provides a downloadable *What Is a Survey* booklet on survey methodology under "Resources" and links to other resources and publications.

REFERENCES CITED

1. Catherine M. Sleezer, Darlene F. Russ-Eft, and Kavita Gupta, *A Practical Guide to Needs Assessment*, 3rd ed. (San Francisco: John Wiley & Sons, 2014), 15–34.
2. Brian M. Ross, Kim Daynard, and David Greenwood, "Medicine for Somewhere: The Emergence of Place in Medical Education," *Educational Research and Reviews* 9, no. 22 (2014): 1250–65, https://doi.org/10.5897/ERR2014.1948.

3. Brian M. Ross, Erin Cameron, and David Greenwood, "Remote and Rural Placements Occurring during Early Medical Training as a Multidimensional Place-Based Medical Education Experience," *Educational Research and Reviews* 15, no. 3 (2020): 150–58, https://doi.org/10.5897/ERR2019.3873.

4. Belinda Y. Chen et al., "From Modules to MOOCs: Application of the Six-Step Approach to Online Curriculum Development for Medical Education," *Academic Medicine* 94, no. 5 (2019): 678–85, https://doi.org/10.1097/ACM.0000000000002580.

5. David T. Stern, "A Hidden Narrative," in *The Hidden Curriculum in Health Professional Education*, ed. Frederic W. Hafferty and Joseph F. O'Donnell (Lebanon, NH: Dartmouth College Press/University Press of New England, 2014), 24.

6. Ralph W. Tyler, *Basic Principles of Curriculum and Instruction*, 1st ed., revised (Chicago: University of Chicago Press, 2013), 63–82.

7. Allan C. Ornstein and Francis P. Hunkins, *Curriculum: Foundations, Principles, and Issues*, 7th ed. (Harlow, Essex, UK: Pearson, 2016), 9–14.

8. Ingrid Philibert et al., "Learning and Professional Acculturation through Work: Examining the Clinical Learning Environment through the Sociocultural Lens," *Medical Teacher* 41, no. 4 (2019): 398–402, https://doi.org/10.1080/0142159X.2019.1567912.

9. Saleem Razack and Ingrid Philibert, "Inclusion in the Clinical Learning Environment: Building the Conditions for Diverse Human Flourishing," *Medical Teacher* 41, no. 4 (2019): 380–84, https://doi.org/10.1080/0142159X.2019.1566600.

10. Cheryl L. Holmes et al., "Harnessing the Hidden Curriculum: A Four-Step Approach to Developing and Reinforcing Reflective Competencies in Medical Clinical Clerkship," *Advances in Health Sciences Education* 20, no. 5 (2015): 1355–70, https://doi.org/10.1007/s10459-014-9558-9.

11. Gail Geller et al., "Tolerance for Ambiguity among Medical Students: Patterns of Change during Medical School and Their Implications for Professional Development," *Academic Medicine* 96, no. 7 (2020): 1036–42, https://doi.org/10.1097/ACM.0000000000003820.

12. Samuel Reis-Dennis, Martha S. Gerrity, and Gail Geller, "Tolerance for Uncertainty and Professional Development: A Normative Analysis," *Journal of General Internal Medicine* 36, no. 8 (2021): 2408–13, https://doi.org/10.1007/s11606-020-06538-y.

13. Sleezer, *A Practical Guide to Needs Assessment*, 117–71.

14. Susan Winslow et al., "Multisite Assessment of Nursing Continuing Education Learning Needs Using an Electronic Tool," *Journal of Continuing Education in Nursing* 47, no. 2 (2016): 75–81, https://doi.org/10.3928/00220124-20160120-08.

15. Patricia C. Henwood et al., "A Practical Guide to Self-Sustaining Point-of-Care Ultrasound Education Programs in Resource-Limited Settings," *Annals of Emergency Medicine* 64, no. 3 (2014): 277–85.e2, https://doi.org/10.1016/j.annemergmed.2014.04.013.

16. Mai A. Mahmoud et al., "Examining Aptitude and Barriers to Evidence-Based Medicine among Trainees at an ACGME-I Accredited Program," *BMC Medical Education* 20 (2020): 414, https://doi.org/10.1186/s12909-020-02341-9.

17. Brian Bronson and Greg Perlman, "The Management Experiences, Priorities, and Challenges of Medical Directors in the Subspecialty of Consultation-Liaison Psychiatry: Results of a Needs Assessment," *Psychosomatics* 62, no. 3 (2021): 309–17, https://doi.org/10.1016/j.psym.2020.09.006.

18. Nancy L. Schoenborn et al., "Current Practices and Opportunities in a Resident Clinic regarding the Care of Older Adults with Multimorbidity," *Journal of the American Geriatrics Society* 63, no. 8 (2015): 1645–51, https://doi.org/10.1111/jgs.13526.

19. Jennifer L. Hale-Gallardo et al., "Telerehabilitation for Rural Veterans: A Qualitative Assessment of Barriers and Facilitators to Implementation," *Journal of Multidisciplinary Healthcare* 13 (2020): 559–70, https://doi.org/10.2147/JMDH.S247267.

20. Example adapted with permission from the curricular project of Amanda Nickles Fader, MD, for the Johns Hopkins Longitudinal Program in Faculty Development, cohort 25, 2011–2012.

21. Lucy Bickerton, Nicolle Siegart, and Crystal Marquez, "Medical Students Screen for Social Determinants of Health: A Service Learning Model to Improve Health Equity," *PRiMER* 4 (2020): 27, https://doi.org/10.22454/PRiMER.2020.225894.

22. Example adapted with permission from the curricular project of Sajida Chaudry, MD, MPH; Clarence Lam, MD, MPH; Elizabeth Salisbury-Afshar, MD, MPH; and Miriam Alexander, MD, MPH, for the Johns Hopkins Longitudinal Program in Faculty Development, cohort 26, 2012–2013.

23. "Master of Education in the Health Professions," Johns Hopkins School of Education, accessed May 23, 2021, https://education.jhu.edu/academics/_mehp/.

24. Amy V. Blue et al., "Changing the Future of Health Professions: Embedding Interprofessional Education within an Academic Health Center," *Academic Medicine* 85, no. 8 (2010): 1290–95, https://doi.org/10.1097/ACM.0b013e3181e53e07.

25. Ghaith Al-Eyd et al., "Curriculum Mapping as a Tool to Facilitate Curriculum Development: A New School of Medicine Experience," *BMC Medical Education* 8, no. 1 (2018): 185, https://doi.org/10.1186/s12909-018-1289-9.

26. "Curriculum Inventory," Association of American Medical Colleges, accessed May 23, 2021, https://www.aamc.org/what-we-do/mission-areas/medical-education/curriculum-inventory.

27. Susan Coffey Zern et al., "Use of Simulation as a Needs Assessment to Develop a Focused Team Leader Training Curriculum for Resuscitation Teams," *Advances in Simulation* (London) 5 (2020): 6, https://doi.org/10.1186/s41077-020-00124-2.

28. Anthony R. Artino et al., "Developing Questionnaires for Educational Research: AMEE Guide No. 87," *Medical Teacher* 36 (2014): 463–74, https://doi.org/10.3109/0142159X.2014.889814.

29. James W. Altschuld, *Bridging the Gap between Asset/Capacity Building and Needs Assessment: Concepts and Practical Applications* (Thousand Oaks, CA: SAGE Publications, 2015), 25–49.

30. John M. Bryson, *Strategic Planning for Public and Nonprofit Organizations*, 5th ed. (Hoboken, NJ: John Wiley & Sons, 2018).

31. John M. Bryson and Farnum K. Alston, *Creating Your Strategic Plan: A Workbook for Public and Nonprofit Organizations*, 3rd ed. (San Francisco: Jossey-Bass, John Wiley & Sons, 2011).

32. Arlene Fink, *How to Conduct Surveys: A Step-by-Step Guide*, 6th ed. (Thousand Oaks, CA: SAGE Publications, 2017), 35–66.

33. Michael J. Peluso et al., "Building Health System Capacity through Medical Education: A Targeted Needs Assessment to Guide Development of a Structured Internal Medicine Curriculum for Medical Interns in Botswana," *Annals of Global Health* 84, no. 1 (2018): 151–59, https://doi.org/10.29024/aogh.22.

34. Allison Crawford et al., "Defining Competencies for the Practice of Telepsychiatry through an Assessment of Resident Learning Needs," *BMC Medical Education* 16 (2016): 28, https://doi.org/10.1186/s12909-016-0529-0.

35. Sleezer, *A Practical Guide to Needs Assessment*, 52–57.

36. David L. Morgan, *Basic and Advanced Focus Groups* (Thousand Oaks, CA: SAGE Publications, 2018).

37. Richard A. Krueger and Mary Anne Casey, *Focus Groups: A Practical Guide for Applied Research*, 5th ed. (Thousand Oaks, CA: SAGE Publications, 2015).

38. Roger Tourangeau, Frederic G. Conrad, and Mick P. Couper, *The Science of Web Surveys* (Oxford: Oxford University Press, 2013), 57–98.

39. Don A. Dillman, Jolene D. Smyth, and Leah Melani Christian, *Internet, Phone, Mail, and Mixed-Mode Surveys: The Tailored Design Method*, 4th ed. (Hoboken, NJ: John Wiley & Sons, 2014), 301–18.

40. Andrew W. Phillips, Shalini Reddy, and Steven J. Durning, "Improving Response Rates and Evaluating Nonresponse Bias in Surveys: AMEE Guide No. 102," *Medical Teacher* 38, no. 3 (2016): 217–28, https://doi.org/10.3109/0142159X.2015.1105945.

41. Fink, *How to Conduct Surveys*, 19–25.

42. Mary C. Schuller, Debra A. DaRosa, and Marie L. Crandall, "Using Just-in-Time Teaching and Peer Instruction in a Residency Program's Core Curriculum: Enhancing Satisfaction, Engagement, and Retention," *Academic Medicine* 90, no. 3 (2015): 384–91, https://doi.org/10.1097/ACM.0000000000000578.

43. Hunter Gehlbach and Anthony R. Artino Jr., "The Survey Checklist (Manifesto)," *Academic Medicine* 93, no. 3 (2018): 360–66, https://doi.org/10.1097/ACM.0000000000002083.

44. Gail M. Sullivan and Anthony R. Artino Jr., "How to Create a Bad Survey Instrument," *Journal of Graduate Medical Education* 9, no. 4 (2017): 411–15, https://doi.org/10.4300/JGME-D-17-00375.1.

45. Anthony R. Artino Jr. et al., "'The Questions Shape the Answers': Assessing the Quality of Published Survey Instruments in Health Professions Education Research," *Academic Medicine* 93, no. 3 (2018): 456–63, https://doi.org/10.1097/ACM.0000000000002002.

46. Sleezer, *A Practical Guide to Needs Assessment*, 59–71.

47. Robert M. Groves et al., *Survey Nonresponse* (Hoboken, NJ: John Wiley & Sons, 2001), 3–26.

48. Andrew W. Phillips, Benjamin T. Friedman, and Steven J. Durning, "How to Calculate a Survey Response Rate: Best Practices," *Academic Medicine* 92, no. 2 (2017): 269, https://doi.org/10.1097/ACM.0000000000001410.

49. David A. Cook et al., "Incentive and Reminder Strategies to Improve Response Rate for Internet-Based Physician Surveys: A Randomized Experiment," *Journal of Medical Internet Research* 18, no. 9 (2016): e244, https://doi.org/10.2196/jmir.6318.

50. John F. Reinisch, Daniel C. Yu, and Wai-Yee Li, "Getting a Valid Survey Response from 662 Plastic Surgeons in the 21st Century," *Annals of Plastic Surgery* 76, no. 1 (2016): 3–5, https://doi.org/10.1097/SAP.0000000000000546.

51. Vincent M. Meyer et al., "Global Overview of Response Rates in Patient and Health Care Professional Surveys in Surgery: A Systematic Review," *Annals of Surgery*, September 15, 2020, https://doi.org/10.1097/SLA.0000000000004078.

52. Michaela Brtnikova et al., "A Method for Achieving High Response Rates in National Surveys of U.S. Primary Care Physicians," *PLOS One* 13, no. 8 (2018): e0202755, https://doi.org/10.1371/journal.pone.0202755.

53. Timothy J. Beebe et al., "Testing the Impact of Mixed-Mode Designs (Mail and Web) and Multiple Contact Attempts within Mode (Mail or Web) on Clinician Survey Response," *Health Services Research* 53, Suppl 1 (2018): 3070–83, https://doi.org/10.1111/1475-6773.12827.

54. Scott E. Kellerman and Joan Herold, "Physician Response to Surveys: A Review of the Literature," *American Journal of Preventive Medicine* 20, no. 1 (2001): 61–67, https://doi.org/10.1016/s0749-3797(00)00258-0.

55. Andrew W. Phillips et al., "Surveys of Health Professions Trainees: Prevalence, Response Rates, and Predictive Factors to Guide Researchers," *Academic Medicine* 92, no. 2 (2017): 222–28, https://doi.org/10.1097/ACM.0000000000001334.

56. Nanxi Zha et al., "Factors Affecting Response Rates in Medical Imaging Survey Studies," *Academic Radiology* 27, no. 3 (2020): 421–27, https://doi.org/10.1016/j.acra.2019.06.005.

57. Tamara Taylor and Anthony Scott, "Do Physicians Prefer to Complete Online or Mail Surveys? Findings from a National Longitudinal Survey," *Evaluation & the Health Professions* 42, no. 1 (2019): 41–70, https://doi.org/10.1177/0163278718807744.

58. Ellen Funkhouser et al., "Survey Methods to Optimize Response Rate in the National Dental Practice-Based Research Network," *Evaluation & the Health Professions* 40, no. 3 (2017): 332–58, https://doi.org/10.1177/0163278715625738.

59. Terry S. Field et al., "Surveying Physicians: Do Components of the 'Total Design Approach' to Optimizing Survey Response Rates Apply to Physicians?," *Medical Care* 40, no. 7 (2002): 596–605, https://doi.org/10.1097/00005650-200207000-00006.

60. Jonathan B. VanGeest, Timothy P. Johnson, and Verna L. Welch, "Methodologies for Improving Response Rates in Surveys of Physicians: A Systematic Review," *Evaluation & the Health Professions* 30, no. 4 (2007): 303–21, https://doi.org/10.1177/0163278707307899.

61. Cathy Thorpe et al., "How to Obtain Excellent Response Rates When Surveying Physicians," *Family Practice* 26, no. 1 (2009): 65–68, https://doi.org/10.1093/fampra/cmn097.

62. Yandara Martins et al., "Increasing Response Rates from Physicians in Oncology Research: A Structured Literature Review and Data from a Recent Physician Survey," *British Journal of Cancer* 106, no. 6 (2012): 1021–26, https://doi.org/10.1038/bjc.2012.28.

63. Jennifer Dykema et al., "Surveying Clinicians by Web: Current Issues in Design and Administration," *Evaluation & the Health Professions* 36, no. 3 (2013): 352–81, https://doi.org/10.1177/0163278713496630.

64. Young Ik Cho, Timothy P. Johnson, and Jonathan B. VanGeest, "Enhancing Surveys of Health Care Professionals: A Meta-Analysis of Techniques to Improve Response," *Evaluation & the Health Professions* 36, no. 3 (2013): 382–407, https://doi.org/10.1177/0163278713496425.

65. Fink, *How to Conduct Surveys*, 135–166.

66. Matthew B. Miles, A. Michael Huberman, and Johnny Saldaña, *Qualitative Data Analysis: A Methods Sourcebook*, 4th ed. (Thousand Oaks, CA: SAGE Publications, 2020).

67. Lyn Richards and Janice M. Morse, *README FIRST for a User's Guide to Qualitative Methods*, 3rd ed. (Thousand Oaks, CA: SAGE Publications, 2013).

68. Marilyn Lichtman, *Qualitative Research in Education: A User's Guide*, (Thousand Oaks, CA: SAGE Publications, 2013).

Step 3
Goals and Objectives

. . . focusing the curriculum

Patricia A. Thomas, MD

DEFINITIONS

Once the needs of the learners have been clarified, it is desirable to target the curriculum to address these needs by setting goals and objectives. *A goal or objective is defined as an end toward which an effort is directed. In this book, the term "goal" will be used when broad educational aims are being discussed. The term "objective" will be used when specific measurable objectives are being discussed.*

> **EXAMPLE:** *Goal versus Specific Measurable Objective.* A *goal* (or broad educational aim) of a longitudinal quality improvement and patient safety preclerkship curriculum is that early medical students will have the knowledge and skills to apply patient safety principles and concepts in clinical practice.[1] The following is an example of a *specific measurable objective* of the curriculum: By the end of the workshop, each student will describe six fundamental principles of patient safety (PS) and quality improvement (QI).[2]

IMPORTANCE

Goals and objectives are important because they

- help direct the choice of curricular content and the assignment of relative priorities to various components of the curriculum;
- suggest what learning methods will be most effective;
- enable evaluation of learners and the curriculum, thus permitting demonstration of the effectiveness of a curriculum;
- suggest what evaluation methods are appropriate;
- set the boundaries of the curriculum within the larger program curriculum;
- facilitate mapping of the curriculum to higher-level program objectives; and
- clearly communicate to others, such as learners, faculty, program directors, department chairs, and accreditation bodies, what the curriculum addresses and hopes to achieve.

Broad educational goals communicate the overall purposes of a curriculum and serve as criteria against which the selection of various curricular components can be judged. The development and prioritization of *specific measurable objectives* permit further refinement of the curricular content and guide the selection of appropriate educational and evaluation methods.

WRITING OBJECTIVES

Writing educational objectives is an underappreciated skill. Despite the importance of objectives, learners, teachers, and curriculum planners frequently have difficulty in formulating or explaining the objectives of a curriculum. Poorly written objectives can result in a poorly focused and inefficient curriculum, prone to "drift" over time from its original goals.

A key to writing useful educational objectives is to make them *specific and measurable. Five basic elements* should be included in such objectives:[3] (1) Who, (2) will do, (3) how much (how well), (4) of what, (5) by when?

> **EXAMPLE:** *Specific Measurable Objective.* The example objective provided at the beginning of the chapter contains these elements: (1) Each student (who), (2) will describe (will do), (3) six (how much/how well), (4) of the fundamental principles of PS and QI (of what), (5) by the end of the workshop (by when)?

In other words, the specific measurable objective should include a verb (will do) and a noun (what) that describe a *performance*, as well as a *criterion* (how much/how well) and *conditions* (who, when) of the performance. (Readers may recognize the similarity to SMART—specific, measurable, assignable, realistic, time-based—objectives used in the business literature.)[4] In writing specific measurable objectives (as opposed to goals), one should *use verbs that are open to fewer interpretations* (e.g., to list or demonstrate) rather than words that are open to many interpretations (e.g., to know or appreciate). Table 4.1 lists more and less precise words to use in writing objectives. It is normal for objectives to go through several revisions. At each revision, asking whether the written objective answers all the elements in the question *"Who will do how much of what by when?"* confirms that it is specific and measurable. Before finalizing, it is important to

Table 4.1.   Verbs Open to More or Fewer Interpretations

Verbs Open to More Interpretations	Verbs Open to Fewer Interpretations	
Verbs that frequently apply to cognitive objectives:		
	Cognitive levels from Bloom's taxonomy of cognitive objectives[8,9]	Verb
know	*Remember* (recall of facts)	identify list recite define recognize retrieve
understand	*Understand*	define contrast interpret classify describe sort explain illustrate
be able know how appreciate	*Apply*	implement execute use (a model, method) complete
	Analyze	differentiate distinguish organize deconstruct discriminate
	Evaluate	detect judge critique test
know how	*Create*	design hypothesize construct produce
Verbs that frequently apply to affective objectives:		
appreciate	rate as valuable, rank as important	
grasp the significance of	rate as valuable, rank as important	
believe, perceive	identify, rate, or rank as a belief or opinion	
enjoy	rate or rank as enjoyable	
internalize	(use one of above terms)	

Table 4.1.   *(continued)*

Verbs Open to More Interpretations	Verbs Open to Fewer Interpretations
Verbs that frequently apply to psychomotor objectives:	
Skill/Competence	
be able	demonstrate
know how	show
Behavior/Performance	
internalize	use or incorporate into performance (as measured by)
Other verbs:	
learn	(use one of the above terms)
teach	(use one of the above terms; do not confuse the teacher and the learner in writing learner objectives)

have people such as content experts and potential learners review the objectives to ensure that others understand what the objectives are intended to convey. Table 4.2 provides some examples of poorly written and better-written objectives.

TYPES OF OBJECTIVES

In constructing a curriculum, one should be aware of the different types and levels of objectives. *Types of objectives* include objectives related to the learning of *learners*, to the educational *process* itself, and to health care and other *outcomes* of the curriculum. These types of objectives can be written at the level of the *individual learner*, the *program*, or all learners in *aggregate*. Table 4.3 provides examples of the different types of objectives for a curriculum on smoking cessation.

Learner Objectives

Learner objectives include objectives that relate to learning in the cognitive, affective, psychomotor/skill, and behavioral domains. The identification of the learning needs in these domains occurred in the general needs assessment part of Step 1, when health care provider knowledge, attitude, and/or skills deficits were articulated for the health problem of interest. Learner objectives that pertain to the *cognitive* domain of learning are often referred to as "knowledge" objectives. The latter terminology, however, may lead to an overemphasis on factual knowledge. Objectives related to the cognitive domain of learning should take into consideration a spectrum of mental skills relevant to the goals of a curriculum, from simple factual knowledge to higher levels of cognitive functioning, such as problem-solving and clinical decision-making.

> **EXAMPLE:** *Cognitive Objective.* By the end of the year 1 lecture, the student will list the nine critical steps in the QI process[5] (factual knowledge).

Table 4.2.   Examples of Poorly Written and Better-Written Objectives

Poorly Written Objectives	Better-Written Objectives
• Residents will learn the techniques of joint injections. [*The types of injection to be learned are not specified. The types of residents are not specified. It is unclear whether cognitive understanding of the technique is sufficient, or whether skills must be acquired. It is unclear by when the learning must have occurred and how proficiency could be assessed. The objective on the right addresses each of these concerns.*]	• By the end of the residency, each family practice resident will have demonstrated at least once (according to the attached protocol) the proper techniques for the following: - subacromial, bicipital, and intra-articular shoulder injection; - intra-articular knee aspiration and/or injection; - injections for lateral and medial epicondylitis; - injections for de Quervain's tenosynovitis; and - aspiration and/or injection of at least one new bursa, joint, or tendinous area, using appropriate references and supervision.
• By the end of the internal medicine clerkship, each third-year medical student will be able to diagnose and manage common ambulatory medical disorders. [*This objective specifies "who" and "by when" but is vague about what it is the medical students are to achieve. The two objectives on the right add specificity to the latter.*]	• By the end of the internal medicine ambulatory medicine clerkship, each third-year medical student will have achieved cognitive proficiency in the diagnosis and management of hypertension, diabetes, angina, chronic obstructive pulmonary disease, hyperlipidemia, alcohol and drug abuse, smoking, and asymptomatic HIV infection, as measured by acceptable scores on interim tests and the final examination. • By the end of the internal medicine clerkship, each third-year medical student will have seen and discussed with the preceptor, or discussed in a case conference with colleagues, at least one patient with each of the above disorders.
• Physician practices whose staff complete the three-session communication skills workshops will have more satisfied patients. [*This objective does not specify the comparison group or what is meant by "satisfied." The objective on the right specifies more precisely which practices will have more satisfied patients, what the comparison group will be, and how satisfaction will be measured. It specifies one aspect of performance as well as satisfaction. One could look at the satisfaction questionnaire and telephone management monitoring instrument for a more precise description of the outcomes being measured.*]	• Physician practices that have ≥50% of their staff complete the three-session communication skills workshops will have lower complaint rates, higher patient experience scores on the yearly questionnaire, and better telephone management, as measured by random simulated calls, than practices that have lower completion rates.

Table 4.3.   Types of Objectives: Examples from a Smoking Cessation Curriculum for Residents

	Individual Learner	Aggregate or Program
Learner		
Cognitive (knowledge)	By the end of the curriculum, each resident will list the five-step approach to effective smoking cessation counseling.	By the end of the curriculum, ≥80% of residents will list the five-step approach to effective smoking cessation counseling, and ≥90% will list the four critical (asterisked) steps.
Affective (attitudinal)	By the end of the curriculum, each primary care resident will rank smoking cessation counseling as an important and effective intervention by primary care physicians (≥3 on a 4-point scale).	By the end of the curriculum, there will have been a statistically significant increase in how primary care residents rate the importance and effectiveness of smoking cessation counseling by primary care physicians.
Psychomotor (skill or competence)	During the curriculum, each primary care resident will demonstrate in role-play a smoking cessation counseling technique that incorporates the attached five steps.	During the curriculum, ≥80% of residents will have demonstrated in role-play a smoking cessation counseling technique that incorporates the attached five steps.
Psychomotor (behavioral)	By 6 months after completion of the curriculum, each primary care resident will have negotiated a plan for smoking cessation with ≥60% of their smoking patients or have increased the percentage of patients with a smoking cessation plan by ≥20% from baseline.	By 6 months after completion of the curriculum, there will have been a statistically significant increase in the percentage of general internal medicine (GIM) residents who have negotiated a plan for smoking cessation with their patients.
Process	Each primary care resident will have attended both sessions of the smoking cessation workshop.	≥80% of primary care residents will have attended both sessions of the smoking cessation workshop.
Patient outcome	By 12 months after completion of the curriculum, the smoking cessation rate (for ≥6 months) for the patients of each primary care resident will have increased twofold or more from baseline or be ≥10%.	By 12 months after completion of the curriculum, there will have been a statistically significant increase in the percentage of primary care residents' patients who have quit smoking (for ≥6 months).

EXAMPLE: *Higher-Level Problem-Solving.* By the end of the workshop, the student will demonstrate QI knowledge by analyzing a health system scenario and describing an aim, a measure, and an appropriate change to address the health system gap[6,7] (application of knowledge measured by validated rubric).

Bloom's taxonomy was the first attempt to describe this potential hierarchy of mental skills.[8] At the time of its development in the mid-twentieth century, Bloom's taxonomy of cognitive learning objectives conceptualized a linear process of learning that occurred through a series of steps, which were referred to as six levels in the cognitive domain: knowledge (i.e., recall of facts), comprehension, application, analysis, synthesis, and evaluation.[8] By the turn of the century, revisions of the taxonomy incorporated modern cognitive psychology's more complex understanding of learning, including the role of motivation, emotions, and metacognition[9–11] (see Chapter 5, "Learning Theory, Principles, and Science").

To some extent, these taxonomies are hierarchical, although cognitive expertise is no longer assumed to develop linearly through these levels.

EXAMPLE: *Cognitive Levels.* The following learning objectives were created for a medical student preclerkship QI and PS curriculum.[2]
By the completion of the curriculum, the student will

- identify common causes of medical errors, with a multiple-choice examination showing latent and active medical errors (recall of facts—lower-order objective); and
- demonstrate the steps of a PDSA (plan-do-study-act) cycle and the use of run-chart analysis as a measure of effectiveness during a PDSA exercise (application/procedural dimension—higher-order objective).[2]

Curriculum planners usually specify the highest-level objective expected of the learner. Documenting the highest level of knowledge to be achieved can also be critical to the accreditation process. In several international accreditation systems, programs must provide evidence that the level of knowledge obtained by learners meets a national standard for the degree, such as "advanced problem-solving skills; the integration and formulation of judgments; self-evaluating and taking responsibility for contribution to professional knowledge and practice."[12,13]

The level of objectives is implied by the choice of verbs. The ability to *explain* and *illustrate*, for example, is a higher-level objective than the ability to *list* or *recite.* Table 4.1 shows an organization of verbs by Bloom's cognitive level; more elaborate lists of verbs can be found and are often organized as a "verb wheel," a pie chart of cognitive levels, with levels at the hub, verbs in the middle, and measures or assessments in the outermost rim.[14] These lists and wheels help the writer of the objective choose a verb and an assessment (measure) that are *congruent* with the cognitive level to be achieved.

Planners should also recognize that there are *enabling objectives* necessary to attain a certain higher-level objective. In the QI example above, learners need to know the steps of the PDSA cycle to demonstrate the run-chart analysis as a measure of the effectiveness of the PDSA cycle. Making these enabling objectives explicit will help learners, especially novices to the content, understand how the higher-order objective will be achieved and facilitate the educational strategies and assessment (Steps 4 and 6). Being explicit needs to be balanced with controlling the number of learner objectives so that learners are not overwhelmed with objectives. In larger curricula, this balance often occurs with lower-level, or enabling, objectives linked to, or nested within, individual events and higher-level objectives linked to the overall course or program.

Health professions curricula are being developed in a time of rapid biomedical information growth and evolving health care environments. One of the challenges in designing curricula in these environments is ascertaining whether the curriculum should focus on a body of factual knowledge that learners need to master (lower-order cognitive objectives) or on the development of conceptual frameworks that can be adapted and elaborated over a lifetime. Understanding the need to address a knowledge gap (reflection and meta-cognition), to collect and evaluate new information, and to apply it to problem-solving is referred to as *adaptive learning*, a process felt to promote innovative and lifelong learners (higher-order objective)[15] (see Chapter 5). The process of writing and prioritizing learner cognitive objectives helps curriculum developers clarify and focus them, ensuring they are aligned with the overall program goals (see "Additional Considerations," below).

Learner objectives that pertain to the *affective* domain are frequently referred to as "attitudinal" objectives. They may refer to specific attitudes, values, beliefs, biases, emotions, or role expectations. Affective objectives are usually more difficult to express and to measure than cognitive objectives.[16] Indeed, some instructional design experts maintain that because attitudes cannot be accurately assessed by observation of behaviors, attitudinal objectives should not be written.[17] Affective objectives, however, are implicit in most health professions' educational programs. Nearly every curriculum, for instance, holds as an affective objective that learners will value the importance of learning the content, which is critical to the attainment of other learner objectives.[18] This "attitude" relates to Marzano and Kendall's "self-system," which includes motivation, emotional response, perceived importance, and self-efficacy, and which they argue is an important underpinning of learning.[11] Even with motivated learners, actual experiences within and outside medical institutions (termed the "informal" and "hidden" curricula) may run counter to what is formally taught.[19,20] Curriculum developers should recognize and address such attitudes and practices (see Chapter 3).

> **EXAMPLE:** *Student Attitudes toward Learning.* A medical school's efforts to introduce the health systems science curriculum received mixed receptivity from preclerkship medical students. Students acknowledged that it was important content but also felt that the educational system valued board scores and grades.[21,22] Additional analysis found that students felt a tension between traditional and evolving health system science–related professional identity, and competition between health systems science and basic and clinical curricula. These factors limited student engagement in the new curricular learning objectives.[22]

To the extent that a curriculum involves learning in the affective domain, having a written objective will help to alert learners to the importance of such learning. If the affective objective is to be measured, it should be specific and narrowly defined.[16] Such objectives can help direct educational strategies, even when there are insufficient resources to objectively assess their achievement.

> **EXAMPLE:** *Affective Objective.* By the end of year 1 in the PS and QI longitudinal curricula, learners will recognize the role of the medical student and other health care team members in improving patient safety, as measured by a reflective writing assignment on summer reading with prompts on the role of the medical student in patient safety.[2]

Learner objectives that relate to the *psychomotor* domain of learning are often referred to as "skill" or "behavioral" objectives. These objectives refer to specific psychomotor tasks or actions that may involve hand or body movements, vision, hearing, speech, or the sense of touch. Medical interviewing, patient education and counseling, interpersonal communication, physical examination, record keeping, and procedural skills fall into this domain. In writing objectives for relevant psychomotor skills, it is helpful to indicate whether learners are expected only to achieve the ability to demonstrate a skill (a "skill" objective) or to incorporate the skill into their actual behavior *in the workplace* (a "behavioral" objective). Although mental procedures and behaviors certainly occur in professional work, this book will use the term "behavioral objective" to mean an observable skill in the workplace environment that is done repeatedly or habitually, such as routinely using a surgery checklist before starting an operating room procedure. Whether a psychomotor skill is written as a skill or behavioral objective has important implications for the choice of evaluation strategies and may influence the choice of educational strategies (see Chapter 5).

> **EXAMPLE:** *Skill Objective.* By the end of the curriculum, each undergraduate nursing student will have demonstrated proficiency in screening for substance abuse using the SBIRT (Screening, Brief Intervention, and Referral to Treatment) intervention[23] during a two-hour practice in the simulation lab with culturally diverse scenarios.[24]

> **EXAMPLE:** *Behavioral Objective.* Each undergraduate nursing student who has completed the curriculum will routinely (>80% of the time) use the SBIRT intervention to screen for substance abuse during clinical rotations. (This behavioral objective is assessed by direct observation of supervising faculty in the clinical rotations.)

Another way to envision the learner objectives related to clinical competence is in the hierarchy implied by Miller's assessment pyramid.[25] The pyramid implies that clinical competence begins with building a knowledge base (knows) and proceeds to learning a related skill or procedure (knows how), demonstrating the skill/procedure (shows how), and finally behavior in actual clinical practice (does). An updated version of this pyramid puts professional identity at the final stage, defined as "consistently demonstrates the attitudes, values, and behaviors expected of one who has come to think, act, and feel like a physician" (health professional).[26] The pyramid emphasizes the importance of assessing observable activities *in the workplace,* such as communications or procedures. Behaviors require multiple enabling objectives—cognitive, affective, and skill—that interact and support the learner's use of a new skill. Because some objectives encompass more than one domain, efficiency may be achieved by clearly articulating the highest-order objective, without separately articulating the underlying cognitive, affective, and skill objectives. This approach is the hallmark of competency-based frameworks (see below) which state the outcomes of educational programs as integrated competencies. Educational strategies, however, must still address the knowledge, attitudes, and skills that the learner needs to perform well (see Chapter 5).

> **EXAMPLE:** *Multidomain Behavioral Objective.* Recognizing that most clinical services for substance-abuse patients are provided by nonphysician providers, educational leaders created discipline-specific SBIRT training[27] for nonphysician graduate health profession students (psychology, nursing, occupational therapy, physical therapy, and physician assistant studies). An objective for this curriculum was that each student, on completion of the training, would incorporate SBIRT into their practice routine. This implies that students have achieved requisite core knowledge, attitudes, and perceived competency in screening and referral.[27]

Process Objectives

Process objectives relate to the implementation of the curriculum. For the learner, process objectives may indicate the degree of participation that is expected from the learners, or learner satisfaction with the curriculum. For the course director, process objectives may describe other indicators that the curriculum was implemented as planned (see Table 4.3).

> **EXAMPLE.** *Learner Process Objective.* Prior to the PS and QI workshop, each learner will complete four of the Institute for Healthcare Improvement (www.ihi.org) QI online modules.[6]

Program process objectives address the success of the implementation at the program level and may be written at the individual learner level or at the aggregated learner level.

> **EXAMPLE:** *Individual Process Objective.* Each physician assistant student will complete the four-hour SBIRT training program, including practice with a standardized patient, interview with a patient during a clinical rotation, and self-assessment with a proficiency checklist.[27] Note that this example describes the completion of the intervention, not the ultimate performance of the learner, and is therefore a *process* objective.

> **EXAMPLE:** *Program (Aggregated Learners) Process Objectives.* By the end of the clinical year, 100% of physician assistant students will have completed the SBIRT self-assessment proficiency checklist.

Outcome Objectives

In this book, we use the term *outcome objectives* to refer to *health*, *health care*, *patient*, and *population outcomes* (i.e., the impact of the curriculum beyond those delineated in its learner and process objectives). In planning program objectives, it is helpful to anticipate how the curriculum will be evaluated (see Figure 1.1 and Table 7.1). Kirkpatrick proposed four levels of educational program evaluation: (1) learner satisfaction, (2) learning achieved (such as aggregated learner achievement measures), (3) learner behaviors adopted in the workplace, and (4) system impact or outcomes.[28] Many curriculum developers focus on Kirkpatrick levels 1 and 2; planning to document achievement of levels 3 and 4, through written objectives, provides stronger evidence for the impact of the curriculum.

Outcomes might include the health outcomes of patients or the career choices of learners. More proximal outcomes might include changes in the behaviors of patients, such as smoking cessation.[29] Outcome objectives relate to the health care problem that the curriculum addresses. Unfortunately, the term "outcome objective" is used inconsistently, and learner cognitive, affective, and psychomotor objectives are sometimes referred to as outcomes (e.g., as knowledge, attitudinal, or skill outcomes). To avoid confusion, it is best to describe the objective using precise language that includes the specific type of outcome that will be measured.

> **EXAMPLE:** *Career Outcome Objective.* A higher percentage of students graduating from one of the consortium schools, Training for Health Equity Network, will be retained in priority, underserved areas of practice.[30]

> **EXAMPLE:** *Behavioral and Health Outcome Objectives.* At one year, clinical practices that host medical students in the Longitudinal Clerkship will document improved influenza vaccination rates across the practice population.[31]

It is often unrealistic to expect medical curricula to have easily measurable effects on quality of care and patient outcomes. Medical students, for example, may not have responsibility for patients until years after completion of a curriculum. However, most medical curricula should be designed to have positive effects on quality of care and patient outcomes. Even if outcomes will be difficult or impossible to measure, the inclusion of some health outcome objectives in a curriculum plan will emphasize the ultimate aims of the curriculum and may influence the choice of curricular content and educational methods.

At this point, it may be useful to review Table 4.3 for examples of each type and level of an objective.

COMPETENCY AND COMPETENCY-BASED EDUCATION

Competency-based education (CBE) is a design model of health professions education that is driven by systems needs rather than learner needs. CBE is outcomes-defined, time-variable, rather than time-defined, outcomes-variable, meaning that the progression of learners through a program is defined by performance achievement and not by the length of time they have been in the program.[32,33]

The goals of a CBE program are the attainment of health system or patient outcomes. Learner outcomes in CBE are articulated as the achievement of *competencies,* which are observable behaviors that result from the integration of knowledge, attitudes, and psychomotor skills. Competencies are often grouped into *domains of competence*, with more specific professional behaviors subsumed in the domain. For example, six competency domains for residency education in the United States were first published as part of the Accreditation Council for Graduate Medical Education (ACGME) Outcome Project in 1999 as Patient Care, Medical Knowledge, Interpersonal and Communication Skills, Practice-Based Learning and Improvement, Professionalism, and Systems-Based Care.[34] These six competencies continue to be refined and enhanced as training programs acquire more experience with them and seek a connection with patient and health systems outcomes.[34,35]

CBE was a major step forward in health professional education, especially in recognizing the importance of noncognitive behaviors of health professionals that are important in the delivery of quality care. As initially written, the competencies were abstract and context-dependent, however, which made teaching and assessment of learners a challenge. For example, a trainee could demonstrate excellent professionalism in one setting and fail in another situation. Communication skills valued in a surgical setting might be very different from those in an ambulatory clinic or on an emergency team.

EPAs and Milestones

Entrustable professional activities (EPAs) describe tasks or units of work for the health provider and are meant to operationalize CBE—that is, translate the theoretical into practice.[36,37] An EPA has a beginning and an end and is observable. One EPA can require proficiency in several competency domains and one competency domain may support several EPAs, so the relationship between EPAs and competencies is often depicted as a matrix. The EPAs are defined by a professional body that describes the core work of a discipline or profession through a complex consensus-building process[38,39] and are, therefore, specialty-specific. Physician graduate medical education programs typically have 20 to 40 EPAs; one challenge is defining the work of the discipline with a manageable number of EPAs.

Learners progress in a training program from novice to "entrustable" by demonstrating appropriate completion of the EPA task through *multiple* observations. Typically, five levels of proficiency are recognized: (1) observe only without performing the activity; (2) may act under full direct supervision; (3) may act under moderate, indirect, supervision; (4) may act without supervision; and (5) may act as instructor and supervisor.[36,38] EPAs describe the expected level of entrustment at different times or phases in a program, but in keeping with the time-variable approach, learners may progress sooner or later than their peers in achieving entrustment (see Chapter 7).

> **EXAMPLE:** *Internal Medicine EPAs at Two Phases in a Residency Training Program.* A consensus group of clinical experts and educational experts developed 29 EPAs for internal medicine residency, grouped into several phases of training. One EPA for the early phase, *Transition to Discipline*, is "Identifying and assessing unstable patients, providing initial management, and obtaining help." One EPA for the advanced phase, *Transition to Practice*, is "Working with other physicians and health care professionals to develop collaborative patient care plans."[39]
>
> Note that while these are learner educational objectives, the written descriptor is far more general than a specific learning objective as defined in this book and fits the definition of a "goal" better than an "objective" in the six-step approach.

To address the need for specific measures of learner progress toward entrustment, specialties have written "*milestones*" to describe the behaviors of learners within the competency domains as they progress through a training program. In this framework, a clinical competency committee uses a variety of observations and evidence to describe a learner's achievements in each of the six domains every six months of training.[40]

> **EXAMPLE:** *Pediatric Residency Milestone.* A subcompetency of the patient care competency in the pediatrics residency is to "gather essential and accurate information about the patient." Level 1 performance is described as follows: "Either gathers too little information or exhaustively gathers information following a template regardless of the patient's chief complaint, with each piece of information gathered seeming as important as the next. Recalls clinical information in the order elicited, with the ability to gather, filter, prioritize, and connect pieces of information being limited by and dependent upon analytic reasoning through basic pathophysiology alone."[41,42]

The developmental milestone is more specific than an EPA but also implies that *habitual and ongoing development of attitudes and skills* has been directly observed by a faculty member and, as written, is not clearly measurable.[43] One strategy to address this is an evaluation system that electronically collects multiple observations by multiple supervisors over time and creates *dashboards* for each resident[43] (see Chapter 7 and "programmatic assessment" under "Step 6: Evaluation and Feedback" in Chapter 10).

Most international health education systems have migrated to CBE.[44–48] A 2013 review of multiple international health profession competency frameworks found surprising consistency in these domains, adding only two to the six ACGME competencies.[49] The additional domains were *Interprofessional Collaboration* and *Personal and Professional Development*. The competencies related to *interprofessionalism and collaborative practice*, defined as multiple health care workers from different professional backgrounds working with patients, families, and communities to deliver the highest quality care,[50] were published as a consensus statement from the Interprofessional Collaborative and revised in 2016.[51] *Professional formation* was defined in the 2010 Carnegie Report as "habits of thought, feeling and action that allow learners to *demonstrate compassionate, communicative, and socially responsible physicianhood*."[52]

Medical education is also moving to standardize the competency language used across the education continuum from medical student to practicing physician. In 2013, the Association of American Medical Colleges published its *Reference List of General Physician Competencies* and requested that all medical schools map their educational program objectives to this taxonomy.[53] The discipline-descriptors of these competencies will continue to be refined and codified by the specialties. EPAs for medical students, the *Core Entrustable Professional Activities for Entering Residency,* were published by the Association for American Medical Colleges in 2013.[54] For curriculum developers, it is most important to be aware of these overarching goals and consider how specific learning objectives for the planned curriculum could support and map to competency development.

> **EXAMPLE**: *Competency Framework across the Continuum.* The AAMC uses a consensus process to describe new and emerging competencies in medicine. For the Quality Improvement and Patient Safety (QIPS) Competency Framework, five domains were described with detailed competencies at three points in the continuum, from medical student to practicing physician.[55] For example, one of 12 competencies within the QI domain is written as follows: One entering residency level (a recent medical graduate) "demonstrates knowledge of basic QI methodologies and quality measures." One entering practice (a recent residency graduate) demonstrates the same, plus "uses common tools (e.g., flow charts, process maps, fishbone diagrams) to inform QI efforts." The final point in the continuum, the experienced faculty physician, demonstrates these, plus "creates, implements, and evaluates common tools (e.g., flow charts, process maps, fishbone diagrams) to inform QI efforts."[55]

ADDITIONAL CONSIDERATIONS

While educational objectives are an important part of any curriculum, it is vital to remember that most educational experiences encompass much more than a list of preconceived objectives. For example, on clinical rotations, much learning derives from unanticipated experiences with individual patients. In many situations, the most useful learning derives from learning needs identified and pursued by individual learners and their mentors. An exhaustive list of objectives in such settings can be overwhelming for learners and teachers alike, stifle creativity, and limit learning related to individual needs and experiences. On the other hand, if no goals or objectives are articulated, learning experiences will be unfocused, and important cognitive, affective, psychomotor/skill or behavioral objectives may not be achieved.

Goals provide desired overall direction for a curriculum. An important and difficult task in curriculum development is to develop a *manageable number of specific measurable objectives* that

- interpret the goals;
- focus and prioritize curricular components that are critical to the realization of the goals; and
- encourage (or at least do not limit) creativity, flexibility, and nonprescribed learning relevant to the curriculum's goals.

> **EXAMPLE:** *Use of Goals and Objectives to Encourage Learning from Experience.* A broad goal for a medicine clerkship rotation in a physician assistant program might be for learners to become proficient in the initial diagnosis and management of common clinical problems. Once these clinical problems have been identified, the patient case-mix can be assessed to determine whether the settings used for training provide the learners with adequate clinical experience and access to relevant resources.

Broad goals for other clinical rotations in the same program might be that trainees develop as self-directed learners, develop sound clinical reasoning skills, and use evidence-based and patient-centered approaches in the care they provide. Specific measurable *process objectives* could promote the achievement of these goals without being unnecessarily restrictive. One such objective might be that each trainee, during a one-month clinical rotation, presents a 15-minute report on a patient management question encountered that month that incorporates principles of clinical epidemiology, evidence-based medicine, clinical decision-making, high-value care, and an assessment of patient or family preferences. A second objective might be that, each week during the rotation, individual trainees identify a question relevant to the care of one of their patients and briefly report to the team the sources used, the search time required, and the answer to their question.

Usually, several cycles of writing objectives are required to achieve a manageable number of specific measurable objectives that truly match the needs of one's targeted learners.

> **EXAMPLE:** *Refining and Prioritizing Objectives.* Faculty developing a curriculum on diabetes for the physician assistant program in the above example might begin with the following objectives:
>
> 1. By the end of the curriculum, each trainee will list the complications of diabetes mellitus.
> 2. By the end of the curriculum, each trainee will list atherosclerotic cardiovascular disease, retinopathy/blindness, nephropathy, neuropathy, and foot problems/amputation as complications of diabetes and list specific medical interventions that prevent each of these complications or their sequelae.
> 3. By the end of the curriculum, each trainee will list all the medical and sensory findings seen in each of the neuropathies that can occur as a complication of diabetes mellitus. (Similar objectives might have been written for other complications of diabetes.)
> 4. By the end of the curriculum, each trainee will analyze the quality of care provided to their outpatient panel.

After reflection and input from others, objective 1 might be eliminated because without prioritizing complications by prevalence or management implications, remembering every complication of diabetes is felt to be of little value. Objective 3 might be eliminated as being too many in number and containing detail unnecessary for this level of learner. Objective 4 might be clarified to include specific measurable terms such as, "analyze . . . using consensus quality indicators of diabetic care." Objective 2 might be retained because it is felt that it is sufficiently detailed and relevant to the goal of training physician assistant students to be proficient in the cost-effective diagnosis and management of clinical problems commonly encountered in medical practice. In the above process, the curriculum team would have reduced the number of objectives while ensuring that the remaining objectives are sufficiently specific and relevant to direct and focus teaching and evaluation.

CONCLUSION

Writing goals and objectives is a critical skill in curriculum development. Well-written goals and objectives define and focus a curriculum. They provide direction to curriculum developers in selecting educational strategies and evaluation methods.

QUESTIONS

For the curriculum you are coordinating, planning, or would like to be planning, please answer or think about the following questions and prompts:

1. Write one to three broad educational goals.

2. Do these goals relate to a defined competency or EPA for the profession?

3. Write one specific measurable educational objective of each type using the template provided.

Level of Objective

	Individual Learner	Aggregate or Program
Learner (cognitive, affective, psychomotor/ skill or behavioral)		
Process		
Health, health care, or patient outcome		

Check each objective to make sure that it includes all five elements of a specific measurable objective (<u>Who</u> <u>will do</u> <u>how much/how well</u> <u>of what</u> <u>by when</u>?). Check to see that the words you used are precise and unambiguous (see Table 4.1). Have someone else read your objectives and see if they can explain them to you accurately.

4. Do your specific measurable objectives support and further define your broad educational goals? If not, you need to reflect further on your goals and objectives and change one or the other.

5. Can you map these objectives to the defined competency set or EPA identified in Question 2, above?

6. Reflect on how your objectives, as worded, will focus the content, educational methods, and evaluation strategies of your curriculum. Is this what you want? If not, you may want to rewrite, add, or delete some objectives.

GENERAL REFERENCES

Anderson, Lorin W., and David R. Krathwohl, eds. *A Taxonomy for Learning, Teaching, and Assessing: A Revision of Bloom's Taxonomy of Educational Objectives.* New York: Longman, 2001.
A revision of Bloom's taxonomy of cognitive objectives that presents a two-dimensional framework for cognitive learning objectives. Written by cognitive psychologists and educators, with many useful examples to illustrate the function of the taxonomy. 302 pages.

Bloom, Benjamin S. *Taxonomy of Educational Objectives: A Classification of Educational Objectives. Handbook 1: Cognitive Domain.* New York: Longman, 1984.
A classic text that presents a detailed classification of cognitive educational objectives. A condensed version of the taxonomy is included in an appendix for quick reference. 207 pages.

Cutrer, William B., Martin V. Pusic, Larry D. Gruppen, Maya M. Haymmoud, and Sally A. Santen, eds. *The Master Adaptive Learner.* Philadelphia: Elsevier, 2021.
This book is based on the premise that twenty-first-century health professionals need to be lifelong learners who adjust and innovate throughout their professional careers. The text presents a theoretical and practical guide to developing curricula that address the development of adaptive expertise.

Green, Lawrence, Marshall W. Kreuter, Sigrid Deeds, and Kay B. Partridge. *Health Education Planning: A Diagnostic Approach.* Palo Alto, CA: Mayfield Publishing, 1980.
This basic text of health education program planning includes the role of objectives in program planning. 306 pages.

Gronlund, Norman E., and Susan M. Brookhart. *Gronlund's Writing Instructional Objectives.* 8th ed. Upper Saddle River, NJ: Pearson, 2009.
A comprehensive and well-written reference that encompasses the cognitive, affective, and psychomotor domains of educational objectives. It provides a useful updating of Bloom's and Krathwohl's texts with many examples and tables.

Krathwohl, David R., Benjamin S. Bloom, and Bertram B. Masia. *Taxonomy of Educational Objectives, Handbook II: Affective Domain.* New York: David McKay Company, 1956.
A classic text that presents a detailed classification of affective educational objectives. A condensed version of the taxonomy is included in an appendix for quick reference.

Mager, Robert F. *Preparing Instructional Objectives: A Critical Tool in the Development of Effective Instruction.* 3rd ed. Atlanta, GA: Center for Effective Performance, 1997.
A readable, practical guidebook for writing objectives. Includes examples. Popular reference for professional educators, as well as health professionals who develop learning programs for their students. 193 pages.

Marzano, Robert J., and John S. Kendall. *The New Taxonomy of Educational Objectives.* 2nd ed. Thousand Oaks, CA: Corwin Press, 2007.
Yet another revision of Bloom's taxonomy. Based on three domains of knowledge: information, mental procedures, and psychomotor procedures. Well-written and thoughtful, this work argues for well-researched models of knowledge and learning. 167 pages.

REFERENCES CITED

1. World Health Organization, *WHO Patient Safety Curriculum Guide for Medical Schools: A Summary* (United Kingdom: WHO Press, 2009).
2. Luba Dumenco et al., "Outcomes of a Longitudinal Quality Improvement and Patient Safety Preclerkship Curriculum," *Academic Medicine* 94, no. 12 (2019): 1980–87, https://doi.org/10.1097/ACM.0000000000002898.
3. Lawrence Green et al., *Health Education Planning: A Diagnostic Approach* (Palo Alto, CA: Mayfield Publishing, 1980).
4. George T. Doran, "There's a S.M.A.R.T. Way to Write Management's Goals and Objectives," *Management Review* 70, no. 11 (1981): 35–36.
5. Mamta K. Singh, Heidi L. Gullett, and Patricia A. Thomas, "Using Kern's 6-Step Approach to Integrate Health Systems Science Curricula into Medical Education," *Academic Medicine* 96 (2021): 1282–90, https://doi.org/10.1097/ACM.0000000000004141.

6. Luba Dumenco et al., "An Interactive Quality Improvement and Patient Safety Workshop for First-Year Medical Students," *MedEdPORTAL* 14 (2018), https://doi.org/10.15766/mep_2374-8265.10734.

7. Mamta K. Singh et al., "The Quality Improvement Knowledge Application Tool Revised (QIKAT-R)," *Academic Medicine* 89 (2014): 1386–91, https://doi.org/10.1097/ACM.0000000000000456.

8. Benjamin S. Bloom, *Taxonomy of Educational Objectives: Cognitive Domain* (New York: Longman, 1984).

9. Lorin W. Anderson and David R. Krathwohl, eds., *A Taxonomy for Learning, Teaching, and Assessing: A Revision of Bloom's Taxonomy of Educational Objectives* (New York: Addison Wesley Longman, 2001).

10. David R. Krathwohl, "A Revision of Bloom's Taxonomy: An Overview," *Theory into Practice* 41, no. 4 (2002): 212–18.

11. Robert J. Marzano and John S. Kendall, *The New Taxonomy of Educational Objectives*, 2nd ed. (Thousand Oaks, CA: Corwin Press, 2007).

12. Bologna Working Group on Qualifications Frameworks, *A Framework for Qualifications for the European Higher Education Area* (Copenhagen: Ministry of Science, Technology and Innovation, 2005).

13. Commission for Academic Accreditation, *QF Emirates Guide for ERTs* (United Arab Emirates: Ministry of Education, 2019).

14. Ashley Tan, "Remaking the Revised Bloom's Taxonomy," 2016, accessed April 30, 2021, http://bit.ly/newbtref.

15. William B. Cutrer et al., "Fostering the Development of Master Adaptive Learners: A Conceptual Model to Guide Skill Acquisition in Medical Education," *Academic Medicine* 92, no. 1 (2017): 70–75, https://doi.org/10.1097/acm.0000000000001323.

16. Marlene E. Henerson, Lynn L. Morris, and Carol T. Fitz-Gibbon, *How to Measure Attitudes*, vol. 6, 2nd ed. (Newbury Park, CA: Sage Publications, 1987).

17. Robert F. Mager, *Preparing Instructional Objectives: A Critical Tool in the Development of Effective Instruction*, 3rd ed. (Atlanta, GA: CEP Press, 1997).

18. David A. Cook and Anthony R. Artino Jr., "Motivation to Learn: An Overview of Contemporary Theories," *Medical Education* 50, no. 10 (2016): 997–1014, https://doi.org/10.1111/medu.13074.

19. Frederick W. Hafferty and Joseph F. O'Donnell, eds., *The Hidden Curriculum in Health Professional Education* (Hanover, NH: Dartmouth College Press, 2015).

20. Maria A. Martimianakis et al., "Humanism, the Hidden Curriculum, and Educational Reform: A Scoping Review and Thematic Analysis," *Academic Medicine* 90, no. 11 Suppl (2015): S5–S13, https://doi.org/10.1097/ACM.0000000000000894.

21. Jed D. Gonzalo and Greg Ogrinc, "Health Systems Science: The 'Broccoli' of Undergraduate Medical Education," *Academic Medicine* 94 (2019): 1425–32, https://doi.org/10.1097/acm.0000000000002815.

22. Jed D. Gonzalo et al., "Unpacking Medical Students' Mixed Engagement in Health Systems Science Education," *Teaching and Learning in Medicine* 32, no. 3, (2019): 250–58, https://doi.org/10.1080/10401334.2019.1704765.

23. Thomas F. Babor, Frances Del Boca, and Jeremy W. Bray, "Screening, Brief Intervention and Referral to Treatment: Implications of SAMHSA's SBIRT Initiative for Substance Abuse Policy and Practice," *Addiction* 112, Suppl 2 (2017): 110–17, https://doi.org/10.1111/add.13675.

24. Betty J. Braxter et al., "Nursing Students' Experiences with Screening, Brief Intervention, and Referral to Treatment for Substance Use in the Clinical/Hospital Setting," *Journal of Addictions Nursing* 25, no. 3 (2014): 122–29, https://doi.org/10.1097/JAN.0000000000000037.

25. G. E. Miller, "The Assessment of Clinical Skills/Competence/Performance," *Academic Medicine* 65, 9 Suppl (1990): S63–S67, https://doi.org/10.1097/00001888-199009000-00045.

26. Richard L. Cruess, Sylvia R. Cruess, and Yvonne Steinert, "Amending Miller's Pyramid to Include Professional Identity Formation," *Academic Medicine* 91, no. 2 (2016): 180–85, https://doi.org/10.1097/ACM.0000000000000913.

27. Ashley T. Scudder et al., "Screening, Brief Intervention, and Referral to Treatment (SBIRT) Expansion of Training to Non-physician Healthcare Graduate Students: Counseling Psychology, Nursing, Occupational Therapy, Physical Therapy, and Physician Assistant Studies," *Substance Abuse* (2019): 1–11, https://doi.org/10.1080/08897077.2019.1695705.

28. James D. Kirkpatrick and Wendy K. Kirkpatrick, *Kirkpatrick's Four Levels of Training Evaluation* (Alexandria, VA: Association for Talent Development Press, 2016).

29. Jean-Paul Humair and Jacques Cornuz, "A New Curriculum Using Active Learning Methods and Standardized Patients to Train Residents in Smoking Cessation," *Journal of General Internal Medicine* 18, no. 12 (2003): 1023–27, https://doi.org/10.1111/j.1525-1497.2003.20732.x.

30. Simone J. Ross et al., "The Training for Health Equity Network Evaluation Framework: A Pilot Study at Five Health Professional Schools," *Education for Health* 27, no. 2 (2014): 116–26, https://doi.org/10.4103/1357-6283.143727.

31. Bruce L. Henschen et al., "Continuity with Patients, Preceptors, and Peers Improves Primary Care Training: A Randomized Medical Education Trial," *Academic Medicine* 95, no. 3 (2020): 425–34, https://doi.org/10.1097/ACM.0000000000003045.

32. Jason R. Frank et al., "Toward a Definition of Competency-Based Education in Medicine: A Systematic Review of Published Definitions," *Medical Teacher* 32, no. 8 (2010): 631–37, https://doi.org/10.3109/0142159x.2010.500898.

33. Nicolas Fernandez et al., "Varying Conceptions of Competence: An Analysis of How Health Sciences Educators Define Competence," *Medical Education* 46, no. 4 (2012): 357–65, https://doi.org/10.1111/j.1365-2923.2011.04183.x.

34. Susan R. Swing, "The ACGME Outcome Project: Retrospective and Prospective," *Medical Teacher* 29, no. 7 (2007): 648–54, https://doi.org/10.1080/01421590701392903.

35. Kelly J. Caverzagie et al., "Overarching Challenges to the Implementation of Competency-Based Medical Education," *Medical Teacher* 39, no. 6 (2017): 588–93, https://doi.org/10.1080/0142159x.2017.1315075.

36. C. El-Haddad et al., "The ABCs of Entrustable Professional Activities: An Overview of 'Entrustable Professional Activities' in Medical Education," *Internal Medicine Journal* 46, no. 9 (2016): 1006–10, https://doi.org/10.1111/imj.12914.

37. Shefaly Shorey et al., "Entrustable Professional Activities in Health Care Education: A Scoping Review," *Medical Education* 53, no. 8 (2019): 766–77, https://doi.org/10.1111/medu.13879.

38. Olle ten Cate et al., "Curriculum Development for the Workplace Using Entrustable Professional Activities (EPAs): AMEE Guide No. 99," *Medical Teacher* 37, no. 11 (2015): 983–1002, https://doi.org/10.3109/0142159x.2015.1060308.

39. David R. Taylor et al., "Creating Entrustable Professional Activities to Assess Internal Medicine Residents in Training: A Mixed-Methods Approach," *Annals of Internal Medicine* 168, no. 10 (2018): 724–29, https://doi.org/10.7326/M17-1680.

40. Thomas J. Nasca et al., "The Next GME Accreditation System—Rationale and Benefits," *New England Journal of Medicine* 366, no. 11 (2012): 1051–56, https://doi.org/10.1056/NEJMsr1200117.

41. Patricia J. Hicks et al., "The Pediatrics Milestones: Conceptual Framework, Guiding Principles, and Approach to Development," *Journal of Graduate Medical Education* 2, no. 3 (2010): 410–18, https://doi.org/10.4300/JGME-D-10-00126.1.

42. "The Pediatrics Milestone Project: A Joint Initiative of the Accreditation Council for Graduate Medical Education and the American Board of Pediatrics," Pediatrics Milestone Working Group, 2017, accessed April 30, 2021, https://www.acgme.org/portals/0/pdfs/milestones/pediatricsmilestones.pdf.

43. Samir Johna and Brandon Woodward, "Navigating the Next Accreditation System: A Dashboard for the Milestones," *Permanente Journal* 19, no. 4 (2015): 61–63, https://doi.org/10.7812/TPP/15-041.

44. "Outcomes for Graduates," General Medical Council, 2018, accessed April 30, 2021, https://www.gmc-uk.org/education/standards-guidance-and-curricula/standards-and-outcomes/outcomes-for-graduates/outcomes-for-graduates.

45. J. G. Simpson, et al., "The Scottish Doctor—Learning Outcomes for the Medical Undergraduate in Scotland: A Foundation for Competent and Reflective Practitioners," *Medical Teacher* 24, no. 2 (2002): 136–43, https://doi.org/10.1080/01421590220120713.

46. Jason R. Frank, Linda Snell, and Jonathan Sherbino, eds., *CanMEDS 2015 Physician Competency Framework* (Ottawa: Royal College of Physicians and Surgeons of Canada, 2015), accessed April 30, 2021, http://canmeds.royalcollege.ca/uploads/en/framework/CanMEDS%202015%20Framework_EN_Reduced.pdf.

47. "Common Program Requirements (Residency)," Accreditation Council for Graduate Medical Education, 2020, accessed April 30, 2021, https://www.acgme.org/what-we-do/accreditation/common-program-requirements.

48. "ACGME International Foundational Program Requirements for Graduate Medical Education," effective July 1, 2020, ACGME-I, accessed April 30, 2021, https://www.acgme-i.org/Accreditation-Process/Requirements/.

49. Robert Englander et al., "Toward a Common Taxonomy of Competency Domains for the Health Professions and Competencies for Physicians," *Academic Medicine* 88, no. 8. (2013): 1088–94, https://doi.org/10.1097/ACM.0b013e31829a3b2b.

50. WHO Study Group on Interprofessional Education and Collaborative Practice, *Framework for Action on Interprofessional Education and Collaborative Practice* (Geneva, Switzerland: World Health Organization, 2010).

51. Interprofessional Education Collaborative, Core Competencies for Interprofessional Collaborative Practice: 2016 Update (Washington, DC: Interprofessional Education Collaborative, 2016), accessed October 8, 2021, https://www.ipecollaborative.org/ipec-core-competencies.

52. Molly Cooke, David Irby, and Bridget C. O'Brien, *Educating Physicians: A Call for Reform of Medical School and Residency* (San Francisco, CA: Jossey-Bass, 2010).

53. Kristen L. Eckstrand et al., "Giving Context to the Physician Competency Reference Set: Adapting to the Needs of Diverse Populations," *Academic Medicine* 91, no. 7 (2016): 930–35, https://doi.org/10.1097/ACM.0000000000001088.

54. Association of American Medical Colleges, *Core Entrustable Professional Activities for Entering Residency: Curriculum Developers' Guide* (Washington, DC: AAMC, 2014), accessed April 30, 2021, https://www.aamc.org/what-we-do/mission-areas/medical-education/cbme/core-epas/publications.

55. Association of American Medical Colleges, *Quality Improvement and Patient Safety Competencies Across the Learning Continuum,* AAMC New and Emerging Areas in Medicine Series (Washington, DC: AAMC, 2019), accessed April 30, 2021, https://www.aamc.org/what-we-do/mission-areas/medical-education/cbme/qips.

Step 4
Educational Strategies

. . . accomplishing educational objectives

Sean A. Tackett, MD, MPH, and Chadia N. Abras, PhD

True teaching is not an accumulation of knowledge; it is an awakening
of consciousness which goes through successive stages.
—From a temple wall inside an Egyptian pyramid

DEFINITIONS

Once the goals and specific measurable objectives for a curriculum have been determined, the next step is to *develop the educational strategies* by which the curricular

objectives will be achieved. Educational strategies include both content and methods. *Content* refers to the specific topics or subject matter to be included in the curriculum. *Methods* are the ways in which learners will engage with the content.

IMPORTANCE

Educational strategies provide the means by which a curriculum's objectives are achieved. They are the heart of the curriculum, the educational intervention itself. There is a natural tendency to think of the curriculum in terms of this step alone. As we shall see, the groundwork of Steps 1 through 3 guides the selection of educational strategies.

GENERAL CONSIDERATIONS

As curriculum developers think through their options for educational strategies, they should be aware of some of the theory, principles, and science that relate to how learning occurs; technologies that can support learning; and other frameworks that can inform the design of educational activities.

It also helps to have in mind a definition of learning. *Teaching* is what educators do, but *learning* is what happens within the learner. Learning can be visible as changes in the cognitive, affective, and/or psychomotor domains of learning and in learner behaviors. The job of curriculum developers is largely to plan experiences that *facilitate* learning in curriculum participants.

Learning Theory, Principles, and Science

There are now numerous frameworks that describe how learning happens. They often have much in common, although no single framework explains every aspect of learning. Learning frameworks tend to focus on what happens within individuals, what happens when individuals or groups interact with each other, or what happens when people interact with material objects. Learning frameworks that focus on what happens within individuals tend to align more closely with one of the cognitive, affective, or psychomotor domains of learning.

Cognitivism is a broad paradigm that aligns closely with the *cognitive* domain of learning. It explains learning based on how information is processed: starting with environmental stimuli, which get filtered through sensory memory into working memory (which has limited capacity), then transitioned to long-term memory (which has virtually unlimited storage), and ultimately transferred to be applied in new situations.[1,2] Cognitive load theory fits within the cognitivist paradigm and emphasizes the need to minimize extraneous cognitive load to make more working memory available for germane cognitive load in order to perform tasks and expand knowledge.[3] Cognitivism also encompasses the cognitive theory of multimedia learning,[4] which has described principles for combining words and pictures to optimize information processing. For example, arranging words and pictures so that they complement one another can allow them to be processed as one whole "chunk" of information rather than as separate pieces, allowing a greater amount of information overall to be held in working memory. Numerous other practical tips have come from experimental evidence related to the cognitivist paradigm,[5] such as incorporating testing, spaced retrieval (e.g., repeating at increasing intervals to avoid forgetting), or interleaving (e.g., mixing concepts instead of studying them in blocks) into curricular design and experiences. *Personal (cognitive) constructivism* is another paradigm that aligns primarily with the cognitive domain of learning. It emerged from Piaget's theory of cognitive development and focuses on how learners create meaning by elaborating on their existing unique schemata.[6] Whereas cognitivist models seek to optimize the quantity of information that can be processed, constructivism focuses on connecting new knowledge to each learners' existing knowledge and assumes that the shape and contours of each learner's cognitive representations are unique. Cognitivism and constructivism share an emphasis on activating prior knowledge when trying to optimize learning.

Theories of motivation attempt to explain how learners' *affective* attributes—such as beliefs about their own capabilities, perceptions that their actions will influence outcomes, and the perceived value of educational experiences—influence their learning.[7,8] These theories emphasize creating supportive learning environments that foster relationships, clarifying the relevance and value of a task in accordance with learners' goals, helping learners calibrate more accurately their beliefs about their own abilities, and seeking opportunities that allow learners to control and direct their learning.[7] *Transformative learning*, where a deep change in meaning and perspective is cultivated, is intended to change one's worldview. This also aligns primarily with the affective domain of learning and can be useful for raising awareness among learners about their unconscious values, emotions, or biases.[9] Changing learners' frames of reference may occur when they reflect on "disorienting dilemmas"[10] or learn by "problem-posing" based on their observations and experiences rather than solving the problems that someone else frames and presents to them.[11]

Deliberate practice is a model that has particular relevance to *psychomotor* learning, as it describes how skills are practiced with effort and focus, with frequent feedback (often from a coach), through cycles where goals become progressively more difficult or complex.[12] *Mastery learning*, in which learners must achieve a fixed standard of performance, is becoming more important in competency-based, time-varying educational models (see Chapter 4, "Competency and Competency-Based Education"). The achievement of mastery performance standards often occurs through repeated cycles of deliberate practice. Once the predefined mastery standard is achieved, learners can advance to a new stage of training and practice toward more demanding standards.[13]

Social learning theories,[14] which focus on how learning happens when individuals interact with each other, naturally span cognitive, affective, and psychomotor domains. These theories attempt to explain how learning occurs when observing others and how knowledge can be generated and shared by groups. Table 5.1 summarizes paradigms for education, adapted from Baker et al.,[15] that are relevant to health professions education (sociomaterialism and behaviorism, included in Table 5.1, are described later in this chapter).

The common aspects across learning models are that all learning requires that individuals (1) engage with new and potentially challenging concepts and/or experiences, (2) believe that what they will learn is important and achievable, (3) feel safe and supported in their learning environments, and (4) have opportunities for practice, feedback, and reflection, with learning cycles repeated as needed. In general, learning is enhanced along a continuum from learners being passive, to active, to constructive, to interactive.[16]

Finally, while there is the tendency to believe that multitasking can enhance efficiency, evidence suggests that instead it can worsen the quality of the multiple tasks that are being performed.[17]

Rest, Well-Being, and Learning

Goal-directed learning experiences require focus and effort from participants, but learning continues between and beyond planned learning experiences. When one's thoughts are not directed to specific goals, spontaneous thoughts, such as mind-wandering or daydreaming episodes,[18] may occur as the brain's "default mode network" switches on, allowing connections to be made between different parts of the brain.[19] These periods of rest are thought to be generative and responsible for novel insights and creativity, rather than an absence of learning. Spending too much time in goal-directed activities can limit learning and creativity.

Learning also improves when individuals adopt generally healthy behaviors. Adequate sleep is critical for memory consolidation.[20,21] Even short episodes of exercise can improve cognitive performance.[22] Sleep, exercise, and social connections can decrease stress and anxiety, which also benefits learning. Curriculum developers can design curricula to ensure sufficient time for rest and encourage participants to engage in healthy behaviors.

Digital and Online Learning

The term digital education can apply to when educational content or methods use digital (electronic) technologies, offline or online.[23] Resources can be accessed by learners at the same time (i.e., synchronously) or at different times (i.e., asynchronously). Almost all traditional face-to-face educational strategies have analogous digital options. New digital educational strategies appear so often that there is no standard terminology that can encompass all of them. Terminology for different types of online curricula is somewhat more uniform and includes the following:[24]

- *Blended learning* curricula combine face-to-face and online instruction.
- *Instructor-led fully online* curricula have all content accessed online with synchronous and asynchronous interactions between instructors and learners.
- *Self-paced modules* are curricula initiated by individual learners and are fully asynchronous.
- *Massive open online courses (MOOCs)* are curricula developed on specialized platforms that support large scale involvement and are asynchronous, although MOOCs often bring students together into cohorts and support peer and instructor interactions.

Digital technologies and online curricula offer the potential advantages of overcoming location and time constraints. They can improve learning quality by standardizing curricular elements and offering flexibility in how students access resources. Digital education has been shown to be comparable to traditional methods for learning in the health professions.[23,25,26]

At the same time, adopting and implementing new technologies requires resources and often introduces complexity into curriculum development and participation in the curriculum.[27] The simple use of new technologies does not necessarily improve learning. Technologies must be used in accordance with theory, principles, and evidence.

Table 5.1. Paradigms for Education in the Health Professions

Paradigm	Claims about Learning	Desired Learning Outcomes	Example Applications	Main Advantages	Main Limitations
Behaviorism	Behavior changes result from positive and negative stimuli in the environment	Observable changes in actions	Checklists; repetition and reinforcement	Simple, intuitive, effective for workplace-based behavior change	Does not account for differences among learners, individual agency, or affective aspects of learning
Cognitivism	Information processing occurs between environmental stimuli (sensory memory), working memory, and long-term memory	Transfer of learning to new and unfamiliar problems and contexts, with eventual development of expertise	Testing, spaced retrieval, interleaving, or linking graphics and words to "chunk" information	Numerous practical tips founded on large and growing evidence base	Does not account for group interactions; less applicable to affective aspects of learning
Personal (cognitive) constructivism	Individuals learn and develop by building on existing knowledge	More elaborate knowledge schemata	Sequenced organization of knowledge and experiences; problem-based learning; self-directed learning	Frequently used in health professions education and still relevant	Does not account for group interactions or context
Transformative learning	Questioning long-held beliefs and assumptions leads to an altered worldview	New frames of reference	Critical reflection; problem-posing	Can lead to disruptive changes in perspective in learners that go beyond traditional incremental changes in abilities	Can be uncomfortable, time-consuming, and difficult to achieve other objectives at the same time

Social learning theories	Individuals learn through observations and interactions with others and participation in communities	Individual abilities that are context-specific; collective creation of knowledge; altered perspective	Role modeling; group reflection; active participation in practice settings and learning groups	Familiar in health professions education with particular relevance to professional identity formation	Summative assessment can be challenging; not well suited for developing new knowledge or specific skills
Sociomaterialism	Physical materials actively influence human interactions	Improved use of materials; recognition of influence of materials on human actions	Attention to physical learning spaces; how medical artifacts influence perceptions and learning; how humans and materials form assemblages	Approach makes influences on learning that are often ignored more visible	Emerging area of study in education without clear guidance on application

Source: Adapted from Baker et al.[15]

Theories that attempt to explain how technology influences learning are being developed; for example, some theories of *sociomaterialism*[28,29] (see Table 5.1) propose that technologies themselves actively influence human interactions (e.g., videoconferencing software flattens people into two dimensions and prohibits direct eye contact).[30] However, no theory currently offers specific guidance for applying technology to optimize learning. Generally, decisions about what educational content and methods to use in online curricula or other curricula with digital aspects can be made using the same principles as those with no digital component.

Games and Gamification

Games and gamification are increasingly popular frameworks to consider when designing educational activities and selecting educational strategies. *Games* are defined as having six features: (1) rules, (2) outcomes that vary and can be quantified, (3) different values assigned to different outcomes, (4) effort from players to influence the outcome, (5) players' emotional attachment to the outcome, and (6) consequences that may or may not have real-life importance.[31] *Serious games* are games designed specifically for nonentertainment purposes and can comprise complete educational experiences or be incorporated as components of educational activities. *Gamification*[32] (in education) refers to applying some elements from game design principles to a learning activity[33] and most often incorporates competition or incentives (e.g., points, leaderboards, or badges).[34] Gamification does not comprise a learning theory or model per se, although it aligns closely with cognitivist theories and theories of motivation.[35] To employ gamification meaningfully, Nicholson proposed the RECIPE framework, that includes *reflection* opportunities for participants, *exposition* (i.e., narratives or stories), *choice* (i.e., participants have control over their experience), *information* (about a game's rules and incentives), *play* (i.e., freedom to explore, experiment, and fail), and *engagement* (in game aspects and with other participants).[36] Evidence suggests serious games and gamification may improve cognitive and psychomotor learning outcomes in health professions education.[37]

> **EXAMPLE:** *Game for Complex Decision-Making.* GeriatriX was developed to train medical students in complex geriatric decision-making, including weighing patient preferences and appropriateness and costs of care. The game was used as a supplement to a geriatric education program and resulted in an increase in self-perceived competence in these topics for the intervention group and better cost-consciousness when selecting diagnostic tests.[38]

> **EXAMPLE:** *Game for Improving Hypertension Treatment.* Primary care providers were randomized to participate in an online game that tested their hypertension knowledge at spaced intervals, showed their progress, and compared them to other providers. The control group reviewed online posts. Those who completed the game showed improved knowledge and shorter time to having their patients' blood pressure under control.[39]

> **EXAMPLE:** *Gamification to Enhance Simulation Practice.* Surgery residents were not using a robotic skill simulator as often as their educators hoped they would, so the educators announced a single-elimination tournament where performance was tracked by leaderboards and prizes were given to winners. Practice with the simulator increased, decreasing the cost per hour of simulator maintenance.[40]

DETERMINATION AND ORGANIZATION OF CONTENT

The content of the curriculum flows from its learning objectives. Listing the nouns (the "of what" component) used in these objectives (see Chapter 4, "Writing Objectives") should outline the content of the curriculum. The amount of material presented to learners should not be too little (lacking key substance) or too much (cluttering rather than clarifying). Curriculum developers should aim to have just the right amount of detail to achieve the desired objectives and outcomes. Given the vast quantity of content that is available for health professions learners, educators should be prepared to curate the highest quality content[41] and consider recommending content resources that extend beyond those required to meet learning objectives. For curricula of significant duration, there may also be opportunities to incorporate spaced repetition of content to enhance retention, or to interleave (mix) concepts, which yields superior long-term learning.[5]

It is usually helpful to construct a *syllabus* for the curriculum that includes (1) an explicit statement of learning objectives and methods, to help focus learners; (2) a schedule of curriculum events and deadlines; (3) curricular resources (e.g., readings, multimedia, cases, questions); (4) plans for assignments and assessments; and (5) other practical information, such as faculty contact information and office hours, locations and directions for face-to-face sessions, guidance for engaging with technology needed for digital elements, and expectations for professional behaviors during the course. The use of learning management systems allows course directors to easily provide and update resources and add interactive components to them.[42] When using software to deliver digital content, curriculum developers should partner with an expert in instructional design to ensure that the organization of content will lead to efficient learning.

CHOICE OF EDUCATIONAL METHODS

General Guidelines

Recognizing that educational strategies should be consistent with the principles of learning discussed above, it is helpful to keep the following additional principles in mind when considering educational methods for a curriculum.

Maintain Congruence between Objectives and Methods. Choose educational methods that are most likely to achieve a curriculum's goals and objectives. One way to approach the selection of educational methods is to group the specific measurable objectives of the curriculum as cognitive, affective, or psychomotor objectives (see Chapter 4) and select educational methods most likely to be effective for the type of objective (Table 5.2).

Use Multiple Educational Methods. All *adult learners* bring a wealth of different *experiences and cultures* to their learning activities. These shape their interpretations of reality and approaches to learning.[43] They also have unique existing proficiencies, needs, and preferences for how they learn, each of which may vary in a given learning context. Ideally, the curriculum would use methods that work best for all individual learners across all of their different contexts. However, few curricula can be that malleable; often, a large number of learners need to be accommodated in a short period of time.

Learners and educators have many educational methods to choose from.[44] Planning to use a *variety* of educational methods can accommodate learner preferences, enhance learner interest and commitment, and reinforce learning. Also, for curricula attempting to achieve higher-order or complex objectives that span several domains, as is often the case with competency-based frameworks, the use of

Table 5.2. Matching Educational Methods to Objectives

Educational Methods*	Type of Objective				
	Cognitive: Lower-Order[†]	Cognitive: Higher-Order[†]	Affective	Psychomotor Skill	Behavioral
Text-based resources	+++	++	+	+	
Audio or video resources	+++	++	++	+	+
Lectures	+++	+	+	+	
Testing or quizzing	+++	++			
Concept-mapping	+++	++	+		
Discussion (large or small groups)	++	+++	++		+
Problem-based learning	++	+++	+		+
Project-based learning	++	+++	+		+
Team-based learning	+++	+++	+		+
Peer teaching	+++	+++	++	+	+
Facilitating supportive learning environments	+	++	+++	+	++
Role modeling	+	+	+++	++	++
Reflection (e.g., writing, discussion)	+	++	+++	+	+
Arts and humanities–based methods		+	+++	+	+
Narrative medicine		+	+++	+	+
Exposure/immersion experiences	+	++	+++	++	++
Supervised clinical experiences	+	+++	++	+++	+++
Demonstrations	++	+	+	++	+
Role-plays[‡]	+	++	+++	+++	++
Simulated clinical scenarios with artificial models[‡]	+	++	++	+++	++
Simulated or standardized patients[‡]	+	++	++	+++	++
Extended reality (virtual or augmented reality)	+	++	++	+++	++
Audio or video review of skills[‡]			++	+++	+++
Behavioral/environmental interventions[§]			+	+	+++

Note: Blank = not recommended; + = appropriate in some cases, usually as an adjunct to other methods; ++ = good match; +++ = excellent match (consensus ratings by author and editors).

*For the purposes of this table, the methods refer to chapter text descriptions.

[†]Lower-order cognitive refers to *acquisition* of knowledge/facts; higher-order cognitive refers to *application* of knowledge/facts (e.g., in problem-solving or clinical decision-making).

[‡]Assumes feedback on performance is integrated into the method.

[§]Removal of barriers to behavior; provision of resources that promote behaviors; reinforcements that promote behaviors.

multiple educational methods can facilitate the integration of several lower-level objectives.

The Universal Design for Learning Guidelines (http://udlguidelines.cast.org/) provide a framework for making learning accessible to all individuals. The guidelines recommend offering options across cognitive, affective, and psychomotor domains with the goal of developing learners who are knowledgeable, motivated, and self-directed. Some online curricula that become disseminated broadly (e.g., self-paced modules or MOOCs) can be required by law to use methods that make content accessible to all learners, including those with visual or hearing impairments.

Choose Educational Methods That Are Feasible in Terms of Resources. Resource constraints may limit implementation of the ideal approach in this step, as well as in other steps. Curriculum developers will need to consider faculty and learner time, physical space and online resources, availability of clinical material and experiences, and costs. Faculty are often a critical resource; faculty development may be an additional consideration, especially if an innovative instructional method is chosen. Use of technology may involve initial cost but save faculty resources over time. Access to instructional design expertise can be beneficial for selecting and implementing digital educational methods. When resource limitations threaten the achievement of curricular outcomes, objectives and/or educational strategies (content and methods) will need to be further prioritized and selectively limited. The question then becomes "What is the most that can be accomplished, given resource limitations?"

When the curriculum developer selects educational methods for a curriculum, it is helpful to weigh the advantages and disadvantages of each method under consideration. Advantages and disadvantages of commonly used educational methods are summarized in Table 5.3. Specific methods are discussed below, in relation to their function.

Methods for Achieving Cognitive Objectives

Methods that are commonly used to achieve cognitive objectives include the following:

- Text-based resources (e.g., readings from journals or web pages)
- Audio or video resources
- Lectures
- Testing or quizzing
- Concept-mapping
- Discussion (large or small groups)
- Problem-based learning
- Project-based learning
- Team-based learning
- Peer teaching

For learners who may not know much about a topic or discipline, new information can be presented through text, static images, audio and/or video, and during lectures. *Text-based resources* (e.g., books, articles, reports, web pages) offer the advantage of familiarity to both learners and faculty and are easy for learners to scan, search, and re-read for the information they are seeking or want to review. Text-based resources can also apply multimedia principles when text and images are presented in complementary

Table 5.3. Summary of Advantages and Disadvantages of Different Educational Methods

Educational Method	Advantages	Disadvantages
Text-based resources	Low cost Covers fund of knowledge Can be quickly scanned or searched	Passive learning Learners must be motivated to complete Readings need updating
Audio or video resources	Low cost Can be engaging Videos can illustrate complex concepts	Passive learning Learners must be motivated to complete Need updating Can be difficult to isolate specific content
Lectures	Low cost Accommodate large numbers of learners Can be transmitted to multiple locations Can be recorded	Passive learning Teacher-centered Quality depends on speaker and media
Testing or quizzing	Low cost Can be integrated into almost any educational experience Consistently shown to enhance learning	Can cause discomfort for learners Limited application to affective objectives
Concept-mapping	Low cost Can be integrated into most educational experiences Can improve learning by putting learning in one's own terms	May be unfamiliar to learners and educators Can be difficult to standardize and assess learning experiences
Discussion, large group	Active learning Permits assessment of learner needs; can address misconceptions Allows learner to apply newly acquired knowledge Suitable for higher-order cognitive objectives Exposes learners to different perspectives Technology can support	More faculty intensive than readings or lectures Cognitive/experience base required of learners Learners need motivation to participate Group-dependent Usually facilitator-dependent Teaching space needs to facilitate with use of microphones, etc.
Discussion, small group	Active learning Reinforces other learning methods Addresses misconceptions Suitable for higher-order cognitive objectives More suitable for discussion of sensitive topics; opportunity to create a "safe environment" for students	Requires more faculty than lecture or large group discussion Faculty development in small-group teaching and in objectives often required Cognitive/experience base required of learners Learners need motivation to participate Teaching space should facilitate (e.g., room configuration)

Educational Method	Advantages	Disadvantages
Problem-based learning (PBL)	Active learning Facilitates higher-order cognitive objectives: problem-solving and clinical decision-making Can incorporate objectives that cross domains, such as ethics, humanism, cost-efficiency Case-based learning provides relevance and facilitates transfer of knowledge to clinical setting	Case development costs Requires faculty facilitators Faculty time to prepare exercises Learners need preparation in method and expectation of accountability for learning
Project-based learning	Active learning Facilitates higher-order cognitive objectives: problem-solving and clinical decision-making Can incorporate objectives that cross domains, such as ethics, humanism, cost-efficiency Can facilitate transfer to work-place settings and lead to lasting change	Project selection may require vetting to increase chances of successful completion Requires mentorship
Team-based learning (TBL)	Active learning Facilitates higher-order cognitive objectives Application exercises are relevant and facilitate transfer of problem-solving skills Collaborative Students are accountable for learning Uses less faculty than PBL and other small-group learning methods	Developmental costs (readiness assurance tests, application exercises) Learners need preparation in method and expectation of accountability for learning Learners may be uncomfortable with ambiguity of application exercises Requires orientation to the process of teamwork and peer evaluation
Peer teaching	Increases teacher-to-student ratio Safe environment for novice learners (more comfortable asking questions) Student/peer teachers are motivated to learn content and practice retrieval Student/peer teachers acquire teaching skills	Student/peer teachers' availability Student/peer teachers need additional development in teaching skills as well as orientation to the curriculum Need to ensure student/peer teachers receive feedback on teaching skills
Facilitating supportive learning environments	Likely to improve every aspect of learning Often leads to enduring memories and relationships	Requires skilled facilitators/teachers and time for a supportive learning environment to be created Some may not be comfortable with vulnerability that can occur with very open learning environments

Table 5.3.   *(continued)*

Educational Method	Advantages	Disadvantages
Role modeling	Faculty are often available Impact often seems profound Can address the hidden curriculum	Requires valid evaluation process to identify effective role models Specific interventions usually unclear Impact depends on interaction between specific faculty member and learner Outcomes multifactorial and difficult to assess
Reflection (e.g., writing, discussion)	Promotes learning from experience Promotes self-awareness/ mindfulness Can be built into discussion/group learning activities Can be done individually through assigned writings/portfolios Can be used with simulation, standardized patients, role-play, and clinical experience	Requires protected time Requires scheduling time with others when discussion is desirable Reflective discussions often facilitator-dependent Learners may need orientation and/or motivation to complete the activity
Arts and humanities–based methods	Can have profound effect in short period of time Effect can be unique for each individual Can make challenging topics more approachable	Selection of work of art may be difficult Requires skill to design and facilitate Learners and faculty may question relevance to clinical practice
Narrative medicine	Relatively easy to explain and engage in Storytelling aspect often enjoyed by all involved	Structure needed to ensure narratives align with learning objectives Time required for developing narratives, review, and reflection
Exposure/immersion	Can have profound effect in short period of time Can motivate learning effort	May not affect all the same way May be difficult to secure immersion experiences
Supervised clinical experiences	Relevant to learner Learners may draw on previous experiences Promotes learner motivation and responsibility Promotes higher-level cognitive, affective, psychomotor, and behavioral learning	May require coordination to arrange opportunities with patients, community, etc. May require clinical material when learner is ready Clinical experiences require faculty supervision and feedback Learner needs basic knowledge or skill Clinical experience needs to be monitored for case-mix, appropriateness Requires reflection, follow-up

Educational Method	Advantages	Disadvantages
Demonstration	Efficient method for detailing steps in skills or a procedure Effective in combination with experience-based learning (e.g., before practicing skill in simulated or real environment)	Passive learning Teacher-oriented Quality depends on teacher or audiovisual material
Role-play	Suitable for objectives that cross domains of knowledge, attitudes, and skill Efficient Low cost Can be structured to be learner-centered Can be done "on the fly"	Requires trained faculty facilitators Learners need some basic knowledge or skills Can be resource-intensive if there are large numbers of learners Artificiality, learner discomfort
Simulated clinical scenarios with artificial models	Excellent environment to demonstrate and practice skills Can approximate clinical situations and facilitate transfer of learning Learners can use at own pace Facilitates deliberate practice Facilitates mastery learning approach Can be used for team skills and team communications	Requires dedicated space and models/simulators, which can be expensive; may not be available Faculty facilitators need training in teaching with simulation Multiple sessions often required to reach all learners
Simulated or standardized patients	Ensures appropriate clinical material Approximates "real life" more closely than role-play and facilitates transfer of learning Safe environment for practice of sensitive, difficult situations with patients, families, etc. Can incorporate deliberate practice Can reuse for ongoing curricula	Cost of patients, trainers, and in some cases, dedicated space Requires an infrastructure to find and train standardized patients and coordinate them with curriculum Faculty facilitators often required to debrief
Extended reality	Can allow skills practice with less equipment than traditional simulations Can make it easier for students to practice independently Permits flexibility in scenario design	May be difficult to access required equipment Technology still evolving Technology may cause discomfort for some (e.g., dizziness, nausea)
Audio or video review of skills	Provides opportunity for self-observation Can be reviewed multiple times by multiple individuals Can be used with simulation, standardized patients, role-play, and clinical experience	Requires reflection, follow-up Requires trained faculty facilitators Requires patients' permission to record, when recording interactions with real patients
Behavioral/environmental interventions*	Influences performance Often simple to implement	Assumes competence has been achieved Requires control over learners' real-life environment

*Removal of barriers to behavior; provision of resources that promote behaviors; reinforcements that promote behaviors.

ways. Audio and video recordings are typically more difficult to scan quickly for information but can be perceived as more engaging. *Audio recordings* (e.g., podcasts) offer the advantage of being listened to during leisure activities. *Video resources* can effectively apply multimedia principles, and video animations can illustrate complex concepts or dynamic systems that are commonly part of medical education. Text-based, audio, and video resources can function as *reusable learning objects* (RLOs). RLOs are digital curricular units that can be accessed and used by individuals across contexts.[45] RLOs can be reviewed before, during, or after a curriculum session. If learners are expected to review text-based, audio, or video resources, however, the time this will take learners and their motivation for doing it must be considered. Such resources should be carefully assessed to ensure that they target a curriculum's objectives before they are assigned, and learners should be made aware of how resources align with objectives so they can use them most efficiently.

> **EXAMPLE:** *Podcasts as RLOs.* Two emergency medicine residency programs in the United States began replacing scheduled teaching sessions with required podcasts that covered the same topics as the scheduled sessions. This allowed residents to learn when it was convenient for them, reduced time in scheduled educational conferences, and allowed conference time to include more discussion.[46]

Perhaps the most universally applied method for addressing cognitive objectives is the *lecture*, which has the advantages of (1) providing many learners, all at once, with access to experts and thoughtfully curated information; (2) ease of delivery in-person and during remote synchronous sessions; and (3) the enduring value lectures can have when they are recorded. In traditional lectures, lecturers provide prepared presentations to an audience without much interaction until the presentation has ended. This manner of lecturing may still be expected or required, especially when audiences are large. Aspects of traditional lectures that are thought to make them more effective include communicating the importance of the topic, clearly stating goals, presenting in a clear and organized manner, using audiovisual aids, monitoring an audience's understanding, and providing a summary or conclusion.[47] However, any lecturer should seek opportunities to engage learners in active learning processes that help them to recognize what they may not know and apply new knowledge as it is learned. One way to accomplish this is to present information to the full group, divide the full group into smaller groups where they can interact, then return to large group instruction.[48,49]

> **EXAMPLE:** *Think-Pair-Share.* During a plenary presentation, the presenter poses a question to the audience. Audience members are asked to think about their own answer, then pair with someone nearby to share answers. The speaker then requests volunteers to share their answers with the rest of the audience to stimulate discussion. The presenter proceeds with more information before pausing again periodically to repeat the think-pair-share process.

Active learning in lectures can also make use of the *testing effect*,[50] which has been shown to enhance learning even before new information is introduced. Lectures can apply the testing effect by polling students using audience response systems or online software. Polling allows faculty to pose questions and solicit answers from learners. Technology employed in *classroom communication systems* has helped to engage individual learners attending large, lecture-based classes in higher education. Faculty using these systems can send tasks or problems to individuals or groups of students, who respond via mobile devices; the faculty can display results in real time and address learning needs immediately.

EXAMPLE: *Online Polling in a Lecture.* Lecturers in an anatomy class for dental students began using an online polling software. After the lecturer presented some information, students received and responded to questions on their mobile devices. The class's answers were displayed and influenced how the rest of the lecture was conducted. At the end of the lecture, polls were done again and lecturers addressed misconceptions. Students reported that polling increased their focus and motivation to learn.[51]

In addition to polling software that permits testing to take place during synchronous sessions, online quizzing software and *question banks* are used by nearly every medical learner. Such assessment items can be effective when integrated in formal curricula synchronously or asynchronously. Retention is enhanced when learners are required to repeatedly retrieve information from memory and further enhanced when that retrieval is spaced over time.[52] There is active research on the optimal timing of that spacing and some digital applications purport to be adaptive, adjusting the timing and type of content that is presented based on an individual's previous use.

EXAMPLE: *Online Spaced Education.* Participants attending a face-to-face continuing medical education course were randomized to receive a spaced education (SE) intervention of 40 questions and explanations covering four clinical topics after the course. Repetition intervals (8-day and 16-day) were adapted to the participants based on performance; questions were retired after being correctly answered twice in a row. Most completed the SE intervention, and at week 18, a survey indicated that participants who completed the SE intervention reported significantly greater change in their clinical behaviors than the controls.[53]

MOOCs and self-paced modules are useful curricular formats for knowledge acquisition and often include text-based, audio, and video resources along with formative assessments. They are best suited for learners with strong motivation and self-regulated learning strategies.[54] They can reach a wide variety of learners and permit learners to proceed at their own pace, identify their own knowledge deficiencies, and receive immediate feedback.

EXAMPLE: *Self-Paced Modular Curriculum.* An ambulatory curriculum for internal medicine residents was developed and delivered online. Each module covered one topic and had a pretest-didactics-posttest format. The didactics included immediate feedback to answers and links to abstracts or full-text articles. The curriculum expanded over time to cover over 50 topics and be used by over 200 residency programs. Comparisons of pre- and posttests of knowledge showed improved knowledge of curricular content[55] and posttest scores correlated with residents' scores on their board exams.[56]

EXAMPLE: *Drug Development MOOC.* A college of pharmacy developed an eight-week MOOC to describe the drug development process, which included content contributed by 29 speakers. The MOOC incorporated elements that allowed participants to make choices about new drugs and receive feedback on their choices. Participants ranged from health professionals to high school students. Reviews of the course were positive, and one participant, who was a journalist, described his own experience in a local newspaper.[57]

Concept-mapping is a method where learners, individually or in groups, visually depict how concepts relate to one another. Authors have proposed that these could be especially useful for integrating concepts from basic and clinical sciences and developing clinical reasoning.[58]

EXAMPLE: *Concept-Mapping to Link Basic and Clinical Science Concepts.* Medical and dental students in a first-year physiology course were randomized to apply concept-mapping to illustrate physiologic mechanisms that explained clinical findings in problem-based learning small-group tutorials. Students in concept-mapping groups reported that concept-mapping helped them think critically about the case and identify areas that they did not fully understand, and they had higher scores on the final course assessment.[59]

Discussion moves the learner further from a passive to an active role, facilitates retrieval of previously learned information, and provides opportunities to add meaning to new information. Much of the learning that occurs in a discussion format depends on the skills of the instructor to create a supportive learning climate, to assess learners' needs, and to effectively use a variety of interventions, such as maintaining focus, questioning, generalizing, and summarizing for the learner. Group discussions are most successful when facilitated by teachers trained in the techniques of small-group teaching[60] and when participants have some background knowledge or experience in discussion facilitation methods. Case-based discussions, as in attending rounds or morning report, is a popular method that allows clinical learners to process new knowledge with faculty and peers, identify specific knowledge deficiencies, and develop clinical reasoning abilities.[61] *Virtual patients* have been defined as "interactive computer simulations of real-life clinical scenarios for the purpose of health professions training, education or assessment"[62] and are frequently used to develop learners' clinical reasoning abilities.[63] While virtual patient cases are typically accessed asynchronously, learning can be enhanced with facilitated discussion that connects the virtual patient scenario to real practice.

> **EXAMPLE:** *Virtual Patient and Discussion.* Faculty developed virtual patient cases to teach medical students about diagnostic error. Case scenarios included multiple-choice and short-answer questions where students responded and received immediate feedback. Faculty met with students afterward to discuss diagnostic errors. All students improved knowledge about diagnostic reasoning and error, and most identified changes they would make in their future diagnostic approaches.[64]

While discussions are usually thought of as being synchronous activities, they can also occur asynchronously through multiple digital media, such as email, discussion boards, or social media. *Social media* consists of technology-mediated platforms that allow individual users to create and distribute content to virtual communities and can range from collaborative authorship platforms such as wikis (e.g., Wikipedia) to single-author dialogue platforms such as microblogging (e.g., Twitter).[65] Many learning management systems have a social media function, but other apps are widely used and available. In health professions education, the use of online discussions has facilitated the interaction of learners across disciplines and geographic boundaries.

> **EXAMPLE:** *Asynchronous Case-Based Discussions.* Faculty created cases that described educational dilemmas and listed them on a website. During the following week, an asynchronous discussion was facilitated on the website and on Twitter. At the end of the week, the crowdsourced responses and editor opinions were listed on the website for download. Individuals from a variety of settings were able to share in the discussion, and downloadable materials could be used for local faculty development.[66]

> **EXAMPLE:** *Virtual Community of Practice.* A geographically distributed cohort of faculty created a virtual community of practice during a 12-month curriculum intended to facilitate their scholarly development. During the curriculum, participants were highly engaged on the social media platform, which was used for file-sharing and messaging. A number of peer-reviewed articles and a book resulted from participation in the curriculum.[67]

The *combination of didactic resources and small-group discussion* can be especially effective in helping learners develop a knowledge foundation and practice the higher-order cognitive skills of understanding complex physiologic and pathophysiologic processes. The use of the *flipped classroom* is one example of this model that has become popular in health professions education. It can take a variety of forms[68] and is frequently used in blended learning. In this model, learners are assigned the task of mastering factual content before participating in formal curricular events, which are designed as active "application exercises," such as problem-solving or discussion activities. In this method, a faculty facilitator monitors and models critical thinking skills rather than serving as an information resource. This method is thought to improve learners' sense of competence, relatedness, and autonomy, and help them better manage cognitive load.[69]

> **EXAMPLE:** *Shared Flipped Classroom Modules.* Faculty teams from four medical schools collectively created 34 modules on microbiology and immunology topics. Each module included videos to be watched before class, facilitator guides for in-class interactive activities, and assessment and evaluation instruments. The modules were incorporated into each school's unique curriculum.[70]

> **EXAMPLE:** *Content for Flipped Classroom and MOOC.* An interprofessional collaboration curriculum was converted to a flipped classroom by a workgroup of faculty and students from schools of dentistry, medicine, nursing, pharmacy, and physical therapy. Students in the course completed online content before quarterly face-to-face skills sessions. The online content was also used to create a six-week MOOC that was accessed by thousands of learners from over 100 countries. Learners who took part in the flipped classroom and those who accessed the MOOC rated their experiences favorably.[57]

Problem-based learning (PBL) is a particular use of small groups that originated in undergraduate medical education[71,72] to help learners become self-directed in their preparation for solving problems in clinical environments.[73] In PBL, learner groups are presented with a case and set their own learning objectives, often dividing the work and teaching each other, guided by a tutor-facilitator. In a case of renal failure in a child, for instance, the learning objectives may include genitourinary anatomy, renal physiology, calcium metabolism in renal failure, and genetic disorders of renal function. Students bring new knowledge back to the PBL group, and the group problem-solves the case together. PBL is highly dependent on the tutor-facilitators and requires intensive faculty and case development. After decades of use in medical education, the efficacy of PBL compared with conventional approaches in achieving cognitive objectives is still debated, although it is generally understood that successful PBL depends on a mix of learner, faculty, and contextual factors.[74]

PBL typically focuses on patient cases, although its principles can be applied to projects.[75] *Project-based learning*, where individuals or groups of learners work collaboratively on a project (defined as extensive activities with clear outcomes[76]), can facilitate learning, especially when accompanied by mentorship. Basing learning on projects can facilitate transfer of learning into workplace activities.[77] Aligning learning with projects that are required or that are consistent with institutional priorities may enhance the feasibility of both the project and its related curriculum. Project-based learning is commonly used to help students develop cognitive skills related to research and evidence-based medicine[78] and for faculty development in a range of settings.[79,80]

> **EXAMPLE**: *Project-Based Faculty Development for Capacity-Building.* To build individual and institutional capacity for health professions education in resource-limited settings, a two-year fellowship for faculty was created. The fellowship required applicants to submit an education innovation project, which would be the basis of their learning. Faculty fellows convened for a one-to-two-week residential session, which included sessions to develop foundational knowledge and skills in education, leadership, and management. They returned to their local institutions and were mentored remotely for the next

11 months. They convened for a second one-to-two-week residential session to share progress with one another and generate ideas for improvement, followed by another 11 months of remote mentorship. Most projects were successfully implemented at fellows' local institutions, leading to improvement in educational quality.[76] This model was replicated from a single institute to include 11 additional institutes and development of an extensive international network of fellow alumni.

Team-based learning (TBL) is another application of small groups but requires fewer faculty than PBL.[81,82] It combines reading, testing, discussion, and collaboration to achieve both lower- and higher-order cognitive learning objectives. The process of TBL is as follows:

Phase I
1.   Students are assigned readings or self-directed learning before class.

Phase II
2.   On arrival to class, students take a brief knowledge test, the *Readiness Assurance Test* (RAT), and are individually scored (IRAT).
3.   Students work in teams of six to seven to retake the RAT and turn in consensus answers for immediate scoring and feedback (Group, or GRAT).

Phase III (may last several class periods)
4.   Groups work on problem-solving or application exercises.
5.   Groups eventually share responses to the exercise with the entire class, and discussion is facilitated by the instructor.

Peer teaching, or near-peer (one or two levels above the learner) teaching, is frequently used in medical education and can have a variety of benefits.[83] Although often initiated to relieve teaching pressures for faculty, there may be significant learning benefits for a peer teaching approach. For learners, peer facilitators may be more effective because they are closer to the learners' fund of knowledge and better able to understand the conceptual challenges that the learners are facing. Learners often find the learning environment to be more comfortable with peers and are more likely to seek clarification with peers than with faculty. For the peer teachers, there is additional effort to learn the material during preparation for teaching, as well as practice with retrieval, which should reinforce retention.

Peer teaching is usually thought of as occurring in formal educational programs, but it can also be thought of as occurring between practicing clinicians. *Project ECHO* (Extension for Community Healthcare Outcomes, https://echo.unm.edu/about-echo /model), for example, has created an educational model that employs peer-mentorship and PBL principles. Specialist physicians educate generalists remotely on specific topics to build generalist knowledge and independence in care of patients with conditions typically managed by specialists. ECHO curricula have been demonstrated to improve patient outcomes.[84] Online curricula that are at the confluence of education and patient care can be considered telehealth.[85]

EXAMPLE: *ECHO for Community and Prison Providers.* Specialists at an urban clinic for hepatitis C virus treatment had weekly video conferences with primary care providers (PCPs) who worked remotely in rural communities and prisons. During their meetings, PCPs presented cases for discussion, which were supplemented by didactics from the specialists. Specialists were also available for ongoing mentorship and support. After PCPs participated in the ECHO curriculum, patient treatment by PCPs was as effective as that at the urban specialist clinic.[86]

Methods for Achieving Affective Objectives

Methods that are commonly used to achieve affective objectives include the following:

- Facilitating supportive learning environments
- Role modeling
- Reflection (e.g., writing, discussion)
- Arts- and humanities-based methods
- Narrative medicine
- Exposure/immersion (e.g., readings, videos, discussions, real or virtual experiences)

Learners' values, beliefs, preferences, moods, and emotions can have profound influence over what they learn and how they perceive an educational experience. Learner motivation to acquire knowledge and skills, retain them, and apply them to their everyday practice is also critical to consider when seeking to improve behaviors that impact patient care. Curricula may need to raise awareness about unconscious affective attributes, such as implicit biases, which can be uncomfortable for learners and educators alike. Failure to consider what learners' affective states may be when a learning experience begins, how these states may evolve throughout the experience, and what they may be at the end of the experience could limit the impact the curriculum will have on learners, their behaviors, and patient care.

Affective change can occur by addressing cognitive objectives (e.g., teaching about growth mindset can improve motivation) and psychomotor objectives (e.g., obtaining a skill can improve self-efficacy beliefs). Addressing long-held or unconscious beliefs can be particularly challenging and require longitudinal efforts, often including consideration of factors in the hidden curriculum. Specifically addressing affective objectives typically requires creating a safe learning environment; exposure to ideas, individuals, environments, or experiences that evoke changes in learners' affective states (e.g., trigger new emotions); and opportunities for reflection.

> **EXAMPLE:** *Implicit Association Test (IAT) to Reveal Implicit Bias.* Social work students were given a presentation on the theoretical underpinnings of stereotypes and were then asked to take the IAT,[87] which detects links between stereotypes and unconscious feelings. They wrote a reflective essay that faculty analyzed, indicating that taking the test took them out of their emotional comfort zones and provided insight into the nature of bias and stereotypes and people's abilities to change them.[88]

Learning environments that optimize psychological safety have been described as those where learners can achieve a state of "flow,"[89,90] which refers to when individuals become immersed in the present with full concentration and without a sense of risk or concern about their personal images.[91] Creating opportunities for learners and educators to engage in appreciative inquiry,[92] where they consider strengths and imagine potential, may develop trusting relationships that foster safe and supportive learning environments and promote learner flourishing.[93] Learning environments that include learners as legitimate participants in a community of practice may further enhance their experiences and professional development (see below on Professional Identity Formation). Orienting educational experiences to emphasize the positive aspects of individual characteristics and experiences may improve their attitudes and well-being.

> **EXAMPLE:** *Coaching for PCPs.* PCPs were assigned to six sessions with individual coaches who solicited the PCPs' goals at each session, had them engage in appreciative activities (such as reflecting on

positive experiences and writing gratitude letters), and helped them create action plans. After the coaching sessions, PCPs had sustained improvements in positive outlook and had reduced burnout.[94]

Selecting educators who are respected and knowledgeable and who can facilitate openness and inclusivity can also help learners feel welcome and motivated.[91,95] Individuals who are perceived to have integrity, a commitment to excellence, a positive outlook, and strong interpersonal skills, and who show interest in learner growth, may become positive role models for learners.[96] *Role models* can have a powerful influence over learner attitudes,[97,98] so increasing exposure to positive role models may benefit learners. Faculty can also be taught to become better role models, which typically requires reflecting on their roles and what they model during longitudinal reflective sessions with a consistent group.[99]

> **EXAMPLE:** *Developing Humanistic Faculty Role Models.* Faculty from five medical schools participated in an 18-month curriculum that included monthly meetings with the same group of faculty clinical teachers. At these meetings, they developed specific skills and reflected on experiences. After completing the curriculum, those who had participated in the program had higher ratings by learners for role modeling humanistic behaviors during their teaching.[100]

Reflection is a complex process, yet is vital for personal and professional growth.[101,102] Reflection has been defined as "the process of engaging the self in attentive, critical, exploratory and iterative interactions with one's thoughts and actions, and their underlying conceptual frame, with a view to changing them and with a view on the change itself."[103] Reflection can occur after an experience (reflection-on-action) or during an experience (reflection-in-action). Individuals can be encouraged to engage in reflection independently or in groups. Reflection is commonly facilitated through discussion about experience and reflective writing. Exposure to challenging or uncomfortable circumstances followed by reflection can evoke powerful emotions and potentially lead to lasting changes in attitudes.

> **EXAMPLE:** *Video Trigger and Reflection.* In a 90-minute faculty development workshop, participants viewed a three-minute video showing a supervising physician making disparaging comments about a patient and resident who were of minority race. Participants discussed their feelings about the video in small groups, then again in the large group, revealing emotions of anger, fear, and shame. In pre-post measures, participants expressed an increased desire to make personal changes to deal with racism in patient care and more confidence to make those changes at their institution and in their teaching.[104]

Integrating *arts and humanities* (A&H) within health professions education is being recommended due to a variety of potential benefits.[105–107] A&H-based educational methods can be effective at facilitating cognitive and psychomotor learning. For example, engaging with historical documents may provide knowledge about the social determinants of health. Visual arts can be effective in improving observation and other clinical skills.[108] A&H-based methods are believed to be especially well suited for affective objectives. They can facilitate perspective-taking (i.e., understanding the perspectives of others), development of personal self-awareness, and critical discussions on social inequities.[109,110] A&H-based methods to facilitate affective change typically involve an experience with literature, visual arts, music, and/or performance arts followed by a reflective exercise (e.g., discussion, writing). A&H-based methods can make difficult subjects approachable for a heterogeneous group of learners.[111]

> **EXAMPLE:** *Visual Arts Reflective Experience.* Patients, clinicians, and policy experts who were gathered to develop a patient safety research agenda began the conference with a visual arts-based reflec-

tive experience. Participants selected a visual image that triggered thoughts related to patient harm, then discussed images with each other. The dialogue unearthed feelings of turmoil and fear and reflections on the healing effects of being heard and the power of human connection. Authors reported that the experience helped create a safe space for further dialogue about emotionally difficult topics as they worked together during the conference.[111]

EXAMPLE: *Theatre of the Oppressed Workshop.* Medical students and providers were invited to participate in a three-day Theatre of the Oppressed workshop. Participants reflected on their own experiences with oppression and, during a live performance, practiced identifying and responding to oppressive acts. Participants described the experience as evoking strong emotions, creating trust and community, and improving their empathy.[112]

Narrative medicine is an A&H-based method that is defined as the competence to recognize, interpret, and be moved by stories of illness. Narrative approaches can take place in discussion and writing, and there is evidence that applying narrative medicine in educational settings can change learner attitudes.[113]

EXAMPLE: *Narrative Medicine and Reflection.* Students on an internal medicine clerkship were introduced to narrative medicine concepts and practiced storytelling. Students then interviewed a patient to elicit their narrative, wrote the narrative, and read the story back to the patient. They reflected on their experience with the patient by writing an essay and sharing their thoughts during a facilitated discussion. Students described feeling a deeper appreciation of the human side of medicine and closer connections to their patients. Patients who were interviewed by students also felt attended to and heard.[114]

Finally, *immersive experiences* where learners are placed into authentic practice environments or completely new environments or roles can affect attitudes.

EXAMPLE: *Four-Year Continuity Experience for Medical Students.* In a curriculum intended to have students feel like participants in patient continuity experiences in ambulatory primary care, students joined an ambulatory clinic for a half day every other week starting in their first year of medical school. First- and second-year students saw patients with third- and fourth-year students under the supervision of an ambulatory attending, participated in panel management, and educated one another.[115] Students described a sense of belonging in the clinic[116] and provided higher ratings of their learning environments and team-centered attitudes.[117]

EXAMPLE: *Attitude toward Socioeconomic Class, Experience Combined with Reflection and Discussion.* Senior nursing students participated in a one-day poverty simulation. In this simulation, participants assumed the roles of different families living in poverty. The families were tasked to provide for basic necessities of food and shelter for one month, consisting of four 15-minute weeks. Exercises included applying for a job, negotiating a delayed utility bill, and applying for welfare assistance. The simulation concluded with facilitated reflection and discussion. Following the simulation, scores on a validated Attitudes about Poverty and Poor Populations Scale showed significant improvement on the factor of stigma of poverty.[118]

Methods for Achieving Psychomotor Objectives

Skill Objectives

Methods commonly used to achieve skill objectives (the ability to perform) include the following:

- Demonstration
- Supervised clinical experience
- Role-plays

- Simulated clinical scenarios with artificial models
- Simulated or standardized patients
- Extended reality (i.e., virtual and augmented reality)
- Audio or video review of skills

Health professional learners need to develop a variety of clinical skills, such as conducting physical examination maneuvers, performing procedures, and communicating with patients and team members. The learning of skills can be facilitated when learners (1) are *introduced* to the knowledge required for the skills by appropriate methods (e.g., didactic presentations, demonstration, and/or discussion); (2) are given the opportunity to *practice* the skill; (3) are given the opportunity to *reflect* on their performance; (4) receive *feedback* on their performance that helps them make adjustments to their practice; and then (5) *repeat the cycle* of practice, reflection, and feedback until mastery is achieved. These cycles can occur during focused deliberate practice, as described above, or experiential learning,[119] which involves having a concrete experience, reflecting on the experience to identify general principles, and adjusting based on those principles in future experiences.

These cycles of learning can occur in *clinical settings when appropriate supervision is available*. Learners can practice clinical skills under observation and have time for reflection, and experts can facilitate feedback.[120–122] Effective clinical teachers can facilitate deliberate practice and experiential learning processes (see General References).

Supervised clinical learning experiences may not always be possible. Increased administrative burdens and work hour limits in high-resource settings can decrease the amount of time learners have to spend with patients and the opportunities that faculty have to observe and share feedback. In lower-resource settings, clinicians may need to limit educational time in order to meet patient care demands. When expert clinicians are not readily available for *demonstration,* or the appropriate clinical situations are not available for skills practice, supplementary methods should be considered. Videos can be used to demonstrate skills before learners practice. They are especially effective when they break down a skill into steps and are relatively short in duration (e.g., less than 10 minutes).[123] *Simulation* in health care has been defined as "a technique that creates a situation or environment to allow persons to experience a representation of a real event for the purpose of practice, learning, evaluation, testing, or to gain understanding of systems or human actions."[124] The use of simulation to train professionals and health care teams has shown dramatically improved outcomes in performance and patient safety indicators, especially when implemented according to mastery learning principles.[13] In simulated clinical scenarios, learners can practice skills and take risks without harming patients. They can also have greater exposure to important scenarios that may not occur frequently (e.g., cardiopulmonary resuscitation). Feedback and debriefing after a simulation augment learning among individuals and teams.[125]

Simulation-based medical education is rapidly becoming more widespread and sophisticated. It is now arguably its own subspecialty within medical education as the Society for Simulation in Healthcare has standards for accreditation and professional certification and has published a dictionary of terms.[124] Guides have been published for integration of simulation-based health care education into curricula[126] and for developing simulation-based[127] and mastery learning curricula[128] according to the six-step approach.

Simulations can take place off site (e.g., in a simulation center) or "in situ," at an actual clinical site (e.g., a team rehearsing before a complicated procedure). In situ simulations may also be announced or unannounced (e.g., a drill).[129]

EXAMPLE: *Unannounced In Situ Simulation: Mock Codes.* To improve the performance of pediatric cardiopulmonary resuscitation interprofessional teams, monthly "mock" cardiac arrests were staged with a human simulator on hospital floor units, without prior notice to the teams. Video recordings of the mock codes were debriefed with a trained facilitator. After 48 months of random mock codes, resuscitation survival increased from 30% to 50% and remained stable for three years of follow-up.[130]

Simulation *fidelity* can vary. Fidelity describes how closely learner experiences during a simulation resemble reality. Fidelity has physical aspects (e.g., equipment, environment), individual learner psychological aspects (e.g., emotions, cognitive processes), and social aspects (e.g., trust, culture).[124] Generally, higher fidelity is believed to enhance learning more than lower fidelity as long as the aspects of fidelity being considered relate to the learning objectives. For example, expensive equipment may not be required when cognitive processes, such as decision-making, are of interest. Simply using simulation technologies that offer greater physical fidelity is unlikely to improve cognitive or psychomotor learning.[131]

Role-playing, during which a learner plays one role (e.g., clinician) and another learner or faculty member plays another role (e.g., patient), is a common and low cost way to provide simulated practice for learners,[132] and it may be as effective as the use of simulated patients.[133] It is efficient, inexpensive, and portable and can be used spontaneously in any setting. Role-play is often useful for teaching physical examination techniques, the recognition of normal physical examination findings, and communication skills.

Limitations to using role-play include variable degrees of artificiality and learner and faculty discomfort with the technique. Facilitators can alleviate students' initial discomfort by discussing it at the outset, fostering a supportive learning environment, and establishing *ground rules for role-play* to prepare learners and structure the activity. These are:

Phase of Role-Play	Facilitator Task
Preparation	Choose a situation that is relevant and readily conceptualized by the learners. Describe the situation and critical issues for each role-player. Choose/assign roles and give learners time to assimilate and add details. Identify observers and clarify their functions. Establish expectations for time-outs by the learner and interruptions by others (e.g., time limits).
Execution	Ensure compliance with agreed-upon ground rules. Ensure that learners emerge comfortably from their roles.
Debriefing	First give the principal learners the opportunity to self-assess what they did well, what they would want to do differently, and what they would like help with. Assess the feelings and experiences of other participants in the role-play. Elicit feedback from all observers on what seemed to go well. Elicit suggestions regarding alternative approaches that might have been more effective.
Replay	Give the principal learners the opportunity to repeat the role-play using alternative approaches.

Simulated or standardized patients (SPs) are actors or real patients trained to play a clearly defined patient role in high-fidelity simulation experiences.[134] As with role-play, the use of SPs ensures that important content areas will be covered and allows learners to try new techniques, make mistakes, and repeat their performance until a skill is achieved. SPs may also provide feedback and be used to assess learners. SPs have become widely incorporated into undergraduate health professions education and can have application for practicing providers.[135] The major limitation is the need to recruit, train, schedule, and pay SPs.

> **EXAMPLE:** *Standardized Patients and Breaking Bad News.* During a four-day residential workshop, oncology fellows practiced relationship building, sharing bad news, and discussing goals of care with standardized patients who progressed from diagnosis of progressive cancer, treatment failure, and transition to hospice care. Evaluation of audio recordings of encounters with standardized patients demonstrated that fellows improved their skills substantially.[136]

Artificial models, such as partial task trainers (e.g., pelvic models, airway management heads) and manikins, can afford high physical fidelity and are commonly used in clinical simulations.

> **EXAMPLE:** *Simulation-Based Mastery Learning for Central Venous Catheter Insertion.* In a fully simulated clinical environment, internal medicine residents attempted central-line insertion into a manikin under ultrasound guidance. None of the residents achieved the mastery standard (defined by a 27-item skills checklist) on their pretest. Residents then had didactic sessions and received specific feedback on their performance as they practiced with the manikin toward the mastery standard. All residents achieved the standard, and subsequent evaluations demonstrated high levels of skill retention and improvement in patient care outcomes related to central-line insertion.[137]

Extended reality refers to any computer-generated reality and includes virtual reality (VR) (completely simulated environment) and augmented reality (AR) (virtual features are superimposed on the real world so both are experienced).[138] VR can be experienced by using a headset and handheld devices that permit practice similar to fully simulated clinical scenarios. Use of virtual cadavers to learn anatomy is the most commonly employed method of AR and can allow for both psychomotor skill development and achievement of cognitive objectives. Extended reality is also becoming more common to allow safe practice of complex clinical procedures and afford practice opportunities that can fit into a busy clinician's schedule.

> **EXAMPLE:** *VR to Practice Surgical Skills.* Surgical residents were video-recorded performing a laparoscopic cholecystectomy to establish their baseline skill level and individualize their learning plans. Residents who performed elements of the surgery below a predetermined level of performance were required to complete practice on a VR simulator for each task performed below a predetermined cutoff level. The VR simulator automatically assessed and provided feedback on performance. The VR group performed better than the control group on a subsequent video-recorded laparoscopic cholecystectomy.[139]

Reviews of recorded (audio or video) performances of role-play or simulated or real clinical encounters can provide opportunities for direct observation from faculty that overcome time and location constraints and provide greater opportunity for reflection. Learners may also observe their own performance and notice aspects of patient behaviors or the environment that escaped them in the moment. Studies suggest that the learning value from video review comes primarily from expert feedback and debriefing on performance, rather than learner self-assessment.[140–142]

> **EXAMPLE:** *Video Recordings and Feedback.* Students participating in a formative objective structured clinical examination (OSCE) with a simulated patient received feedback by a supervisor who directly observed them or who viewed a video recording. Analysis of audio-recorded feedback from supervisors

indicated that video-based feedback covered more topics overall with greater discussion of communication skills, clinical reasoning, and professionalism. Students rated video-based feedback more positively than feedback based on direct observation.[143]

Behavioral Objectives

Methods commonly used to achieve behavioral objectives (performance in practice) include the following:

- Removal of barriers to the behavior
- Provision of resources that facilitate the behavior
- Provision of reinforcements for the behavior

Changing learners' behaviors can be one of the more challenging aspects of a curriculum. There is no guarantee that helping learners develop new skills and/or improved attitudes will result in the desired behaviors when learners are in actual clinical situations. *Behaviorism* (see Table 5.1) is an orientation to learning that has been influential in instructional design[144] and focuses on the observable actions of individuals and how behaviors change in relationship to stimuli and reinforcements in the external environment. The original formulations of behaviorism are similar to the concepts of *habits*, which are routines that are triggered by an environmental cue. Changing behaviors may involve breaking old habits and/or seeking cues that trigger new habits.[145] Curriculum developers may need to address *barriers to behaviors* in the learners' physical environments, provide material *resources that promote behaviors*, and design *reinforcements* that will encourage the continued use of newly acquired skills. Attention to the learners' subsequent environments can reduce or eliminate the decay of performance that often occurs after an educational intervention.

Theories of behavior change have become increasingly sophisticated over time. Models of behavior change now place greater emphasis on addressing the affective domain of learning to foster learners' motivation and intention to apply their knowledge and skills in a given situation. These include learners' self-efficacy and perceived control, how the behavior relates to the norms of their peers and the culture (e.g., hidden curriculum), and the salience of the behavior in a specific context.[146]

Ultimately, behavior change requires learners to have the knowledge and skills required to be able to perform the behavior, believe that the behavior is important enough to initiate and to overcome potential obstacles to performing it, and have the necessary materials in the physical environment to make the behavior possible.

EXAMPLE: *Systems Improvements and Feedback.* Pediatric residents were expected to use a standardized template to facilitate safe transfer of patient care. In one program, trainees were introduced to a template with an interactive workshop that included presentation of relevant communication theory, case-based examples emphasizing the importance of handoffs, and video demonstration of appropriate handoffs. A pocket card reminder of the standardized template was provided. Trainees were evaluated by residents also trained to use the template with a Handoff CEX (clinical evaluation exercise), based on the Mini-CEX. Finally, trainees received feedback in the workplace on the efficacy of observed written and verbal handoffs.[147]

EXAMPLE: *Reminders and Simulation Integrated into Practice to Reduce Neonatal Mortality.* In an effort to reduce preventable neonatal mortality in low-resource settings, a simulation-based curriculum was developed.[148] Educators created a small package that could be shipped to remote locations and that contained all elements needed for simulated practice (including a manikin that could be filled with water before use). In one instance, midwives, nurse students, operating nurses, and physicians in a labor ward in Tanzania received one-day training with the manikin and were required to practice with the manikin daily. Manikins were placed in the labor ward. Posters with resuscitation actions were placed in labor rooms and in practice settings. Follow-up training sessions were conducted periodically and facilitators provided feedback to correct skills. Recommended resuscitative behavior improved, and neonatal mortality decreased during the intervention period.[149]

Remediation

Ideally, when a curriculum is well designed and implemented, all learners would be able to achieve its objectives during the planned period of time, and remediation would not be necessary. Even in well-designed curricula, however, some learners may not meet educational objectives. In health professions education, achieving objectives often has important consequences for patients, so it becomes imperative that all objectives are met before advancement. The reasons that learners may not achieve objectives are often complex.[150,151] Attention to some curricular structures and processes may help avoid the need for remediation, such as admission and selection processes and the early identification of and provision of additional support for struggling learners.

Factors within a curriculum that may lead to learner remediation include challenges that are specific to the curriculum's educational content and methods, faculty, and learning environment.[152,153] Events or situations in learners' personal lives, such as those affecting their own health or their loved ones, can also influence their performance in a curriculum. For individuals who require remediation, diagnosing the reason(s) a learner did not achieve objectives is the place to begin, because there is a growing evidence base that can guide remediation strategies based on the underlying cause.[153] However, some competency domains, such as professionalism, lack evidence-based remediation strategies.[154] One can generally expect that remediation will require additional time and resources to support learning.[152] Ultimately, some learners may not be able to achieve the expected objectives despite remediation efforts. If failure to meet expectations has significant consequences, such as inability to remain in an educational program, it is important to counsel the learner regarding alternative career paths and to provide credit for their accomplishments (e.g., a master's degree for those who cannot complete a doctorate program).[155]

Methods for Promoting Achievement of Selected Curricular Goals

As health system and patient needs continue to evolve, health professions education must also evolve to anticipate and meet those needs. Here we emphasize educational methods related to newer concepts in health profession education: adaptive expertise, professional identity formation, and interprofessionalism and teamwork.

Adaptive Expertise

Methods for promoting adaptive expertise include the following:

- Problem-based and case-based learning
- Simulated clinical scenarios
- Personal learning portfolios
- Reflection
- Coaching and formative feedback on performance

As learners develop knowledge and skills that are increasingly complex (often through cycles of deliberate practice), they develop *expertise*.[156] Performing complex tasks may be difficult or impossible for novice learners when they are not given strict rules to follow. However, over time they can develop more complex mental models, schemata, or heuristics, which allow them to perform complex tasks intuitively and automatically. They rely less on rules or guidelines, and they slow down when a situation does not fit a pattern they have seen in the past. *Routine expertise* is the rapid and effortless performance of complex tasks that remain similar each time they are performed. *Adaptive expertise* is when individuals display expertise and innovate in their practice without sacrificing efficiency or safety so that they can continue to learn from each new variation.[157-159] Health care providers must apply adaptive expertise to develop original solutions when confronted with unique clinical scenarios and to facilitate lifelong learning processes.

Adaptive expertise requires a habit of *inquiry*—the ability to ask relevant questions, identify resources to answer them, and apply new knowledge to practice.[160] It also requires sophisticated metacognitive abilities. *Metacognition*, the awareness or analysis of one's own learning or thinking processes, is critical to effectively recognize one's own limitations and direct one's own development.

Principles for educational strategies to support learners' development of adaptive expertise[161,162] include (1) encouraging learners to think about the mechanisms that link causes with their effects, which can engender integration of concepts (*cognitive integration*), (2) intentionally exposing learners to multiple contrasting *variations*, and (3) providing opportunities for "*productive failure*,"[163] where learners are asked to solve problems for which they have not been prepared, and then providing instruction after they attempt to generate solutions.

In nonclinical settings, adaptive expertise can be promoted through careful organization of content and using methods such as problem-based learning. Learners may be encouraged to think of innovative solutions by engaging in thought experiments (e.g., "what if?" questions). *Personal learning portfolios,*[164] which can serve as a record of learning and stimulate reflection, can help strengthen metacognitive abilities.

Traditional clinical learning often exposes learners to regular variation and challenging problems that present opportunities for productive failure. Simulations can allow learners to practice variations in rapid succession, and simulations can be adjusted based on learner performance. *Coaching* combines (1) mutual engagement with a shared orientation toward growth, (2) ongoing reflection and involvement of both learners and coaches, and (3) embracing failure or suboptimal performance as a catalyst for learning.[165] Coaching is becoming more popular in medical education and may be an intuitive model when considering how to foster adaptive expertise.

EXAMPLE: *Preclinical Curriculum to Foster Adaptive Expertise.* A medical school with a four-year curriculum revised its first two years to encourage adaptive expertise. Each week for 72 weeks, students worked independently through virtual patient cases that allowed students to explore concepts in basic and clinical sciences and experience productive struggle. Cases were reviewed in small groups facilitated by faculty who could reinforce the relationships and mechanisms that linked concepts. Personal e-portfolios collated assessment data and included student reflections and plans for learning; these were used as the basis for guidance and coaching from faculty.[161]

Professional Identity Formation

Methods for promoting professional identity formation include the following:

- Methods for cognitive objectives to learn about the concept of professional identity formation
- Faculty role modeling
- Fostering safe, supportive learning environments
- Methods that facilitate reflection on experiences (e.g., discussion, writing, learning portfolios)
- Coaching and formative feedback
- Exposure to new practice environments that can change perspectives

Professionalism includes respect for others, compassion, cross-cultural sensitivity, effective communication, shared decision-making, honesty and integrity, self-awareness, responsiveness to the needs of patients and society that supersede self-interest, accountability, sense of duty, a commitment to ethical principles, confidentiality, appropriate management of conflicts of interest, and a commitment to excellence, scientific knowledge, and ongoing professional development.[166,167] It has become especially salient as skepticism and the erosion of trust in professions and institutions have been increasing in many areas of the world.

Professional identity formation has been used to describe the continuous development of professional characteristics during training and the incorporation of those characteristics into one's sense of self. Professional identity formation is a more complicated construct than professionalism because of its developmental nature, and it includes elements of social learning and identity formation.[168] During professional identity formation, individuals link and reconcile their unique personal identities that existed before their formal health professions education with their developing professional identities. Professional identities form as learners move from "legitimate peripheral participation" to full participation in a *"community of practice."*[169] A community of practice forms around (1) mutual engagement (i.e., social interactions), (2) joint enterprise (i.e., shared goals), and (3) shared repertoire (e.g., common language and routines).[170] Individuals often belong to more than one community of practice in medicine's landscapes of practice[170] and demonstrate multiple professional identities that can be expressed differently depending on the context.

To promote professional identity formation, educators can inform learners and faculty about the facets and processes of professional identity formation through educational methods appropriate for cognitive objectives.[169] They can also aid learners' identity development and sense of belonging by using methods appropriate for affective objectives, such as cultivating safe and supportive learning environments, being attentive to and addressing unprofessional behaviors that may be encountered in the hidden curriculum, and role modeling professional behaviors.[169] Faculty can serve as coaches who orient toward learners' growth, share formative feedback, and facilitate reflection.[171] Exposure to patient care in different communities or cultures, such as international settings, may effect transformative learning that leads to a new understanding of one's professional identity.[172]

EXAMPLE: *Critical Reflection on Patient Interactions.* In order to facilitate professional identity formation, medical students on a family medicine clerkship were required to complete two reflective essays describing patient interactions that "struck" them and to submit the essays to faculty.[173] Faculty then facilitated small-group discussions, during which they emphasized the group as a safe space for students to reflect on and process their narratives. Afterward, students received written formative feedback from faculty. Evaluation of student essays illustrated the thoughts and emotions that students experienced as they reconciled idealized visions of professionalism with their lived realities, thus informing development of their own professional identities.[174]

EXAMPLE: *Summer Internship with Seminars and Community Experience.* A summer internship for medical students included seminars related to professionalism and clinical experience in community-based organizations with community mentors. Students reported that the internship taught them about influences on professionalism, especially that of pharmaceutical companies; the role of physician advocacy for patients; and the experience of vulnerable populations with the health care system.[175]

Interprofessionalism and Teamwork

Methods for promoting and reinforcing team skills include the following:

- Focused curricula on team functioning and related skills
- Involvement of trainees in collaborative versus competitive approaches to learning, such as team-based learning (TBL)
- Learner participation in multidisciplinary teams and in work environments that model effective teamwork
- Having learners assess and discuss the functioning of the teams in which they are involved

As medical knowledge has increased, and as societal expectations for high-quality, cost-effective care have risen, the mechanisms for providing the best health care have become more complex. Health care professionals have to work effectively in teams to accomplish desired goals of access, quality, and cost-effectiveness. Traditional medical curricula that have fostered a competitive approach to learning, or an autocratic approach to providing care, need to foster collaborative approaches to learning and to prepare learners to be effective team members.

Effective interprofessional education has been described as a *"wicked problem,"* which unlike a "tame problem," does not have clear agreement among stakeholders on what the problem is, resists a linear-analytic problem-solving approach, and defies solutions that are objectively right or wrong.[176] Interprofessional competencies have been described and include a breadth of knowledge, attitudes, and skills to achieve collaborative practice with other health professionals.[177] Health care professionals need to become knowledgeable about and skilled in facilitating group process, running and participating in meetings, being appropriately assertive, managing conflict, facilitating organizational change, motivating others, delegating to and supervising others, and providing feedback, in addition to having effective general communication skills.

The World Health Organization has emphasized that the development of interprofessional competencies is best done when interprofessional students learn together. Successful models include introduction to the competencies in didactic formats and discussions, followed by actual practice.[178] Finding the optimal timing to do this is difficult in the crowded curricula of modern health education programs. Ideally, clinical rotations would occur in model collaborative practice sites, but those may also be challenging for some programs to identify.

Baker et al.[179] elucidated a framework of principles that characterize effective teamwork, including leadership skills, articulation of shared goals and objectives, effective communication, trust, task sharing and backup behavior, adaptability, and performance monitoring/feedback. TeamSTEPPS, an evidence-based teamwork system that emphasizes team leadership, situational monitoring, mutual support, and communication behaviors, is being used in health professions education.[180,181]

EXAMPLE: *Focused Curricula on Team Skills: TeamSTEPPS Training.* A half-day workshop with first-year nursing students and third-year medical students used TeamSTEPPS as an educational intervention. Following a didactic introduction and simulation training exercise, students were better able to identify the presence and quality of team skills in video vignettes.[182]

EXAMPLE: *Online Discussion and Problem-Solving.* A longitudinal program for medical students and nursing students began with completion of online modules on teamwork, conflict resolution, and communication. Interprofessional teams of students worked together on solving problems using an instant messaging platform. In the second half of the curriculum, pairs of medical and nursing students were assigned a virtual ambulatory patient and managed that patient through acute and chronic illness.[183]

EXAMPLE: *Interprofessional Student-Run Free Clinic.* First- and second-year medical students (MS), undergraduate nursing students (NS), and social work students partnered to design and implement a weekend urban student-run free clinic. The students designed a process that included intake by a case manager (NS), evaluation by a junior (MS or NS) and a senior (MS or NS) clinician, presentation to a faculty preceptor, and then sign-out by a social work student. In both the design and the implementation of the clinic, students expressed respect for the other professions, comfort with interprofessional teams, and increased understanding of roles and responsibilities of the other professions.[184]

CONCLUSION

The challenge of Step 4 is to devise educational strategies that achieve the curricular objectives set out in Step 3, within the resource constraints of available people, time, facilities/materials, and funding. The need to align educational strategies with learning theory, principles, and science, and thoughtful application of emerging technologies while seeking to foster learner behaviors that address health problems, are additional considerations. Creativity in the development of educational strategies is an opportunity for facilitating meaningful, enduring learning and for scholarship, particularly if the curriculum is carefully evaluated, as we shall see in Chapter 7.

QUESTIONS

For the curriculum you are coordinating, planning, or would like to be planning, please answer or think about the following questions and prompts:

1. In the table below, write one important, specific measurable objective in each of the following domains: cognitive, affective, and psychomotor.

2. Review Table 5.1 and consider what learning framework might relate to your response to the prompt above.

3. Choose educational methods from Tables 5.2 and 5.3 to achieve each of your educational objectives and write them in the table below.

4. Is each educational method congruent with the domain of its objective (see Table 5.2)?

5. Are you concerned that there will be decay over time in the achievement of any of your objectives?

6. From Tables 5.2 and 5.3, choose an additional method for each objective that would most likely prevent decay after its achievement. Write those methods in the table below.

7. Identify the resources that you will need to implement your educational methods. Consider available teachers in your institution, costs for simulations or clinical experiences, time in the training program or elective, and space. Write them in the table below. Are your methods feasible?

	Cognitive (Knowledge)	Affective (Attitudinal)	Psychomotor (Skill or Behavior)
Specific measurable objectives			
Educational method to achieve objective			
Educational method to prevent decay			
Resources required			

8. Will your curriculum include educational strategies that promote adaptive expertise? Why or why not? If yes, what are these strategies?

9. Will your curriculum include educational strategies that promote professionalism, professional identity formation, or interprofessionalism/teamwork? Why or why not? If yes, what are these strategies?

10. Have the methods you suggested in your answers to Questions 8 and 9 affected your need for resources? How? Are your methods feasible?

GENERAL REFERENCES

Ambrose, Susan A., Michael W. Bridges, Michele DiPietro, Marsha C. Lovett, and Marie K. Norman. *How Learning Works: Seven Research-Based Principles for Smart Teaching*. San Francisco: Jossey-Bass, 2010.
  Popular book that provides numerous practical tips for teaching in alignment with seven principles. 301 pages.

Brown, Peter C., Henry L. Roediger, and Mark A. McDaniel. *Make It Stick*. Cambridge, MA: Belknap Press of Harvard University Press, 2014.
  Popular and accessible book that summarizes how our intuition can be misleading and how testing, spaced retrieval, and interleaving can enhance learning. 313 pages.

Chen, Belinda Y., David E. Kern, Robert M. Kearns, Patricia A. Thomas, Mark T. Hughes, and Sean Tackett. "From Modules to MOOCs: Application of the Six-Step Approach to Online Curriculum Development for Medical Education." *Academic Medicine* 94, no. 5 (2019): 678–85. https//doi.org/10.1097/ACM.0000000000002580.
Brief guide of the six-step approach for application to online curriculum development.

Cleland, Jennifer, and Steven J. Durning, eds. *Researching Medical Education*. Oxford: Wiley Blackwell, 2015.
First edition of a book on scholarship in health professions education that includes 16 chapters on theories related to learning. 296 pages.

Dent, John A., Ronald M. Harden, and Dan Hunt, eds. *A Practical Guide for Medical Teachers*, 5th ed. Edinburgh: Churchill Livingstone, 2017.
Includes 101 international contributors and provides global perspectives on curriculum development and instructional design. 428 pages.

Mayer, Richard E., ed., *The Cambridge Handbook of Multimedia Learning*. 2nd ed. New York: Cambridge University Press, 2014.
Compendium covering a wealth of information related to multimedia principles across its 34 chapters. 930 pages.

McGaghie, William C., Jeffrey H. Barsuk, and Diane B. Wayne, eds., *Comprehensive Healthcare Simulation: Mastery Learning in Health Professions Education*. Cham, Switzerland: Springer, 2020.
Places simulation for learning in the health professions into historical context, summarizes evidence related to its use, and includes advice of overall curricular design and specific tips for applying for cognitive and psychomotor skill development. 399 pages.

Swanwick, Tim, Kirsty Forrest, and Bridget C. O'Brien, eds. *Understanding Medical Education: Evidence, Theory, and Practice*. 3rd ed. Hoboken, NJ: John Wiley & Sons, 2019.
Excellent resource developed through the Association for the Study of Medical Education that covers relevant theory spanning teaching and learning, assessment, scholarship, and faculty development. 580 pages.

REFERENCES CITED

1. John Sweller, Jeroen J. G. van Merriënboer, and Fred Paas, "Cognitive Architecture and Instructional Design: 20 Years Later," *Educational Psychology Review* 31, no. 2 (2019): 261–92, https://doi.org/10.1007/s10648-019-09465-5.
2. Stoo Sepp et al., "Cognitive Load Theory and Human Movement: Towards an Integrated Model of Working Memory," *Educational Psychology Review* 31, no. 2 (2019): 293–317, https://doi.org/10.1007/s10648-019-09461-9.
3. Adam Szulewski et al., "From Theory to Practice: The Application of Cognitive Load Theory to the Practice of Medicine," *Academic Medicine* 96, no. 1 (2021): 24–30, https://doi.org/10.1097/acm.0000000000003524.
4. Richard E. Mayer, ed., *The Cambridge Handbook of Multimedia Learning*, 2nd ed. (Cambridge: Cambridge University Press, 2014), https://doi.org/10.1017/CBO9781139547369.
5. John Dunlosky et al., "Improving Students' Learning with Effective Learning Techniques: Promising Directions from Cognitive and Educational Psychology," *Psychological Science in the Public Interest* 14, no. 1 (2013): 4–58, https://doi.org/10.1177/1529100612453266.
6. Karen Mann and Anna MacLeod, "Constructivism: Learning Theories and Approaches to Research," in *Researching Medical Education*, ed. Jennifer Cleland and Steven J. Durning (Oxford: Wiley Blackwell, 2015), 49–66.

7. David A. Cook and Anthony R. Artino Jr., "Motivation to Learn: An Overview of Contemporary Theories," *Medical Education* 50, no. 10 (2016): 997–1014, https://doi.org/10.1111/medu.13074.

8. Anthony R. Artino et al., "Control-Value Theory: Using Achievement Emotions to Improve Understanding of Motivation, Learning, and Performance in Medical Education: AMEE Guide No. 64," *Medical Teacher* 34, no. 3 (2012): e148–60, https://doi.org/10.3109/0142159x.2012.651515.

9. Javeed Sukhera, Christopher J. Watling, and Cristina M. Gonzalez, "Implicit Bias in Health Professions: From Recognition to Transformation," *Academic Medicine* 95, no. 5 (2020): 717–23, https://doi.org/10.1097/acm.0000000000003173.

10. Andrew Kitchenham, "The Evolution of John Mezirow's Transformative Learning Theory," *Journal of Transformative Education* 6 (2008): 104–23, https://doi.org/10.1177/1541344608322678.

11. Alice Cavanagh, Meredith Vanstone, and Stacey Ritz, "Problems of Problem-Based Learning: Towards Transformative Critical Pedagogy in Medical Education," *Perspectives in Medical Education* 8, no. 1 (2019): 38–42, https://doi.org/10.1007/s40037-018-0489-7.

12. K. Anders Ericsson, "Acquisition and Maintenance of Medical Expertise: A Perspective from the Expert-Performance Approach with Deliberate Practice," *Academic Medicine* 90, no. 11 (2015): 1471–86, https://doi.org/10.1097/acm.0000000000000939.

13. William C. McGaghie, "Mastery Learning: Origins, Features, and Evidence from the Health Professions," in *Comprehensive Healthcare Simulation: Mastery Learning in Health Professions Education,* ed. William C. McGaghie, Jeffrey H. Barsuk, and Diane B. Wayne (Cham, Switzerland: Springer, 2020), 27–46.

14. Dario Torre and Steven J. Durning, "Social Cognitive Theory: Thinking and Learning in Social Settings," in *Researching Medical Education* (Oxford: Wiley Blackwell, 2015), 105–16.

15. Lindsay Baker et al., "Aligning and Applying the Paradigms and Practices of Education," *Academic Medicine* 94, no. 7 (2019): 1060. https://doi.org/10.1097/ACM.0000000000002693.

16. Micheline T. Chi, "Active-Constructive-Interactive: A Conceptual Framework for Differentiating Learning Activities," *Topics in Cognitive Science* 1, no. 1 (2009): 73–105, https://doi.org/10.1111/j.1756-8765.2008.01005.x.

17. L. Mark Carrier et al., "Causes, Effects, and Practicalities of Everyday Multitasking," *Developmental Review* 35 (2015): 64–78, https://doi.org/10.1016/j.dr.2014.12.005.

18. Kalina Christoff et al., "Mind-Wandering as Spontaneous Thought: A Dynamic Framework," *Nature Reviews Neuroscience* 17, no. 11 (2016): 718–31, https://doi.org/10.1038/nrn.2016.113.

19. Mary Hellen Immordino-Yang, Joanna A. Christodoulou, and Vanessa Singh, "Rest Is Not Idleness: Implications of the Brain's Default Mode for Human Development and Education," *Perspectives on Psychological Science* 7, no. 4 (2012): 352–64, https://doi.org/10.1177/1745691612447308.

20. Bjorn Rasch and Jan Born, "About Sleep's Role in Memory," *Physiological Reviews* 93, no. 2 (2013): 681–766, https://doi.org/10.1152/physrev.00032.2012.

21. Susanne Diekelmann and Jan Born, "The Memory Function of Sleep," *Nature Reviews Neuroscience* 11, no. 2 (2010): 114–26, https://doi.org/10.1038/nrn2762.

22. Julia C. Basso and Wendy A. Suzuki, "The Effects of Acute Exercise on Mood, Cognition, Neurophysiology, and Neurochemical Pathways: A Review," *Brain Plasticity* 2, no. 2 (2017): 127–52, https://doi.org/10.3233/bpl-160040.

23. World Health Organization. *Digital Education for Building Health Workforce Capacity* (Geneva: World Health Organization, 2020), accessed May 24, 2021, https://www.who.int/publications/i/item/dfigital-education-for-building-health-workforce-capacity-978-92-4-000047-6.

24. Belinda Y. Chen et al., "From Modules to MOOCs: Application of the Six-Step Approach to Online Curriculum Development for Medical Education," *Academic Medicine* 94, no. 5 (2019): 678–85, https://doi.org/10.1097/acm.0000000000002580.

25. Leisi Pei and Hongbin Wu, "Does Online Learning Work Better Than Offline Learning in Undergraduate Medical Education? A Systematic Review and Meta-Analysis," *Medical Education Online* 24, no. 1 (2019): 1666538, https://doi.org/10.1080/10872981.2019.1666538.

26. Alexandre Vallée et al., "Blended Learning Compared to Traditional Learning in Medical Education: Systematic Review and Meta-Analysis," *Journal of Medical Internet Research* 22, no. 8 (2020): e16504, https://doi.org/10.2196/16504.

27. David A. Cook, "The Value of Online Learning and MRI: Finding a Niche for Expensive Technologies," *Medical Teacher* 36, no. 11 (2014): 965–72, https://doi.org/10.3109/0142159x.2014.917284.

28. Paul M. Leonardi, "Theoretical Foundations for the Study of Sociomateriality," *Information and Organization* 23, no. 2 (2013): 59–76, https://doi.org/10.1016/j.infoandorg.2013.02.002.

29. Anna MacLeod et al., "Sociomateriality: A Theoretical Framework for Studying Distributed Medical Education," *Academic Medicine* 90, no. 11 (2015): 1451–56, https://doi.org/10.1097/acm.0000000000000708.

30. Anna MacLeod et al., "Technologies of Exposure: Videoconferenced Distributed Medical Education as a Sociomaterial Practice," *Academic Medicine* 94, no. 3 (2019): 412–18, https://doi.org/10.1097/acm.0000000000002536.

31. Jesper Juul, "The Game, the Player, the World: Looking for a Heart of Gameness," in *Level Up: Digital Games Research Conference Proceedings*, ed. Marinka Copier and Joost Raessens (Utrecht: Utrecht University, 2003), 30–45, accessed June 6, 2021, https://www.jesperjuul.net/text/gameplayerworld/.

32. Sebastian Deterding et al., "From Game Design Elements to Gamefulness: Defining 'Gamification,'" (Proceedings of the 15th International Academic MindTrek Conference: Envisioning Future Media Environments, Tampere, Finland, Association for Computing Machinery, 2011), https://doi.org/10.1145/2181037.2181040.

33. Chrystal Rutledge et al., "Gamification in Action: Theoretical and Practical Considerations for Medical Educators," *Academic Medicine* 93, no. 7 (2018): 1014–20, https://doi.org/10.1097/acm.0000000000002183.

34. Julie A. Noyes et al., "A Systematic Review of Digital Badges in Health Care Education," *Medical Education* 54, no. 7 (2020): 600–615, https://doi.org/10.1111/medu.14060.

35. Jan L. Plass, Bruce D. Homer, and Charles K. Kinzer, "Foundations of Game-Based Learning," *Educational Psychologist* 50 no. 4 (2015): 258–83, https://doi.org/10.1080/00461520.2015.1122533.

36. Scott Nicholson, "A RECIPE for Meaningful Gamification," in *Gamification in Education and Business*, ed. Torsten Reiners and Lincoln C. Wood (Cham, Springer, 2015), https://doi.org/10.1007/978-3-319-10208-5_1.

37. Sarah V. Gentry et al., "Serious Gaming and Gamification Education in Health Professions: Systematic Review," *Journal of Medical Internet Research* 21, no. 3 (2019): e12994, https://doi.org/10.2196/12994.

38. Joep Lagro et al., "A Randomized Controlled Trial on Teaching Geriatric Medical Decision Making and Cost Consciousness with the Serious Game GeriatriX," *Journal of the American Medical Directors Association* 15, no. 12 (2014): 957.e1-6, https://doi.org/10.1016/j.jamda.2014.04.011.

39. B. Price Kerfoot et al., "An Online Spaced-Education Game among Clinicians Improves Their Patients' Time to Blood Pressure Control: A Randomized Controlled Trial," *Circulation: Cardiovascular Quality and Outcomes* 7, no. 3 (2014): 468–74, https://doi.org/10.1161/circoutcomes.113.000814.

40. B. Price Kerfoot and Nicole Kissane, "The Use of Gamification to Boost Residents' Engagement in Simulation Training," *JAMA Surgery* 149, no. 11 (2014): 1208–9, https://doi.org/10.1001/jamasurg.2014.1779.

41. Deborah K. Simpson et al., "Job Roles of the 2025 Medical Educator," *Journal of Graduate Medical Education* 10, no. 3 (2018): 243–46, https://doi.org/10.4300/jgme-d-18-00253.1.

42. Madara Mason, "iTeach+: The Interactive Syllabus," University of Alaska Fairbanks, 2017, accessed May 24, 2021, https://iteachu.uaf.edu/iteach-the-interactive-syllabus/.

43. Malcolm S. Knowles et al., *The Adult Learner: The Definitive Classic in Adult Education and Human Resource Development*, 9th ed. (London: Routledge, 2020).

44. John Hattie, "The Applicability of Visible Learning to Higher Education," *Scholarship of Teaching and Learning in Psychology* 1 (2015): 79–91, https://doi.org/10.1037/stl0000021.

45. David Wiley, "The Learning Objects Literature," *Handbook of Research on Educational Communication and Technology* 16 (2007): 345–54.

46. Kevin R. Scott et al., "Integration of Social Media in Emergency Medicine Residency Curriculum," *Annals of Emergency Medicine* 64, no. 4 (2014): 396–404, https://doi.org/10.1016/j.annemergmed.2014.05.030.

47. Lori R. Newman et al., "Developing Expert-Derived Rating Standards for the Peer Assessment of Lectures," *Academic Medicine* 87, no. 3 (2012): 356–63, https://doi.org/10.1097/ACM.0b013e3182444fa3.

48. Avraham Z. Cooper and Jeremy B. Richards, "Lectures for Adult Learners: Breaking Old Habits in Graduate Medical Education," *American Journal of Medicine* 130, no. 3 (2017): 376–81, https://doi.org/10.1016/j.amjmed.2016.11.009.

49. Henk G. Schmidt et al., "On the Use and Misuse of Lectures in Higher Education," *Health Professions Education* 1, no. 1 (2015): 12–18, https://doi.org/10.1016/j.hpe.2015.11.010.

50. Henry L. Roediger III, Adam L. Putnam, and Megan A. Smith, "Ten Benefits of Testing and Their Applications to Educational Practice," in *Psychology of Learning and Motivation*, ed. Jose P. Mestre and Brian H. Ross (San Diego: Academic Press, 2011), 1–36.

51. Abdel Meguid and Megan Collins, "Students' Perceptions of Lecturing Approaches: Traditional versus Interactive Teaching," *Advances in Medical Education and Practice* 8 (2017): 229–241, https://doi.org/10.2147/AMEP.S131851.

52. Emilie Gerbier and Thomas C. Toppino, "The Effect of Distributed Practice: Neuroscience, Cognition, and Education," *Trends in Neuroscience and Education* 4, no. 3 (2015): 49–59, https://doi.org/10.1016/j.tine.2015.01.001.

53. Timothy A. Shaw et al., "Impact on Clinical Behavior of Face-to-Face Continuing Medical Education Blended with Online Spaced Education: A Randomized Controlled Trial," *The Journal of Continuing Education in the Health Professions* 31, no. 2 (2011): 103–8, https://doi.org/10.1002/chp.20113.

54. Daeyeoul Lee, Sunnie Lee Watson, and William R. Watson, "Systematic Literature Review on Self-Regulated Learning in Massive Open Online Courses," *Australasian Journal of Educational Technology* 35, no. 1 (2019), https://doi.org/10.14742/ajet.3749.

55. Stephen D. Sisson et al., "Effect of an Internet-Based Curriculum on Postgraduate Education: A Multicenter Intervention," *Journal of General Internal Medicine* 19, no. 5 (2004): 505–9, https://doi.org/10.1111/j.1525-1497.2004.30097.x.

56. Stephen D. Sisson et al., "Concurrent Validity between a Shared Curriculum, the Internal Medicine In-Training Examination, and the American Board of Internal Medicine Certifying Examination," *Journal of Graduate Medical Education* 7, no. 1 (2015): 42–47, https://doi.org/10.4300/jgme-d-14-00054.1.

57. Whitney D. Maxwell et al., "Massive Open Online Courses in U.S. Healthcare Education: Practical Considerations and Lessons Learned from Implementation." *Currents in Pharmacy Teaching and Learning* 10, no. 6 (2018): 736–43, https://doi.org/10.1016/j.cptl.2018.03.013.

58. Barbara Daley, Steven Durning, and Dario Torre, "Using Concept Maps to Create Meaningful Learning in Medical Education," *MedEdPublish* 5, no. 1 (2016): 19, https://doi.org/10.15694/mep.2016.000019.

59. Carolina Veronese et al., "A Randomized Pilot Study of the Use of Concept Maps to Enhance Problem-Based Learning among First-Year Medical Students," *Medical Teacher* 35, no. 9 (2013): e1478–84, https://doi.org/10.3109/0142159x.2013.785628.

60. Annette Burgess et al., "Facilitating Small Group Learning in the Health Professions," *BMC Medical Education* 20, no. Suppl 2 (2020): 457, https://doi.org/10.1186/s12909-020-02282-3.

61. Henk G. Schmidt and Silvia Mamede, "How to Improve the Teaching of Clinical Reasoning: A Narrative Review and a Proposal," *Medical Education* 49, no. 10 (2015): 961–73, https://doi.org/10.1111/medu.12775.

62. Andrzej Kononowicz et al., "Virtual Patient Simulations in Health Professions Education: Systematic Review and Meta-Analysis by the Digital Health Education Collaboration," *Journal of Medical Internet Research* 21, no. 7 (2019): e14676, https://doi.org/10.2196/14676.

63. Andrzej Kononowicz et al., "Virtual Patients—What Are We Talking About? A Framework to Classify the Meanings of the Term in Healthcare Education," *BMC Medical Education* 15 (2015): 11, https://doi.org/10.1186/s12909-015-0296-3.

64. Rabih Geha et al., "Teaching about Diagnostic Errors through Virtual Patient Cases: A Pilot Exploration," *Diagnosis (Berl)* 5, no. 4 (2018): 223–27, https://pubmed.ncbi.nlm.nih.gov/30285947/.

65. Teresa M. Chan et al., "Social Media in Knowledge Translation and Education for Physicians and Trainees: A Scoping Review," *Perspectives in Medical Education* 9, no. 1 (2020): 20–30, https://doi.org/10.1007/s40037-019-00542-7.

66. Teresa M. Chan, Brent Thoma, and Michelle Lin, "Creating, Curating, and Sharing Online Faculty Development Resources: The Medical Education in Cases Series Experience," *Academic Medicine* 90, no. 6 (2015): 785–89, https://doi.org/10.1097/acm.0000000000000692.

67. Teresa M. Chan et al., "The ALiEM Faculty Incubator: A Novel Online Approach to Faculty Development in Education Scholarship," *Academic Medicine* 93, no. 10 (2018): 1497–502, https://doi.org/10.1097/acm.0000000000002309.

68. Gökçe Akçayır and Murat Akçayır, "The Flipped Classroom: A Review of Its Advantages and Challenges," *Computers & Education* 126 (2018): 334–45, https://doi.org/10.1016/j.compedu.2018.07.021.

69. Lakmal Abeysekera and Phillip Dawson, "Motivation and Cognitive Load in the Flipped Classroom: Definition, Rationale and a Call for Research," *Higher Education Research & Development* 34, no. 1 (2015): 1–14, https://doi.org/10.1080/07294360.2014.934336.

70. Sharon F. Chen et al., "A Multi-Institution Collaboration to Define Core Content and Design Flexible Curricular Components for a Foundational Medical School Course: Implications for National Curriculum Reform," *Academic Medicine* 94, no. 6 (2019): 819–25. https://doi.org/10.1097/acm.0000000000002663.

71. Alan Neville, Geoff Norman, and Robert White, "McMaster at 50: Lessons Learned from Five Decades of PBL," *Advances in Health Sciences Education* 24, no. 5 (2019): 853–63, https://doi.org/10.1007/s10459-019-09908-2.

72. Virginie F. Servant and Henk G. Schmidt, "Revisiting 'Foundations of Problem-Based Learning: Some Explanatory Notes,'" *Medical Education* 50, no. 7 (2016): 698–701, https://doi.org/10.1111/medu.12803.

73. Alan J. Neville and Geoff R. Norman, "PBL in the Undergraduate MD Program at McMaster University: Three Iterations in Three Decades," *Academic Medicine* 82, no. 4 (2007): 370–74, https://doi.org/10.1097/ACM.0b013e318033385d.

74. Woei Hung et al., "A Review to Identify Key Perspectives in PBL Meta-Analyses and Reviews: Trends, Gaps and Future Research Directions," *Advances in Health Sciences Education* 24, no. 5 (2019): 943–57, https://doi.org/10.1007/s10459-019-09945-x.

75. Diana Stentoft, "Problem-Based Projects in Medical Education: Extending PBL Practices and Broadening Learning Perspectives," *Advances in Health Sciences Education* 24, no. 5 (2019): 959–69, https://doi.org/10.1007/s10459-019-09917-1.

76. William P. Burdick, Stacey R. Friedman, and Deborah Diserens, "Faculty Development Projects for International Health Professions Educators: Vehicles for Institutional Change?" *Medical Teacher* 34, no. 1 (2012): 38–44, https://doi.org/10.3109/0142159x.2011.558538.

77. Francois J. Cilliers and Ara Tekian, "Effective Faculty Development in an Institutional Context: Designing for Transfer," *Journal of Graduate Medical Education* 8, no. 2 (2016): 145–49, https://doi.org/10.4300/jgme-d-15-00117.1.

78. Marian Cornett et al., "A Realist Review of Scholarly Experiences in Medical Education," *Medical Education* 55, no. 2 (2021): 159–66, https://doi.org/10.1111/medu.14362.

79. Maryellen E. Gusic et al., "The Essential Value of Projects in Faculty Development," *Academic Medicine* 85, no. 9 (2010): 1484–91, https://doi.org/10.1097/ACM.0b013e3181eb4d17.

80. William P. Burdick, "Global Faculty Development: Lessons Learned from the Foundation for Advancement of International Medical Education and Research (FAIMER) Initiatives," *Academic Medicine* 89, no. 8 (2014): 1097–99, https://doi.org/10.1097/acm.0000000000000377.

81. Diana Dolmans et al., "Should We Choose between Problem-Based Learning and Team-Based Learning? No, Combine the Best of Both Worlds!," *Medical Teacher* 37, no. 4 (2015): 354–59, https://doi.org/10.3109/0142159x.2014.948828.

82. Tyler Reimschisel et al., "A Systematic Review of the Published Literature on Team-Based Learning in Health Professions Education," *Medical Teacher* 39, no. 12 (2017): 1227–37, https://doi.org/10.1080/0142159x.2017.1340636.

83. Joanna Tai et al., "Same-Level Peer-Assisted Learning in Medical Clinical Placements: A Narrative Systematic Review," *Medical Education* 50, no. 4 (2016): 469–84, https://doi.org/10.1111/medu.12898.

84. Carrol Zhou et al., "The Impact of Project ECHO on Participant and Patient Outcomes: A Systematic Review," *Academic Medicine* 91, no. 10 (2016): 1439–61. https://doi.org/10.1097/acm.0000000000001328.

85. Rebecca Stovel et al., "Curricular Needs for Training Telemedicine Physicians: A Scoping Review," *Medical Teacher* 42, no. 11 (2020): 1234–42, https://doi.org/10.1080/0142159x.2020.1799959.

86. Sanjeev Arora et al., "Outcomes of Treatment for Hepatitis C Virus Infection by Primary Care Providers," *The New England Journal of Medicine* 364, no. 23 (2011): 2199–207, https://doi.org/10.1056/NEJMoa1009370.

87. Javeed Sukhera et al., "The Implicit Association Test in Health Professions Education: A Meta-Narrative Review," *Perspectives on Medical Education* 8, no. 5 (2019): 267–75, https://doi.org/10.1007/s40037-019-00533-8.

88. Yochay Nadan and Marina Stark, "The Pedagogy of Discomfort: Enhancing Reflectivity on Stereotypes and Bias," *British Journal of Social Work* 47, no. 3 (2016): 683–700, https://doi.org/10.1093/bjsw/bcw023.

89. Jeanne Nakamura and Mihaly Csikszentmihalyi, "The Concept of Flow," in *Flow and the Foundations of Positive Psychology: The Collected Works of Mihaly Csikszentmihalyi* (New York: Springer, 2014), 239–63.

90. Sydney McQueen et al., "Cognitive Flow in Health Care Settings: A Systematic Review," *Medical Education* 55, no.7 (2021): 782–94, https://doi.org/10.1111/medu.14435.

91. Sian Hsiang-Te Tsuei et al., "Exploring the Construct of Psychological Safety in Medical Education," *Academic Medicine* 94, no. 11S (2019): S28-S35, https://doi.org/10.1097/acm.0000000000002897.

92. John Sandars and Deborah Murdoch-Eaton. "Appreciative Inquiry in Medical Education," *Medical Teacher* 39, no. 2 (2017): 123–27, https://doi.org/10.1080/0142159x.2017.1245852.

93. Tyler J. VanderWeele, Eileen McNeely, and Howard K. Koh, "Reimagining Health-Flourishing," *JAMA* 321, no. 17 (2019): 1667–68, https://doi.org/10.1001/jama.2019.3035.

94. Alyssa K. McGonagle et al., "Coaching for Primary Care Physician Well-Being: A Randomized Trial and Follow-up Analysis," *Journal of Occupational Health Psychology* 25, no. 5 (2020): 297–314, https://doi.org/10.1037/ocp0000180.

95. Christy K. Boscardin, "Reducing Implicit Bias through Curricular Interventions," *Journal of General Internal Medicine* 30, no. 12 (2015): 1726–28, https://doi.org/10.1007/s11606-015-3496-y.

96. Vimmi Passi et al., "Doctor Role Modelling in Medical Education: BEME Guide No. 27," *Medical Teacher* 35, no. 9 (2013): e1422–36, https://doi.org/10.3109/0142159x.2013.806982.

97. Jochanan Benbassat, "Role Modeling in Medical Education: The Importance of a Reflective Imitation," *Academic Medicine* 89, no. 4 (2014): 550–54, https://doi.org/10.1097/acm.0000000000000189.

98. Sylvia R. Cruess, Richard L. Cruess, and Yvonne Steinert, "Role Modelling—Making the Most of a Powerful Teaching Strategy," *BMJ* 336, no. 7646 (2008): 718–21, https://doi.org/10.1136/bmj.39503.757847.BE.

99. Karen V. Mann, "Faculty Development to Promote Role-Modeling and Reflective Practice," in *Faculty Development in the Health Professions*, ed. Yvonne Steinert (Springer Netherlands, 2014), 245–64.

100. William T. Branch Jr. et al., "A Good Clinician and a Caring Person: Longitudinal Faculty Development and the Enhancement of the Human Dimensions of Care," *Academic Medicine* 84, no. 1 (2009): 117–25, https://doi.org/10.1097/ACM.0b013e3181900f8a.

101. Stella L. Ng et al., "Reclaiming a Theoretical Orientation to Reflection in Medical Education Research: A Critical Narrative Review," *Medical Education* 49, no. 5 (2015): 461–75, https://doi.org/10.1111/medu.12680.

102. Edvin Schei, Abraham Fuks, and J. Donald Boudreau, "Reflection in Medical Education: Intellectual Humility, Discovery, and Know-How," *Medicine, Health Care, and Philosophy* 22, no. 2 (2019): 167–78, https://doi.org/10.1007/s11019-018-9878-2.

103. Quoc Dinh Nguyen et al., "What Is Reflection? A Conceptual Analysis of Major Definitions and a Proposal of a Five-Component Model," *Medical Education* 48, no. 12 (2014): 1176–89, https://doi.org/10.1111/medu.12583.

104. Tanya White-Davis, "Addressing Racism in Medical Education an Interactive Training Module," *Family Medicine* 50, no. 5 (2018): 364–68, https://doi.org/10.22454/FamMed.2018.875510.

105. National Academies of Sciences, Engineering, and Medicine, *The Integration of the Humanities and Arts with Sciences, Engineering, and Medicine in Higher Education: Branches from the Same Tree*, ed. David Skorton and Ashley Bear (Washington, DC: National Academies Press, 2018), https://doi.org/10.17226/24988.

106. Lisa Howley, Elizabeth Gaufberg, and Brandy King, *The Fundamental Role of Arts and Humanities in Medical Education* (Washington, DC: Association of American Medical Colleges, 2020).

107. Daisy Fancourt and Saoirse Finn, "What Is the Evidence on the Role of the Arts in Improving Health and Well-Being? A Scoping Review," in *WHO Evidence Network Synthesis Reports* (Copenhagen: WHO Regional Office for Europe, 2019).

108. Margaret S. Chisolm, Margot Kelly-Hedrick, and Scott M. Wright, "How Visual Arts–Based Education Can Promote Clinical Excellence," *Academic Medicine* 96, no. 8 (2021): 1100–1104, https://doi.org/10.1097/acm.0000000000003862.

109. Tracy Moniz et. al., "The Prism Model for Integrating the Arts and Humanities into Medical Education," *Academic Medicine* 96, no. 8 (2021): 1225, https://doi.org/10.1097/acm.0000000000003949.

110. Silke Dennhardt et. al., "Rethinking Research in the Medical Humanities: A Scoping Review and Narrative Synthesis of Quantitative Outcome Studies," *Medical Education* 50, no. 3 (2016): 285–99, https://doi.org/10.1111/medu.12812.

111. Elizabeth Gaufberg, Molly Ward Olmsted, and Sigall K. Bell, "Third Things as Inspiration and Artifact: A Multi-Stakeholder Qualitative Approach to Understand Patient and Family Emotions after Harmful Events," *Journal of Medical Humanities* 40, no. 4 (2019): 489–504, https://doi.org/10.1007/s10912-019-09563-z.

112. Satendra Singh et al., "Transformational Learning for Health Professionals through a Theatre of the Oppressed Workshop," *Medical Humanities* 46, no. 4 (2020): 411–16, https://doi.org/10.1136/medhum-2019-011718.

113. Megan Milota, Ghislaine van Thiel, and Johannes J. M. van Delden, "Narrative Medicine as a Medical Education Tool: A Systematic Review," *Medical Teacher* 41, no. 7 (2019): 802–10, https://doi.org/10.1080/0142159X.2019.1584274.

114. Katherine C. Chretien et al., "Tell Me Your Story: A Pilot Narrative Medicine Curriculum during the Medicine Clerkship," *Journal of General Internal Medicine* 30, no. 7 (2015): 1025–28, https://doi.org/10.1007/s11606-015-3211-z.

115. Bruce L. Henschen et al., "The Patient Centered Medical Home as Curricular Model: Perceived Impact of the 'Education-Centered Medical Home,'" *Journal of General Internal Medicine* 28, no. 8 (2013): 1105–9, https://doi.org/10.1007/s11606-013-2389-1.

116. Blair P. Golden et al., "Learning to Be a Doctor: Medical Students' Perception of Their Roles in Longitudinal Outpatient Clerkships," *Patient Education and Counseling* 101, no. 11 (2018): 2018–24, https://doi.org/10.1016/j.pec.2018.08.003.

117. Bruce L. Henschen et al., "Continuity with Patients, Preceptors, and Peers Improves Primary Care Training: A Randomized Medical Education Trial," *Academic Medicine* 95, no. 3 (2020): 425–34, https://doi.org/10.1097/ACM.0000000000003045.

118. Nena Patterson and Linda J. Hulton, "Enhancing Nursing Students' Understanding of Poverty through Simulation," *Public Health Nursing* 29, no. 2 (2012): 143–51, https://doi.org/10.1111/j.1525-1446.2011.00999.x.

119. Sarah Yardley, Pim W. Teunissen, and Tim Dornan, "Experiential Learning: AMEE Guide No. 63," *Medical Teacher* 34, no. 2 (2012): e102–15, https://doi.org/10.3109/0142159x.2012.650741.

120. Jack Ende, "Feedback in Clinical Medical Education," JAMA 250, no. 6 (1983): 777–81.

121. Jennifer R. Kogan et al., "Guidelines: The Do's, Don'ts and Don't Knows of Direct Observation of Clinical Skills in Medical Education," *Perspectives on Medical Education* 6, no. 5 (2017): 286–305, https://doi.org/10.1007/s40037-017-0376-7.

122. Subha Ramani et al., "Twelve Tips to Promote a Feedback Culture with a Growth Mind-Set: Swinging the Feedback Pendulum from Recipes to Relationships," *Medical Teacher* 41, no. 6 (2019): 625–31, https://doi.org/10.1080/0142159x.2018.1432850.

123. Komal Srinivasa, Yan Chen, and Marcus A. Henning, "The Role of Online Videos in Teaching Procedural Skills to Post-graduate Medical Learners: A Systematic Narrative Review," *Medical Teacher* 42, no. 6 (2020): 689–97, https://doi.org/10.1080/0142159x.2020.1733507.

124. Lori Lioce et al., eds., *Health Care Simulation Dictionary*, 2nd ed. (Rockville, MD: Agency for Healthcare Research and Quality, 2020), AHRQ Publication No. 20-0019, https://doi.org/10.23970/simulationv2.

125. Nahzinine Shakeri et al., "Feedback and Debriefing in Mastery Learning," in McGaghie, *Comprehensive Healthcare Simulation*, 139–53.

126. Ivette Motola et al., "Simulation in Healthcare Education: A Best Evidence Practical Guide. AMEE Guide No. 82," *Medical Teacher* 35, no. 10 (2013): e1511–30, https://doi.org/10.3109/0142159x.2013.818632.

127. Nehal Khamis et al., "A Stepwise Model for Simulation-Based Curriculum Development for Clinical Skills, a Modification of the Six-Step Approach," *Surgical Endoscopy* 30, no. 1 (2016): 279–87, https://doi.org/10.1007/s00464-015-4206-x.

128. Jeffrey H. Barsuk et al., "Developing a Mastery Learning Curriculum," in McGaghie, *Comprehensive Healthcare Simulation*, 47–69.

129. Jette Led Sørensen et al., "Design of Simulation-Based Medical Education and Advantages and Disadvantages of In Situ Simulation versus Off-Site Simulation," *BMC Medical Education* 17, no. 1 (2017): 20, https://doi.org/10.1186/s12909-016-0838-3.

130. Pamela Andreatta et al., "Simulation-Based Mock Codes Significantly Correlate with Improved Pediatric Patient Cardiopulmonary Arrest Survival Rates," *Pediatric Critical Care Medicine* 12, no. 1 (2011): 33–38, https://doi.org/10.1097/PCC.0b013e3181e89270.

131. Stanley J. Hamstra et al., "Reconsidering Fidelity in Simulation-Based Training." *Academic Medicine* 89, no. 3 (2014): 387–92, https://doi.org/10.1097/acm.0000000000000130.

132. Debra Nestel and Tanya Tierney, "Role-Play for Medical Students Learning About Communication: Guidelines for Maximising Benefits," *BMC Medical Education* 7 (2007): 3, https://doi.org/10.1186/1472-6920-7-3.

133. Claire Lane and Stephen Rollnick, "The Use of Simulated Patients and Role-Play in Communication Skills Training: A Review of the Literature to August 2005," *Patient Education and Counseling* 67, no. 1–2 (2007): 13–20, https://doi.org/10.1016/j.pec.2007.02.011.

134. Jennifer A. Cleland, Keiko Abe, and Jan-Joost Rethans, "The Use of Simulated Patients in Medical Education: AMEE Guide No 42," *Medical Teacher* 31, no. 6 (2009): 477–86, https://doi.org/10.1080/01421590903002821.

135. Kerry Wilbur, Alaa Elmubark, and Sara Shabana, "Systematic Review of Standardized Patient Use in Continuing Medical Education," *Journal of Continuing Education in the Health Professions* 38, no. 1 (2018): 3–10, https://doi.org/10.1097/ceh.0000000000000190.

136. Anthony L. Back et al., "Efficacy of Communication Skills Training for Giving Bad News and Discussing Transitions to Palliative Care," *Archives of Internal Medicine* 167, no. 5 (2007): 453–60, https://doi.org/10.1001/archinte.167.5.453.

137. William C. McGaghie, Diane B. Wayne, and Jeffrey H. Barsuk, "Translational Science and Healthcare Quality and Safety Improvement from Mastery Learning," in *Comprehensive Healthcare Simulation*, 289–307.

138. Sara M. Zweifach and Marc M. Triola, "Extended Reality in Medical Education: Driving Adoption through Provider-Centered Design," *Digital Biomarkers* 3, no. 1 (2019): 14–21, https://doi.org/10.1159/000498923.

139. Vanessa N. Palter and Teodor P. Grantcharov, "Individualized Deliberate Practice on a Virtual Reality Simulator Improves Technical Performance of Surgical Novices in the Operating Room: A Randomized Controlled Trial," *Annals of Surgery* 259, no. 3 (2014): 443–48, https://doi.org/10.1097/sla.0000000000000254.

140. Maya Hammoud et al., "Is Video Review of Patient Encounters an Effective Tool for Medical Student Learning? A Review of the Literature," *Advances in Medical Education and Practice* 3 (2012): 19–30, https://doi.org/10.2147/amep.S20219.

141. Adam Cheng et al., "Debriefing for Technology-Enhanced Simulation: A Systematic Review and Meta-Analysis," *Medical Education* 48, no. 7 (2014): 657–66, https://doi.org/10.1111/medu.12432.

142. Knut M. Augestad et al., "Video-Based Coaching in Surgical Education: A Systematic Review and Meta-Analysis," *Surgical Endoscopy* 34, no. 2 (2020): 521–35, https://doi.org/10.1007/s00464-019-07265-0.

143. Noelle Junod Perron et al., "Feedback in Formative OSCEs: Comparison between Direct Observation and Video-Based Formats," *Medical Education Online* 21 (2016): 32160, https://doi.org/10.3402/meo.v21.32160.

144. Peggy Ertmer and Timothy Newby, "Behaviorism, Cognitivism, Constructivism: Comparing Critical Features from an Instructional Design Perspective," *Performance Improvement Quarterly* 6 (2008): 50–72, https://doi.org/10.1111/j.1937-8327.1993.tb00605.x.

145. James Clear, *Atomic Habits: An Easy & Proven Way to Build Good Habits & Break Bad Ones* (New York: Penguin Publishing House, 2018).

146. Francois Cilliers, Lambert Schuwirth, and Cees Van Der Vleuten, "Health Behaviour Theories: A Conceptual Lens to Explore Behaviour Change," in *Researching Medical Education*, 141–53.

147. Jeanne Farnan et al., "Hand-Off Education and Evaluation: Piloting the Observed Simulated Hand-Off Experience (OSHE)," *Journal of General Internal Medicine* 25, no. 2 (2010): 129–34, https://doi.org/10.1007/s11606-009-1170-y.

148. Sarah M. Morris et al., "Implementation of the Helping Babies Breathe Training Program: A Systematic Review," *Pediatrics* 146, no. 3 (2020), https://doi.org/10.1542/peds.2019-3938.

149. Estomih Mduma et al., "Frequent Brief On-Site Simulation Training and Reduction in 24-H Neonatal Mortality—an Educational Intervention Study," *Resuscitation* 93 (2015): 1–7, https://doi.org/10.1016/j.resuscitation.2015.04.019.

150. Gisele Bourgeois-Law, Pim W. Teunissen, and Glenn Regehr, "Remediation in Practicing Physicians: Current and Alternative Conceptualizations," *Academic Medicine* 93, no. 11 (2018): 1638–44, https://doi.org/10.1097/acm.0000000000002266.

151. Linda Prescott-Clements et al., "Rethinking Remediation: A Model to Support the Detailed Diagnosis of Clinicians' Performance Problems and the Development of Effective Remedia-

tion Plans," *Journal of Continuing Education in the Health Professions* 37, no. 4 (2017): 245–54, https://doi.org/10.1097/ceh.0000000000000173.

152. Calvin L. Chou et al., "Guidelines: The Do's, Don'ts and Don't Knows of Remediation in Medical Education," *Perspectives on Medical Education* 8, no. 6 (2019): 322–38, https://doi.org /10.1007/s40037-019-00544-5.

153. Miriam Lacasse et al., "Interventions for Undergraduate and Postgraduate Medical Learners with Academic Difficulties: A BEME Systematic Review: BEME Guide No. 56," *Medical Teacher* 41, no. 9 (2019): 981–1001, https://doi.org/10.1080/0142159x.2019.1596239.

154. Nicola Brennan et al., "Remediating Professionalism Lapses in Medical Students and Doctors: A Systematic Review," *Medical Education* 54, no. 3 (2020): 196–204, https://doi.org/10 .1111/medu.14016.

155. Lisa M. Bellini, Adina Kalet, and Robert Englander, "Providing Compassionate Off-Ramps for Medical Students Is a Moral Imperative," *Academic Medicine* 94, no. 5 (2019): 656–58. https://doi.org/10.1097/acm.0000000000002568.

156. Geoffrey R. Norman et al., "Expertise in Medicine and Surgery," in *The Cambridge Handbook of Expertise and Expert Performance*, ed. K. Ericsson et al. (Cambridge: Cambridge University Press, 2018), 331–55, https://doi.org/10.1017/9781316480748.019.

157. Daniel L. Schwartz, John D. Bransford, and David Sears, "Efficiency and Innovation in Transfer," in *Transfer in Learning from a Modern Multidisciplinary Perspective,* ed. Jose P. Mestre (Greenwich, CT: Information Age Publishing, 2005), 1–51.

158. Maria Mylopoulos and Nicole N. Woods, "When I Say . . . Adaptive Expertise," *Medical Education* 51, no. 7 (2017): 685–86, https://doi.org/10.1111/medu.13247.

159. Martin V. Pusic et al., "Learning to Balance Efficiency and Innovation for Optimal Adaptive Expertise," *Medical Teacher* 40, no. 8 (2018): 820–27, https://doi.org/10.1080/0142159x.2018 .1485887.

160. Gustavo Valbuena et al., "Inquiry in the Medical Curriculum: A Pedagogical Conundrum and a Proposed Solution," *Academic Medicine* 94, no. 6 (2019): 804–8, https://doi.org/10.1097 /acm.0000000000002671.

161. Kulamakan Kulasegaram et al., "The Alignment Imperative in Curriculum Renewal," *Medical Teacher* 40, no. 5 (2018): 443–48, https://doi.org/10.1080/0142159x.2018.1435858.

162. Maria Mylopoulos et al., "Twelve Tips for Designing Curricula That Support the Development of Adaptive Expertise," *Medical Teacher* 40, no. 8 (2018): 850–54, https://doi.org/10.1080 /0142159x.2018.1484082.

163. Manu Kapur, "Examining Productive Failure, Productive Success, Unproductive Failure, and Unproductive Success in Learning," *Educational Psychologist* 51, no. 2 (2016): 289–99, https://doi.org/10.1080/00461520.2016.1155457.

164. J. Van Tartwijk and Erik W. Driessen, "Portfolios for Assessment and Learning: AMEE Guide No. 45," *Medical Teacher* 31, no. 9 (2009): 790–801, https://doi.org/10.1080/01421590903139201.

165. Christopher J. Watling and Kori A. LaDonna, "Where Philosophy Meets Culture: Exploring How Coaches Conceptualise Their Roles," *Medical Education* 53, no. 5 (2019): 467–76, https://doi.org/10.1111/medu.13799.

166. Thomas S. Inui, *Flag in the Wind: Educating for Professionalism in Medicine* (Washington, DC: Association of American Medical Colleges, 2003).

167. Jody S. Frost et al., "The Intersection of Professionalism and Interprofessional Care: Development and Initial Testing of the Interprofessional Professionalism Assessment (IPA)," *Journal of Interprofessional Care* 33, no. 1 (2019): 102–15, https://doi.org/10.1080/13561820.2018.1515733.

168. Richard L. Cruess et al., "Reframing Medical Education to Support Professional Identity Formation," *Academic Medicine* 89, no. 11 (2014): 1446–51 https://doi.org/10.1097/acm .0000000000000427.

169. Sylvia R. Cruess, Richard L. Cruess, and Yvonne Steinert, "Supporting the Development of a Professional Identity: General Principles," *Medical Teacher* 41, no. 6 (2019): 641–49, https:// doi.org/10.1080/0142159x.2018.1536260.

170. Nathan Hodson, "Landscapes of Practice in Medical Education," *Medical Education* 54, no. 6 (2020): 504–9, https://doi.org/10.1111/medu.14061.

171. Adam P. Sawatsky, Brandon M. Huffman, and Frederic W. Hafferty, "Coaching versus Competency to Facilitate Professional Identity Formation," *Academic Medicine* 95, no. 10 (2020): 1511–14, https://doi.org/10.1097/acm.0000000000003144.

172. Adam P. Sawatsky et al., "Transformative Learning and Professional Identity Formation during International Health Electives: A Qualitative Study Using Grounded Theory," *Academic Medicine* 93, no. 9 (2018): 1381–90, https://doi.org/10.1097/acm.0000000000002230.

173. Hedy S. Wald et al., "Professional Identity Formation in Medical Education for Humanistic, Resilient Physicians: Pedagogic Strategies for Bridging Theory to Practice," *Academic Medicine* 90, no. 6 (2015): 753–60, https://doi.org/10.1097/acm.0000000000000725.

174. Hedy S. Wald et al., "Grappling with Complexity: Medical Students' Reflective Writings about Challenging Patient Encounters as a Window into Professional Identity Formation," *Medical Teacher* 41, no. 2 (2019): 152–60, https://doi.org/10.1080/0142159x.2018.1475727.

175. Thomas P. O'Toole et al., "Teaching Professionalism within a Community Context: Perspectives from a National Demonstration Project," *Academic Medicine* 80, no. 4 (2005): 339–43, https://doi.org/10.1097/00001888-200504000-00006.

176. Lara Varpio, Carol Aschenbrener, and Joanna Bates, "Tackling Wicked Problems: How Theories of Agency Can Provide New Insights," *Medical Education* 51, no. 4 (2017): 353–65, https://doi.org/10.1111/medu.13160.

177. Interprofessional Education Collaborative, *Core Competencies for Interprofessional Collaborative Practice: 2016 Update* (Washington, DC: Interprofessional Educational Collaborative, 2016), accessed May 31, 2021, https://www.ipecollaborative.org/ipec-core-competencies.

178. Sioban Nelson, Maria Tassone, and Brian D. Hodges, *Creating the Health Care Team of the Future: The Toronto Model for Interprofessional Education and Practice* (Ithaca, NY: Cornell University Press, 2014).

179. David P. Baker et al., "The Role of Teamwork in the Professional Education of Physicians: Current Status and Assessment Recommendations," *The Joint Commission Journal on Quality and Safety* 31, no. 4 (2005): 185–202, https://doi.org/10.1016/s1553-7250(05)31025-7.

180. Carolyn M. Clancy and David N. Tornberg, "TeamSTEPPS: Assuring Optimal Teamwork in Clinical Settings," *American Journal of Medical Quality* 34, no. 5 (2019): 436–38, https://doi.org/10.1177/1062860619873181.

181. Celeste M. Mayer et al., "Evaluating Efforts to Optimize TeamSTEPPS Implementation in Surgical and Pediatric Intensive Care Units," *Joint Commission Journal on Quality and Patient Safety* 37, no. 8 (2011): 365–74, https://doi.org/10.1016/s1553-7250(11)37047-x.

182. Bethany Robertson et al., "The Use of Simulation and a Modified TeamSTEPPS Curriculum for Medical and Nursing Student Team Training," *Simulation in Healthcare* 5, no. 6 (2010): 332–7. https://doi.org/10.1097/SIH.0b013e3181f008ad.

183. Maja Djukic et al., "NYU3T: Teaching, Technology, Teamwork: A Model for Interprofessional Education Scalability and Sustainability," *Nursing Clinics of North America* 47, no. 3 (2012): 333–46, https://doi.org/10.1016/j.cnur.2012.05.003.

184. Tammy Wang and Hiren Bhakta, "A New Model for Interprofessional Collaboration at a Student-Run Free Clinic," *Journal of Interprofessional Care* 27, no. 4 (2013): 339–40, https://doi.org/10.3109/13561820.2012.761598.

CHAPTER SIX

Step 5
Implementation

. . . making the curriculum a reality

Mark T. Hughes, MD, MA

IMPORTANCE

For a curriculum to achieve its potential, careful attention must be paid to issues of implementation. The curriculum developer must ensure that sufficient resources, political and financial support, and administrative structures have been developed to successfully implement the curriculum (Table 6.1).

Table 6.1.   Checklist for Implementation

_____ Identify resources
     _____ People: curriculum director(s), curriculum coordinator, faculty, administrative and other support staff (audiovisual, computing, information technology), learners, patients, virtual patients, standardized patients
     _____ Time: curriculum director, faculty, support staff, learners
     _____ Facilities/materials: space, clinical sites, clinical equipment, educational equipment (audio/visual, simulators), virtual space (servers, content management software)
     _____ Funding/costs: direct financial costs, hidden or opportunity costs, faculty compensation, costs of scholarship

_____ Obtain support
     _____ From: those with administrative authority (dean's office, health system administration, department chair, program director, division director, etc.), community partners, faculty, learners, other stakeholders
          _____ For: curricular time, personnel, resources, political support
     _____ From: government, professional societies, philanthropic organizations or foundations, accreditation bodies, other entities (e.g., health systems), individual donors
          _____ For: political support, external requirements, curricular or faculty development resources

_____ Develop administrative mechanisms to support the curriculum
     _____ Administrative structure: to delineate responsibilities and decision-making
     _____ Communication
           Content: rationale; goals and objectives; information about the curriculum, learners, faculty, facilities and equipment, scheduling; changes in the curriculum; evaluation results; etc.
           Mechanisms: websites, social media, memos, meetings, syllabus materials, site visits, reports, etc.
     _____ Operations: preparation and distribution of schedules and curricular materials; collection, collation, and distribution of evaluation data; curricular revisions and changes; integration with larger institutional program; etc.
     _____ Scholarship and educational research: plans for presenting and publishing about curriculum; human subjects protection considerations; approval from institutional review board, if necessary

_____ Anticipate and address barriers
     _____ Financial and other resources
     _____ Competing demands
     _____ People: attitudes, job/role security, power and authority, etc.

_____ Plan to introduce the curriculum
     _____ Pilot
     _____ Phase in and design thinking
     _____ Full implementation

_____ Plan for curriculum enhancement and maintenance
     _____ Continuous quality improvement

In many respects, Step 5 requires that the curriculum developer become a project manager, overseeing the people and operations that will successfully implement the curriculum.[1] Implementation involves generating support, planning for change, operationalizing the plan, and ensuring viability. Step 5 brings all the other steps in the curriculum development process to fruition. After problem identification, the general and targeted needs assessments (see Chapters 2 and 3) must be implemented with the aid of relevant stakeholders. Curricular goals, objectives, and educational strategies have to be clearly articulated to stakeholders (see Chapters 4 and 5). The actual implementation of the curriculum must attend to operational issues so that curriculum developers, learners, faculty, coordinators, and other support staff remain invested in the curriculum. Curriculum developers must assess for readiness to change, identify barriers and facilitators, engage influencers, and create collaborations to determine the best approaches for implementation.[2,3] Implementation must ensure viability of the curriculum by establishing procedures for evaluation and feedback, obtaining ongoing financial and administrative support, and planning for curriculum maintenance and enhancement (see Chapters 7 and 8). To successfully create and maintain a new curriculum or modify an established curriculum, curriculum developers can draw upon the lessons from diffusion of an innovation (see Chapter 9). Attention to the many aspects of implementation is critical when integrating multiple curricular components in a large program (see Chapter 10).

IDENTIFICATION OF RESOURCES

The curriculum developer must realistically assess the resources that will be required to implement the educational strategies (Chapter 5) and the evaluation (Chapter 7) planned for the curriculum. Resources include people, time, and facilities/materials. Funding is an important ingredient for all of these—without it, delivery of the curriculum may not be possible. Curriculum developers must not neglect their own cachet as a resource, because if it is expended, they and their curriculum can lose support.

People

The people involved in curriculum implementation include curriculum directors, curriculum coordinators, support staff, faculty, instructors, students, and patients. The curriculum developers often become the *curriculum directors* and need to have sufficient time dedicated in their schedules to oversee implementation of the curriculum. For large curricula involving many learners or extending over a long period of time, curriculum developers may need to hire a dedicated *curriculum coordinator*. For instance, in residency education, the Accreditation Council for Graduate Medical Education (ACGME) defines different role responsibilities for a program director and a program coordinator.[4] Coordinators, administrative assistants, and other support staff are usually needed to prepare budgets, curricular materials, and evaluation reports; coordinate and communicate schedules; collect evaluation data; and support learning activities. The curriculum team may need staff knowledgeable in learning management software, computing and information technology (IT) assistance, and audiovisual support.

Ideally, *faculty* and *instructors* will be available and skilled in both teaching and content. Faculty may be drawn from other disciplines, especially in interprofessional education. If there are insufficient numbers of skilled faculty, one must contemplate hiring new faculty or developing existing faculty.

EXAMPLE: *Hiring New Faculty in Response to the Needs Assessment.* A Master of Social Work program in the Four Corners region of Colorado created a partnership with the local Native Peoples community. An advisory council was formed to help inform the curriculum. Council members recommended that students get exposed to specialized knowledge and skills to serve the Native Peoples. The needs assessment also learned that students wanted more content on Native culture and practice. Two courses were developed, and in order to be true to the Native experience, stakeholders emphasized the need for the course to be taught by Native instructors. To accomplish this, the program brought in Native instructors from across the country, which has led to greater depth and understanding than what would have been possible with non-Native faculty.[5]

EXAMPLE: *Faculty Development to Deliver a High-Stakes Curriculum.* A curriculum to address racism, discrimination, and microaggressions uses a dramaturgical approach by developing scripts to depict real-life scenarios of discriminatory behavior. Learners use the "Observe/Why?/Think/Feel/Desire" communication tool to understand how to respond to a challenging situation. The curriculum requires skilled facilitators to create a safe space for open discussion. Curriculum developers emphasize the critical need to develop and recruit faculty with expertise in equity who can also create a trusting environment for dialogue, as good intentions without expertise or experience can cause damage to a fragile conversation.[6]

If properly trained, students can become another resource by serving as peer educators or facilitating learning sessions for junior colleagues.

The most important people to consider for the implementation of a curriculum are the learners. The targeted needs assessment should provide guidance on the best implementation approaches for the particular learners of a curriculum. The curriculum team and its partners may need to account for additional learners who will have access to the curriculum (e.g., making sure the online platform is robust enough to accommodate an increased number of learners) (see Chapter 3). Curriculum developers should also expect that some students will have difficulties and should therefore anticipate what resources will be needed to help students requiring remediation[7] (see Chapter 5).

For clinicians in training, *patients* may also be important people in the delivery of a curriculum. Depending on the goals and objectives, a clinical curriculum must have a suitable mix of patients.

EXAMPLE: *Case-Mix.* A musculoskeletal curriculum was developed for internal medicine residents. In a rheumatology rotation, the case-mix was concentrated on patients with inflammatory arthritis and connective tissue disease. Experiences in an orthopedic clinic involved a case-mix that included many postoperative patients. The general and targeted needs assessments found that residents needed to learn about musculoskeletal conditions commonly encountered in a primary care practice (e.g., shoulder pain, back pain, knee pain). In addition, learners wanted to practice examination maneuvers and diagnostic/therapeutic skills (e.g., arthrocentesis) that did not require specialist training. Therefore, curriculum developers created a musculoskeletal clinic for primary care patients with common joint and muscle complaints. The musculoskeletal clinic was staffed by attending general internists, who precepted residents as they saw patients referred by their usual general internal medicine provider.[8]

If the clinical environment is not conducive to the right mix of patients, or if learners have variable exposure to the right kind of clinical cases, an alternative strategy learned from Step 4 could be use of virtual patients. The curriculum development team will have to account for the costs associated with developing its own bank of virtual patients or subscribing to a known bank. For example, Regenstrief Institute has used profiles of 10,000 patients to create a teaching electronic medical record implemented in a variety of training programs.[9–11]

Sometimes, standardized patients (SPs) can help meet the need for a range of clinical experiences and can augment education by providing opportunities for practice and feedback. The decision to include SPs usually incurs costs for recruitment, training, and hourly compensation, and therefore requires careful planning.

EXAMPLE: *Identifying SP Needs for a New Curriculum.* Evaluations from an existing course preparing fourth-year medical students for internship indicated that the informed consent lecture was not meeting students' needs. Consequently, a new skills-based curriculum was developed using SPs in the clinical scenario of informed consent for placement of a central venous access device. SPs portray a patient newly admitted to the intensive care unit and are trained on how to respond to the student's disclosure of information. To deliver the curriculum to 120 students in two days during the course (six hours per day), 15 SPs were recruited and trained. Ten encounters between an SP and student run concurrently each hour. After the encounter, the SPs provide the students with performance feedback and then each group of 10 students meets with a faculty facilitator to debrief the session for take-home points.

Time

Curriculum developers need time to develop the curriculum, and they often become curriculum directors once it is developed. In implementing the curriculum, curriculum directors need time to coordinate management of the curriculum, which includes working with support staff to be sure that faculty are teaching, learners are participating, and process objectives are being met.

Faculty require time to prepare and teach. Generally, for each increment of contact time with a learner (in-person or asynchronous), at least several times that amount of time will be needed to develop the content and educational strategy. Time should also be budgeted for faculty to provide formative feedback to learners and summative evaluations of the learners and of the curriculum to curriculum developers. As much as possible, curriculum directors should ease the amount of work required of faculty. If curriculum directors or their staff manage the logistics of the curriculum (scheduling, distribution of electronic or paper-based curricular materials, training of SPs, etc.), then faculty can concentrate on delivering the curriculum articulated in the goals and objectives.

For curriculum directors and faculty who have other responsibilities (e.g., meeting clinical productivity expectations), the implementation plan must include ways to compensate, reward, and/or accommodate faculty for the time they devote to the curriculum. Volunteer medical faculty may be most motivated by the personal satisfaction of giving back to the profession, but they may also appreciate opportunities for continuing education, academic appointments, awards or other forms of recognition, or compensation for lost clinical productivity.[12,13] For salaried faculty, educational relative value units (RVUs) can be one way to acknowledge their time commitment to educational endeavors (see below).

Learners require time not only to attend scheduled learning activities but also to read, reflect, do independent learning, and apply what they have learned. As part of the targeted needs assessment (Chapter 3), curriculum developers should become familiar with the learners' schedule and understand what barriers exist for participation in the curriculum. For instance, postgraduate medical trainees may have to meet expectations on regulatory work hour limits.

Support staff members need time to perform their functions. Clearly delineating their responsibilities can help to budget the amount of time they require for curriculum implementation.

If educational research is to be performed as part of the general or targeted needs assessment (see Chapters 2 and 3) or curriculum evaluation (see Chapter 7), curriculum developers should budget time for review and approval of the research plans by an institutional review board (IRB). Curriculum developers should anticipate sufficient lead time to work through the IRB application process, with an awareness of the usual amount of time needed to work with the IRB (or multiple IRBs) and ongoing communication with IRB staff (see below).

Facilities/Materials

Curricula require facilities (physical or virtual space) and materials (ranging from books to clinical equipment). The simplest curriculum may require only a room in which to meet or lecture. Other physical spaces could include lecture halls, laboratory spaces, simulation centers, or clinical settings. Physical facilities may need to be equipped with technology. For virtual meeting spaces, curriculum developers must account for implementation of necessary hardware or software and the bandwidth and internet capabilities of remote learners (e.g., are they accessing the curriculum on mobile devices, tablets, or laptops?). Accommodations may be needed so all learners can participate fully in the curriculum (e.g., including closed captioning for deaf and hard of hearing students). Curriculum developers should prepare for unexpected events and consider optional facilities for delivery of the curriculum.

With the increasing use of online learning, the curriculum team will need to know what resources are necessary to deliver content synchronously or asynchronously and how much IT support is required. The rationale for online learning should be carefully considered, and its advantages should be harnessed—it is not a prime use of technology to just deliver content remotely that would otherwise be provided in person. The implementation team may need to involve subject matter experts, project managers, instructional designers, multimedia technicians, and web designers to provide end-user support.[14] Copyright issues for online content or format may require legal guidance. Online learning platforms may need to be licensed.

> **EXAMPLE:** *Identification and Use of Learning Management System.* Based on accreditation standards and a targeted needs assessment, curriculum developers designed online modules to highlight key concepts in clinical teaching. They secured funding from the medical school for salary support and production of modules on the one-minute preceptor, chalk talks, and coaching. The curriculum developers worked with an instructional designer to identify an appropriate online learning platform that integrated video content and didactic and assessment methods.[15]

The educational strategies may include development or integration of a massive open online course (MOOC).[16,17] Use of a MOOC entails building capacity in the targeted learning environment at four levels: (1) structures, systems, and roles, (2) staff and facilities, (3) skills, and (4) tools.[18]

Clinical curricula often require access to patients and must provide learners with clinical facilities and equipment. A curriculum that addresses acquisition of clinical knowledge or skills may need a clinical site that can accommodate learners and provide the appropriate volume and mix of patients to ensure a valuable clinical experience. Logistical planning for use of a clinical site should include attention to issues such as the need for credentialing, regulatory requirements (e.g., HIPAA training), background checks, immunizations, and mode of travel to the site. Enough time should be budgeted to ensure clinical sites are ready to receive learners.

EXAMPLE: *Logistical Issues in Implementing an Interprofessional Curriculum at a Clinical Site.* To teach nurse practitioner (NP) and physician trainees how to practice together effectively, a dyad model was established in an ambulatory setting. Implementation of the curriculum took four months and involved creation of workgroups with representatives from medicine, nursing, evaluation, and medical center administration. Logistical issues were worked out through a pilot program. Curricular staff pair one NP student with one resident physician. Ambulatory clinic schedules are coordinated to permit the dyad to see four patients in hour-long visits during a half-day clinic session. Normally a resident physician would be expected to see six patients per session. An NP student may be paired with four different residents in a 12-month period. By having residents serve as teachers to the NP students, clinics were able to increase the number of learners without increasing the number of preceptors.[19]

Other curricula may need special educational resources, such as audio or video equipment, computers, software, clinical devices, simulators, or artificial models to teach clinical skills.

EXAMPLE: *Training in Point-of-Care Ultrasound (POCUS).* An internal medicine training program developed a curriculum in POCUS. Ultrasound sessions were integrated into trainees' academic half-days and were taught by subspecialists with POCUS expertise. Six ultrasound machines with appropriate ultrasound probes for several different examinations were stationed in three simulation rooms. Standardized patients and interactive manikins were used for the small-group scanning exercises.[20]

Implementing simulation-based health care education may require facilities such as a simulation center or materials such as manikins that can give learners hands-on experience with realistic clinical scenarios.

EXAMPLE: *Use of Simulation.* The Simulated Trauma and Resuscitation Team Training (STARTT) curriculum teaches crisis resource management skills using simulation.[21] To teach communication skills in handoffs, curriculum developers included prehospital personnel (a helicopter flight nurse and paramedic) in the trauma team simulations. Four scenarios were developed, ranging from picking up a trauma patient at a rural center to mass casualty events. To simulate traveling to or from a remote site, participants moved to different rooms in the simulation center and communicated with trauma teams by handheld radio. High-fidelity trauma simulations were delivered using a simulation manikin.[22]

Use of video as an educational strategy, whether "homemade" or from a reliable source, will need to account for production value, file size, duration, and accessibility.[23] Producing one's own video can entail cost and time commitment, and curriculum developers will need to consider implementation factors, such as video equipment, scripting, sound-proof location, editing, and hosting capabilities.[24]

EXAMPLE: *Creation of Videos for Faculty Development.* As part of a curriculum on conflict resolution for fourth-year medical students in a transition-to-residency course, curriculum developers created videos of simulated encounters. In the curriculum, students conduct a simulated encounter that is videotaped, and they then watch it with a faculty coach for self-reflection and mentored feedback. To prepare faculty on how to provide feedback about conflict resolution styles and best strategies, curriculum developers recruited volunteer students to enact an encounter involving a conflict with a nurse. Practicing nurses trained as SPs played the role of nurse. Video-recorded encounters were debriefed by faculty to reach consensus on entrustable behaviors.[25]

EXAMPLE: *Integration of Virtual Reality.* As part of a curriculum on health equity for medical school and health system leaders, faculty, and staff who interact with learners, curriculum developers incorporated a virtual reality (VR) experience into the training. In addition to attending a large group discussion about microaggressions, each participant individually experienced a 20-minute VR module. The immersive module *1000 Cut Journey* follows the protagonist at three points in his life when he experiences racism. To implement the VR experience, the curriculum team needed to put in place a small, quiet room with electrical outlets, a desk for a laptop, the VR software, the mobile headset and handheld controllers, and a traIned VR staff person.[20]

Appendix A describes the development of a neurology graduate training program, detailing the extensive resources needed, including clinical facilities, didactic facilities, personal hotspots for trainees to access virtual resources, and cloud accounts to store and deliver didactic material.

Funding/Costs

Curriculum developers must consider both financial and opportunity costs in implementing the curriculum. Some of these costs will have been identified in the targeted needs assessment and in the identification of the people, time, facilities, and materials needed for implementation. These costs need to be accounted for to determine how a curriculum is to be funded and implemented. The Association of American Medical Colleges (AAMC) adapted a model from the business industry to encourage undergraduate medical educators to assess the relative costs of all aspects of the intervention and steward resources prudently. The Business Model Canvas for Medical Educators challenges educators to consider, in a systematic fashion, the return on their investment.[27] In addition to identifying key resources and their costs, the model encourages educators to consider funding opportunities such as grants and student tuition. Sometimes, curricula can be accomplished by redeploying existing resources. If this appears to be the case, one should ask what will be given up in redeploying the resources (i.e., what is the hidden or opportunity cost of the curriculum?).

> **EXAMPLE:** *Financial Support and Opportunity Costs of a New Curriculum.* In creating a two-day patient safety course for second-year medical students as preparation for their clinical clerkships, curriculum developers sought internal funding from the hospital's Center for Innovation and Safety. The curriculum recruited faculty to lead discussions of hospital patient safety initiatives, the strengths of high-reliability teamwork, and effective team communications. Simulation center activities included stations dedicated to basic cardiac life support, sterile technique, infection control procedures, and isolation practices. In addition to obtaining financial support, curriculum developers had to obtain permission from faculty leaders in the medical students' pathophysiology course to allow students to attend the clerkship preparation course (opportunity cost).

When additional resources are required, they must be provided from somewhere. If additional funding is requested, it is necessary to develop and justify a budget.

As a project manager, the curriculum developer will need to oversee the budgetary process. The curriculum team will need to itemize facility fees, equipment and supply costs, and personnel compensation. Costs for personnel, including curriculum directors, curriculum coordinators, faculty, administrative staff, and others, often represent the biggest budget item. Often, compensation will be based on the percentage of time devoted to curricular activities relative to full-time equivalents (FTEs). Researchers and consensus panels have attempted to define amount of effort and adequate compensation for various curricular roles.[28-31] One important consideration for faculty support is whether they are being compensated through other funding sources—for basic science faculty, this can come in the form of research grants or school investments;[32] for clinical faculty, the funding may come from billable patient care revenues.[33] Educational or academic RVUs serve as a method to quantify the effort educators put toward curricular activities.[34-36] Calculating educational RVUs can take into account factors such as the time required by the activity, the level of learner, the complexity of the teaching, the level of faculty expertise, and the quality of teaching.[34] Financially compensating faculty for educational RVUs can incentivize them to complete tasks such as filling out learner evaluations and attending didactic sessions.[37–39] The curriculum developer can present a sound budget justification if these factors are considered in the implementation plan.

Curriculum developers must also be cognizant of the financial costs of conducting educational scholarship (see Chapter 9). In addition to whatever funds are needed to deliver the curriculum, funds may also be necessary to perform robust curriculum evaluation with a view toward dissemination of the curriculum. It has been shown that manuscripts reporting on well-funded curricula are of better quality and have higher rates of acceptance for publication in a peer-reviewed journal.[40,41]

Research and development grants may be available from one's own institution. Summer student stipends can support student assistance in curricular development or evaluation activities. Sometimes there are insufficient institutional resources to support part or all of a curriculum or to support its further development or expansion. In these situations, developing a sound budget and seeking a source of external support are critical.

Potential sources of *external funding* (see Appendix B) include government agencies, professional societies, private funders like philanthropic organizations or foundations, corporate entities, and individual donors.

EXAMPLE: *Initial Philanthropic Support Leading Stakeholder to Expand Program.* With a visionary philanthropic gift, the Center for Innovative Medicine, at the Johns Hopkins Bayview Medical Center, launched the Aliki Initiative. By assigning one inpatient medical housestaff team a lower patient census, residents had more time to focus on patient-centered care activities, such as enhanced communication skills, help with transitions of care, and more attention to medication adherence. Higher satisfaction rates among patients and housestaff and improved clinical outcomes were observed compared with standard housestaff teams.[42] Due to the early success of the initiative, hospital and residency program administrators supported incorporation of the patient-centered housestaff team as an important component in the overall residency curriculum.[43]

External funding may be more justifiable when the funding is legitimately not available from internal sources. External funds are more likely to be obtained when there has been a request for proposals, or a funding source has specific focus areas. For example, the Josiah Macy Jr. Foundation has three priority areas: promoting diversity, equity, and belonging; increasing collaboration among future health professionals; and preparing future health professionals to navigate ethical dilemmas.[44] Curriculum developers may also find success with external funding when support is requested for an innovative or particularly needed curriculum.

EXAMPLE: *Combination of Internal and External Support.* The Urban Health Residency Primary Care Track of the Johns Hopkins University Osler Medical Housestaff Training Program was developed to help train physician primary care leaders whose focus would be on the medical and social issues affecting underserved and vulnerable populations in urban settings. The school of medicine program partnered with the schools of nursing and public health, the university's Urban Health Institute, the county health department, community-based organizations, and multiple community-based health centers to provide this novel training experience. In addition to hospital and departmental financial support, initial funding came from a university-based foundation, the Osler Center for Clinical Excellence, and the Josiah Macy Jr. Foundation. Subsequent funding came from federal grants through the Affordable Care Act to cover the costs of resident salaries and insurance and other residency-related expenditures.[45]

A period of external funding can be used to build a level of internal support that may sustain the curriculum after cessation of the external funding.

> **EXAMPLE:** *Foundation Support for Faculty Leading to Internal Support.* Bioethics faculty who were designing clinical ethics curricula in postgraduate education obtained philanthropic support from two foundations for their work. The salary support lasted several years, during which time the faculty members successfully implemented curricula for residency programs in medicine, pediatrics, surgery, obstetrics-gynecology, and neurology. The funding also allowed them time to publish educational research about their work. The success of their curricular program led to institutional financial support as an annual line item in the hospital budget, permitting the faculty to sustain and expand their curricular efforts once one of the foundational grants expired.

Finally, professional societies or other institutions may have *curricular or faculty development resources* that can be used by curriculum developers to defray some of the costs of developing a curriculum (see Appendix B). It may be necessary to get legal permission or purchase a subscription to use an established learning platform, but this may be less costly than creating the curriculum de novo.

OBTAINING SUPPORT FOR THE CURRICULUM

Stakeholders

A curriculum is more likely to be successful in achieving its goals and objectives if it has broad support. It is important that curriculum developers and coordinators recognize who the stakeholders are in a curriculum and foster their support. Stakeholders are those individuals who directly affect, or are directly affected by, a curriculum. For most curricula, stakeholders include the learners, the faculty who will deliver the curriculum, and individuals with administrative power within the institution. Community partners may also be supportive of curricular efforts.

Having the support of *learners* when implementing the curriculum can make or break the curriculum. They can be change agents for a curriculum.[27] Adult learners, in particular, need to be convinced that the goals and objectives are important to them and that the curriculum has the means to achieve their personal goals.[46,47] Diffusion of a biomedical innovation requires triggering a demand through a combination of "push" and "pull" — the "push" is the evidence-based knowledge, and the "pull" is the need and desire of the health care provider to change their practice.[48] Once a curriculum is established, learners serve a vital role in its maintenance and enhancement by providing feedback.[49,50]

> **EXAMPLE:** *Feedback from Learners to Modify Course.* Based on pharmacy student feedback and evaluation over a five-year period, a Top Drugs course evolved from poor ratings to high ratings. The course started as a self-paced course covering 200 drugs with no alignment to other coursework. Free text comments in evaluations and verbal feedback from student leaders reflected negative perceptions of the course's relevance and value. Course directors redesigned the course to cover a smaller number of drugs each week, increase the number of examinations, conduct review sessions to reinforce concepts, and introduce active learning strategies. The school's curriculum committee moved the course from first year to second year to better align it with pharmacology course work. Students reported enhanced learning and greater satisfaction.[51]

Learners' opinions can influence those with administrative power.

> **EXAMPLE:** *Support of Learners.* Curriculum developers created a capstone course for fourth-year medical students to prepare them at the start of their professional lives to acquire the knowledge, skills, and

attitudes necessary to be successful physicians. The curriculum was initially offered as an elective and then refined over a several-year period based on learner feedback. Overall, students who elected to take the course rated it highly, convincing school administrators to make it a mandatory course for all fourth-year students before graduation.

Curricular faculty can devote varying amounts of their time, enthusiasm, and energy to the curriculum. Gaining broad faculty support may be important for some innovative curricula, especially when the curriculum will cross disciplines or specialties.

EXAMPLE: *Fostering Faculty Champions for an Interprofessional Curriculum.* In developing an interdisciplinary training program for substance use disorder screening and treatment, curriculum developers used implementation science to create a council of directors. The council was composed of department heads from participating disciplines and served as a steering committee for the curriculum. Inclusion of program leaders facilitated cross-departmental collaborations and communication. The project implementation team conducted site visits to talk with local faculty about their capacity to implement the training. Faculty champions for the curriculum were identified, and their partnership fostered greater interprofessional collaboration, allowing faculty to teach across specialties.[52]

Other faculty who have administrative influence or who also need curricular space or time in the broader educational mission should be sought as partners in the curriculum.

Those with administrative authority (e.g., dean, hospital administrators, department chair, program director, division director) can allocate or deny the funds, space, faculty time, curricular time, and political support that are critical to a curriculum.

EXAMPLE: *Administrative Support of a New Curriculum.* A task force of university faculty from multiple specialties was convened by the dean of the school and tasked with developing curricular innovations in graduate medical education (GME). The task force identified patient handoffs as a focus area. The targeted needs assessment found that nearly half of residents felt that patient information was lost during shift changes and that unit-to-unit transfers were a source of problems. It was also recognized that duty-hour restrictions would increase the number of handoffs between residents. Consequently, the task force met regularly to discuss educational strategies. Funding did not permit direct observation and feedback of patient handoffs, but the task force obtained funding from the GME office and dean's office to develop a curriculum to be delivered during intern orientation.[53]

Negotiation

Curriculum developers may need to *negotiate* with key stakeholders to obtain the political support and resources required to implement their curriculum successfully. Development of skills related to negotiation can therefore be useful. There are five generally recognized modes for conflict management.[54,55] A *collaborative* or principled negotiation style that focuses on interests, not positions, is most frequently useful.[56] When negotiating with those who have power or influence, this model would advise the curriculum developer to find areas of common ground, to understand the needs of the other party, and to focus on mutual interests, rather than negotiating from fixed positions. Most of the examples provided in this section have ingredients of a collaborative approach, in which the goal is a win-win solution. Sometimes one must settle for a *compromise* (less than ideal, better than nothing) solution. Occasionally, the curriculum developer may need to *compete* for resources and support, which creates the possibility of either winning or losing. At other times, *avoidance* or *accommodation* may be the most reasonable approach, at least for certain aspects of the curriculum implementation. By engaging stakeholders, addressing their needs, providing a strong rationale, providing needs assessment and evaluation data, and building broad-based political support, curriculum developers put themselves in an advantageous bargaining position.

Change Agency

In some situations, the curriculum developer must be a *change agent* to champion curricular innovation at an institution. It helps if a new curriculum is consistent with the institution's mission, goals, and culture and if the institution is open to educational innovation.[57] When this alignment is not in place or resistance is met, the curriculum developer must become an agent of change[58-60] (see Chapter 10).

> **EXAMPLE:** *Developing Faculty as Agents of Change.* San Francisco State University partnered with the University of California at San Francisco to create SF BUILD, a program to build institutional infrastructure leading to increased diversity in the sciences. Rather than "fixing the student," SF BUILD aims to "fix the institution" by cultivating a community of change agents. In addition to training faculty about the effects of stereotyping on the experiences of underrepresented students, the program established the Faculty Agents of Change Initiative. The initiative consists of faculty groups who are committed to be communities of transformation. They collaborate to advance curricular change for social justice pedagogy in science and shift the culture of science in teaching and research.[61]

Organizational change can occur when the curriculum developer is intentional about creating a vision but also flexible in how the vision comes to fruition.[58,59]

Individuals who feel that a curriculum is important, effective, and popular, who believe that a curriculum positively affects them or their institution, and who have had input into that curriculum are more likely to support it. It is, therefore, helpful to *encourage input* from stakeholders as the curriculum is being planned, as well as to *provide* stakeholders with the appropriate *rationale* (see Chapters 2 and 3) and *evaluation data* (Chapter 7) to address their concerns.

Curriculum developers can also look outside their institution to find support for the curriculum. Government, professional societies, and other entities may have *influence*, through their political or funding power, that can affect the degree of internal support for a curriculum. Accrediting bodies may support innovative curricula through demonstration projects or provide previously developed curricular resources (see Appendix B). The curriculum developer may want to bring guidelines or requirements of such bodies to the attention of stakeholders within their own institution.

> **EXAMPLE:** *Accreditation Standards.* The Interprofessional Education Collaborative (IPEC) was formed in 2009 with representation from six health professions, and nine other professions joined the collaborative in 2016. IPEC has published core competencies for interprofessional collaborative practice to guide curriculum development across health professions schools.[62] Guidelines for medical schools published by the Liaison Committee on Medical Education (LCME) support medical student preparation to function as members of health care teams. Curricular experiences should include participation by students and/or practitioners from the other health professions.[63] The guidelines promulgated by these organizations provide a strong impetus for health professional schools to work together in delivering mutually advantageous, collaborative, interprofessional curricula.

ADMINISTRATION OF THE CURRICULUM

Administrative Structure

A curriculum does not operate by itself. It requires an administrative structure to assume responsibility, to maintain communication, and to make operational and policy decisions. Often these functions are performed by the curriculum director, but it may be helpful to have a curriculum team consisting of core faculty, an administrator, a coordinator, and other support staff. Larger curricula naturally need more administrative support. Some types of decisions can be delegated to a curriculum administrator for segments of the curriculum. Operation of a curriculum can be managed by a curriculum coordinator. Major policy or operational changes may best be made with the help of a core faculty group and input from other stakeholders. A structure for efficient communication and decision-making should be established and made clear to faculty, learners, and support staff.

The administrative structure of the curriculum must be responsive to larger institutional governance and policy considerations (see Chapter 10). The curriculum team must understand how the curriculum integrates with the overall educational program. Standards may be established across curricula for timing and availability of syllabi, curricular hours (e.g., scheduling limits for clinical activities), use of external learning sites (e.g., clinical or community venues), examination and evaluation structures, and performance outcomes. An institution or program may have centralized evaluation personnel or software that the curriculum team will need to use. The curriculum team may need to have representation on institutional committees that address curricular performance, feedback, learner promotion, and remediation.

Communication

The rationale, goals, and objectives of the curriculum, evaluation results, and changes in the curriculum need to be communicated in appropriate detail to all involved stakeholders. Lines of communication need to be open to and from stakeholders. Therefore, the curriculum coordinator needs to establish *mechanisms for communication*, such as a website, social media memos, periodic meetings, syllabi, presentations, site visits or observations, and annual reports. Curriculum coordinators should establish a policy regarding their accessibility to learners, faculty, and other stakeholders.

Operations

Mechanisms need to be developed to ensure that important functions that support the curriculum are performed. Such functions include preparing and distributing schedules and curricular materials, collecting and collating evaluation data, supporting the communication function of the curriculum director, and implementing contingency plans when the need arises. The operations component of the curriculum implementation is where decisions by the curriculum director or administrators are put into action (e.g., whom should one talk to about a problem with the curriculum? When should syllabus material be distributed? When, where, and how will evaluation data be collected? Should there be a midpoint change in curricular content? Should a learner be assigned to a different faculty member?). Some functions can be delegated to support staff, but they still need to be supervised in their performance.

EXAMPLE: *Operation of a School-Wide Curriculum*. A course on research ethics for principal investigators and members of the research team in a medical school is coordinated through the combined efforts of the Office of Research Administration and the Office of Continuing Medical Education. An overall course director delegates operational functions to support staff from both offices while serving as a point person for learners and faculty. Support staff in the Office of Research Administration administer the online curricular materials, while a course administrator in the Office of Continuing Medical Education communicates with learners and coordinates the course logistics (registering learners, distributing syllabus materials, scheduling classroom space or synchronous online sessions, confirming faculty availability, collecting and analyzing evaluations, obtaining annual certification of the course, etc.).

Scholarship and Educational Research

As discussed in Chapter 9, curriculum developers may wish to disseminate, through presentation or publication, information related to their curricula, such as the needs assessment, curricular methods, or curricular evaluations. When dissemination is a goal, additional resources and administration may be required for more rigorous needs assessments, educational methodology, evaluation designs, data collection and analysis, and/or assessment instruments.

Curriculum developers also must address ethical issues related to research (see Chapter 7). Issues such as informed consent of learners, confidentiality, and the use of incentives to encourage participation in a curriculum all need to be considered.[64,65] An important consideration is whether learners are to be classified as human research subjects. Federal regulations governing research in the United States categorize many educational research projects as exempt from the regulations if the research involves the study of normal educational practices or records information about learners in such a way that they cannot be identified.[66] However, IRBs may differ in their interpretation of what is exempt under the regulations.[67,68] Some IRBs may want to ensure additional safeguards for learners besides those that the regulations require. It is, therefore, prudent for curriculum developers to seek guidance from their IRBs about how best to protect the rights and interests of learners who are also research subjects.[69–71] Failure to consult one's IRB before implementation of the curriculum can have adverse consequences for the curriculum developer who later tries to publish research about the curriculum.[72]

ANTICIPATING BARRIERS

Before initiating a new curriculum or making changes in an old curriculum, it is helpful to anticipate and address any potential barriers. Barriers can relate to finances, other resources, people, or unforeseen circumstances (e.g., competing demands for resources; unsupportive attitudes of learners or other faculty; issues of job or role security, credit, and political power; weather or health emergencies). Time can also pose a barrier, such as carving out curricular time when health professional students are dispersed at different clinical sites or residents are not available to attend teaching sessions because of duty-hour restrictions.

EXAMPLE: *Competition.* In planning the ambulatory component of the internal medicine clerkship for third-year medical students, the curriculum developer anticipated resistance from the inpatient clerkship director, based on loss of curricular time and responsibility/power. The curriculum developer built a well-reasoned argument for the ambulatory component based on external recommendations and current needs. She ensured student support for the change and the support of critical faculty. She gained support from the dean's office and was granted additional curricular time for the ambulatory component, which addressed some of the inpatient director's concerns about loss of curricular time for training on the inpatient services. She invited the inpatient coordinator to be on the planning committee for the ambulatory component to increase his understanding of needs, to promote his sense of ownership and responsibility for the ambulatory component, and to promote coordination of learning and educational methodology between the inpatient and ambulatory components.

EXAMPLE: *Resistance.* The developers of a tool to evaluate the surgical skills of plastic surgery residents anticipated incomplete faculty evaluations if they were required after each surgery. They created a brief, web-accessible tool to document the trainee's level of operative autonomy. Using a smartphone, tablet, or computer, the resident completes a self-assessment score postoperatively, and then the attending can submit the evaluator score immediately after the resident or at a later time.[73] It was found that the faculty evaluation maintained its reliability if completed within two weeks of the resident self-assessment.[74]

INTRODUCING THE CURRICULUM

Piloting

It is important to pilot critical segments of a new curriculum on friendly or convenient audiences before formally introducing it. Critical segments might include needs assessment and evaluation instruments, as well as educational methods. Piloting on a small group of people before rolling out the segment or entire curriculum to learners enables curriculum developers to receive critical feedback and to make important revisions that increase the likelihood of successful implementation.

> **EXAMPLE:** *Piloting a Holographic Anatomy Program to Supplement Cadaveric Dissection.* Volunteer first-year medical students were recruited to pilot test holographic software covering three anatomic dissections (thorax, abdomen, and pelvis and perineum). The learning material supplemented reviews conducted by faculty facilitators for each anatomic block, and the students were asked to rate and provide open-ended feedback on the instructional value of the software and hardware. Students expressed enthusiasm for the program and a desire to use it to supplement their anatomy reviews. Piloting revealed physical complaints with viewing the holographic images, including headache, nausea, eye fatigue, and neck strain. Image brightness, pupillary distance, and time spent viewing images needed to be adjusted to optimize the learning experience.[75]

Phasing In and Design Thinking

Phasing in a complex curriculum one part at a time, or the entire curriculum on a segment of the targeted learners, permits a focusing of initial efforts as faculty and staff learn new procedures. When the curriculum represents a cultural shift in an institution or requires attitudinal changes in the stakeholders, introducing the curriculum one step at a time, rather than all at once, can lessen resistance and increase acceptance, particularly if the stakeholders are involved in the process.[58] Like piloting, phasing in affords the opportunity to have a cycle of experience, feedback, evaluation, and response before full implementation.

> **EXAMPLE:** *Phasing In a New Interprofessional Curriculum.* Curriculum developers designing a curriculum in spiritual care for medical residents and chaplain trainees viewed involvement of the chaplain trainees in medical rounds as a key educational strategy. This strategy was introduced on a medical service dedicated to a more holistic approach to patient care. Two successive groups of chaplain trainees rotated through the medical service, attending rounds with the resident team, before the entire curriculum was fully implemented in the following year.[76]

Use of design thinking principles can be another means of phasing in curricular ideas through creativity and teamwork[2,3,77–79] (see Chapter 8). Among the five stages of design thinking are experimentation (developing and testing prototypes) and evolution (selecting most promising approaches based on feedback).[80]

> **EXAMPLE:** *Using Design Thinking to Develop a Well-Being Intervention.* Interested internal medicine residents were invited to participate in a program to learn and apply the design thinking approach. Residents interviewed stakeholders (other residents and friends/family members of residents) to gain a deeper understanding of well-being. Field notes led to themes, and then design teams of four to five residents brainstormed solutions. Prototypes were developed and refined based on feedback. The residency program phased in support communities, which were later adapted to one-on-one peer support pairings.[81]

Both the piloting and phasing-in approaches to implementing a curriculum advertise it as a curriculum in development, increase participants' tolerance and desire to help, decrease faculty resistance to negative feedback, increase the chance for success on full implementation, and set the stage for continuous quality improvement once the curriculum is established.

Full Implementation

In general, full implementation should follow a piloting and/or phasing-in experience. Sometimes, however, the demand for a full curriculum for all learners is so pressing, or a curriculum is so limited in scope, that immediate full implementation is preferable. In this case, the first cycle of the curriculum can be considered a "pilot" cycle. Evaluation data on educational outcomes (i.e., achievement of goals and objectives) and processes (i.e., milestones of curriculum delivery) from initial cycles of a curriculum can then be used to refine the implementation of subsequent cycles (see Chapter 7). Of course, a successful curriculum should always be in a stage of continuous quality improvement (CQI), as described in Chapter 8 and Chapter 10.

> **EXAMPLE**: *Implementing a Curriculum to Teach Surgeons High-Stakes Communication Skills.* Curriculum developers created a curriculum to teach surgeons how to conduct preference-sensitive, shared decision-making conversations in the setting of critical illness. They developed a communication tool called Best Case/Worst Case (BC/WC), which is a graphic aid to illustrate treatment options, express uncertainty, and provide prognostic information. They trained three cohorts of surgery residents and fellows and iteratively revised the curriculum based on process evaluations, performance data, coaches' debriefing, and learner feedback.[82] Curriculum developers subsequently created and disseminated training materials to other institutions.[83]

Full implementation of an entire school curriculum involves coordination of multiple moving parts (see Chapter 10). For instance, at Johns Hopkins University School of Medicine, the governance structure includes an integration committee to oversee implementation and evaluation of the four-year curriculum, a committee to manage clinical portions of the curriculum, and the Student Assessment and Program Evaluation (SAPE) Committee to verify program objectives are implemented and assessed effectively and to facilitate curricular CQI in response to evaluation data.[84]

INTERACTION WITH OTHER STEPS

On thinking through what is required to implement a curriculum, the curriculum developer should use the insights about the targeted learners and their learning environment from Step 2 to prioritize and focus the curricular objectives (Step 3), educational strategies (Step 4), and/or evaluation and feedback methods (Step 6) based on the available resources and administrative structure. It is better to anticipate problems than to discover them too late.

Curriculum development is an interactive, cyclical process, and each step affects the others. It may be more prudent to start small and build on a curriculum's success than to aim too high and watch the curriculum fail due to unachievable goals, insufficient resources, or inadequate support. The curriculum developer should also appreciate that the iterative process permits some degree of failure if one can learn from the mistakes and stay committed to moving the curriculum forward. *Implementation is the step that converts a mental exercise to reality.*

QUESTIONS

For the curriculum you are coordinating, planning, or would like to be planning, please answer or think about the questions below. If your thoughts about a curriculum are just beginning, you may wish to answer these questions in the context of a few educational strategies, such as the ones you identified in your answers to the questions at the end of Chapter 5.

1. What *resources* are required for the curriculum you envision, in terms of people, time, and facilities? Will your faculty need specialized training before implementation? Did you remember to think of patients as well as faculty and support staff? What is the anticipated budget for the curriculum? What are the costs of this curriculum? Is there a need for external funding? Finally, are your curricular plans feasible in terms of the required resources?

2. What is the degree of *support* within your institution for the curriculum? Where will the resistance come from? How could you increase support and decrease resistance? How likely is it that you will get the support necessary? Will external support be necessary? If so, what are some possible sources and what is the nature of the support that is required (e.g., resource materials, accreditation requirements, political support)?

3. What sort of *administration*, in terms of *administrative structure, communications, operations, and scholarship*, is necessary to implement and maintain the curriculum? How will decisions be made, how will communication take place, and what operations are necessary for the smooth functioning of the curriculum (e.g., preparation and distribution of schedules, curricular and evaluation materials, evaluation reports)? Are IRB review and approval of an educational research project needed?

4. What *barriers* do you anticipate to implementing the curriculum? Develop plans for addressing them.

5. Develop plans to *introduce* the curriculum. What are the most critical segments of the curriculum that would be a priority for *piloting*? On whom would you pilot it? Can the curriculum be *phased in*, or must it be implemented all at once on all learners? How will you learn from piloting and phasing in the curriculum and apply this learning to the curriculum? If you are planning on full implementation, what structures are in place to provide feedback on the curriculum for further improvements?

6. Given your answers to Questions 1 through 5, is your curriculum likely to be feasible and successful? Do you need to go back to the drawing board and alter your approach to some of the steps?

GENERAL REFERENCES

Glanz, Karen, Barbara K. Rimer, and K. Viswanath, eds. *Health Behavior and Health Education: Theory, Research, and Practice*. 5th ed. San Francisco: Jossey-Bass, 2015.
    This book reviews theories and models for behavioral change important in delivering health education. Health education involves an awareness of the impact of communication, interpersonal relationships, and community on those who are targeted for behavioral change. For the curriculum

developer, the chapters on diffusion of innovations and change theory are particularly relevant. Chapter 16 (pp. 301–26) describes theories about diffusion of innovations, dissemination and implementation, and how to operationalize innovations. Chapter 19 (pp. 359–87) discusses change theory and methods, including the PRECEDE-PROCEED method and intervention mapping. 486 pages.

Heagney, Joseph. *Fundamentals of Project Management*. 5th ed. New York: American Management Association, 2016.
An introduction to the principles and practice of project management, offering a step-by-step approach and useful tips in planning and executing a project. The suggestions on how to function as a project leader can be helpful for the curriculum developer to enable successful implementation of a curriculum. 231 pages.

Kalet, Adina, and Calvin L. Chou, eds. *Remediation in Medical Education: A Mid-course Correction*. New York: Springer, 2014.
This text focuses on competency-based education and steps that should be taken throughout a curriculum to assess and remediate difficulties students may experience in achieving academic success. For curriculum implementation, the book provides examples and strategies from a variety of institutions and perspectives. 367 pages.

Kotter, John P. *Leading Change*. Boston: Harvard Business Review Press, 2012.
An excellent book on leadership, differentiating between leadership and management, and outlining the qualities of a good leader. The author discusses eight steps critical to creating major change in an organization: (1) establishing a sense of urgency, (2) creating the guiding coalition, (3) developing a vision and strategy, (4) communicating the change vision, (5) empowering employees for broad-based action, (6) generating short-term wins, (7) consolidating gains and producing more change, and (8) anchoring new approaches in the culture. 208 pages.

Larson, Erik W., and Clifford F. Gray. *Project Management: The Managerial Process*. 8th ed. New York: McGraw-Hill, 2020.
A book written for the professional or student business manager but of interest to anyone overseeing the planning and implementation of a project. It guides the reader through the steps in project management, from defining the problem and planning an intervention to executing the project and overseeing its impact. 704 pages.

Rogers, Everett M. *Diffusion of Innovations*. 5th ed. New York: Free Press, 2003.
Classic text describing all aspects and stages of the process whereby new phenomena are adopted and diffused throughout social systems. The book contains a discussion of the elements of diffusion, the history and status of diffusion research, the generation of innovations, the innovation-decision process, attributes of innovations and their rate of adoption, innovativeness and adopter categories, opinion leadership and diffusion networks, the change agent, innovations in organizations, and consequences of innovations. Among many other disciplines, education, public health, and medical sociology have made practical use of the theory with empirical research of Rogers's work. Implementation is addressed specifically in several pages (pp. 179–88, 430–32), highlighting the great importance of implementation to the diffusion process. 551 pages.

Viera, Anthony J., and Robert Kramer, eds. *Management and Leadership Skills for Medical Faculty: A Practical Handbook*. New York: Springer, 2016.
This book provides guidance to medical school faculty on personal self-development and leadership development. Directed at faculty in academic medical centers, the book reviews management principles and offers practical skills for communicating effectively, navigating conflict, creating change, and thinking strategically. 286 pages.

Westley, Frances, Brenda Zimmerman, and Michael Q. Patton. *Getting to Maybe: How the World Is Changed*. Toronto: Random House Canada, 2006.
Richly illustrated with real-world examples, this book focuses on complex organizations and social change. Change can come from the bottom up as well as from the top down. The authors contend that an agent of change needs to have intentionality and flexibility, must recognize that achieving

success can have peaks and valleys, should understand that relationships are key to engaging in social intervention, and must have a mindset framed by inquiry rather than certitude. With this framework, the book outlines the steps necessary to achieve change for complex problems. 258 pages.

REFERENCES CITED

1. Erik W. Larson and Clifford F. Gray, *Project Management: The Managerial Process*, 8th ed. (New York: McGraw-Hill, 2020).
2. Kylie Porritt et al., eds., *JBI Handbook for Evidence Implementation* (JBI, 2020), accessed May 23, 2021, https://doi.org/10.46658/JBIMEI-20-01.
3. JoAnn E. Kirchner et al., "Getting a Clinical Innovation into Practice: An Introduction to Implementation Strategies," *Psychiatry Research* 283, (2020): 112467, https://doi.org/10.1016/j.psychres.2019.06.042.
4. "Additional Resources," Accreditation Council in Graduate Medical Education, accessed May 23, 2021, https://www.acgme.org/Program-Directors-and-Coordinators/Welcome/Additional-Resources.
5. Wanda Ellingson, Susan Schissler Manning, and Janelle Doughty, "Native Peoples as Authors of Social Work Curriculum," *Journal of Evidence-Based Social Work* 17, no. 1 (2019): 90–104, https://doi.org/ 10.1080/26408066.2019.1636331.
6. Sylk Sotto-Santiago et al., "'I Didn't Know What to Say': Responding to Racism, Discrimination, and Microaggressions with the OWTFD Approach," *MedEdPORTAL* 16, (2020): 10971, https://doi.org/10.15766/mep_2374-8265.10971.
7. Miriam Lacasse et al., "Interventions for Undergraduate and Postgraduate Medical Learners with Academic Difficulties: A BEME Systematic Review: BEME Guide No. 56," *Medical Teacher* 41, no. 9 (2019): 981–1001, https://doi.org/10.1080/0142159X.2019.15962398.
8. Thomas K. Houston et al., "A Primary Care Musculoskeletal Clinic for Residents: Success and Sustainability," *Journal of General Internal Medicine* 19, no. 5, pt. 2 (2004): 524–29, https://doi.org/10.1111/j.1525-1497.2004.30173.x.
9. "Helping Transform Medical Education: The Teaching EMR," Regenstrief Institute, July 25, 2016, https://www.regenstrief.org/article/helping-transform-medical-education-teaching-emr/.
10. Olga O. Vlashyn et al., "Pharmacy Students' Perspectives on the Initial Implementation of a Teaching Electronic Medical Record: Results from a Mixed-Methods Assessment," *BMC Medical Education* 20, no. 1 (2020): 187, https://doi.org/10.1186/s12909-020-02091-8.
11. Joshua Smith et al., "A Pilot Study: A Teaching Electronic Medical Record for Educating and Assessing Residents in the Care of Patients," *Medical Education Online* 23, no. 1 (2018): 1447211, https://doi.org/10.1080/10872981.2018.1447211.
12. Ashir Kumar, David J. Kallen, and Thomas Mathew, "Volunteer Faculty: What Rewards or Incentives Do They Prefer?" *Teaching and Learning in Medicine 14*, no. 2 (2002): 119–23, https://doi.org/10.1207/S15328015TLM1402_09.
13. Tobias Deutsch et al., "Willingness, Concerns, Incentives and Acceptable Remuneration regarding an Involvement in Teaching Undergraduates—a Cross-Sectional Questionnaire Survey among German GPs," *BMC Medical Education* 19, no. 1 (2019):33, https://doi.org/10.1186/s12909-018-1445-2.
14. Belinda Y. Chen et al., "From Modules to MOOCs: Application of the Six-Step Approach to Online Curriculum Development for Medical Education," *Academic Medicine* 94, no. 5 (2019): 678–85, https://doi.org/10.1097/ACM.0000000000002580.
15. Example adapted with permission from the curricular projects of Michael Melia, MD; Lauren Block, MD, MPH; Lorrel Brown, MD; and Deepa Rangachari, MD, for the Johns Hopkins Longitudinal Program in Faculty Development, cohort 26, 2012–2013, and cohort 27, 2013–2014.

16. James D. Pickering et al., "Twelve Tips for Developing and Delivering a Massive Open Online Course in Medical Education," *Medical Teacher* 39, no. 7 (2017): 691–96, https://doi.org/10.1080/0142159X.2017.1322189 17.

17. Peter G. M .de Jong et al., "Twelve Tips for Integrating Massive Open Online Course Content into Classroom Teaching," *Medical Teacher* 42, no. 4 (2020): 393–97, https://doi.org/10.1080/0142159X.2019.1571569.

18. Cole Hooley et al., "The TDR MOOC Training in Implementation Research: Evaluation of Feasibility and Lessons Learned in Rwanda," *Pilot and Feasibility Studies* 6, (2020): 66, https://doi.org/10.1186/s40814-020-00607-z19.

19. Annette L. Gardner et al., "The Dyad Model for Interprofessional Academic Patient Aligned Care Teams," *Federal Practitioner: For the Health Care Professionals of the VA, DoD, and PHS* 36, no. 2 (2019): 88–93.

20. Thomas E. Mellor et al., "Not Just Hocus POCUS: Implementation of a Point of Care Ultrasound Curriculum for Internal Medicine Trainees at a Large Residency Program," *Military Medicine* 184, no. 11–12 (2019): 901–6, https://doi.org/10.1093/milmed/usz124.

21. Lawrence M. Gillman et al. "Simulated Trauma and Resuscitation Team Training Course: Evolution of a Multidisciplinary Trauma Crisis Resource Management Simulation Course," *American Journal of Surgery* 212, no. 1 (2016): 188–193.e3, https://doi.org/10.1016/j.amjsurg.2015.07.024.

22. Lawrence M. Gillman et al., "S.T.A.R.T.T. Plus: Addition of Prehospital Personnel to a National Multidisciplinary Crisis Resource Management Trauma Team Training Course," *Canadian Journal of Surgery* 59, no. 1 (2016): 9–11, https://doi.org/10.1503/cjs.010915.

23. Kristina Dzara et al., "The Effective Use of Videos in Medical Education," *Academic Medicine* 95, no. 6 (2020): 970, https://doi.org/10.1097/ACM.0000000000003056.

24. Chaoyan Dong and Poh Sun Goh, "Twelve Tips for the Effective Use of Videos in Medical Education," *Medical Teacher* 37, no. 2 (2015): 140–45, https://doi.org/10.3109/0142159X.2014.943709.

25. Rathnayaka Mudiyanselage Gunasingha et al., "Vital Conversations: An Interactive Conflict Resolution Training Session for Fourth-Year Medical Students," *MedEdPORTAL* 17, (2021): 11074, https://doi.org/10.15766/mep_2374-8265.11074.

26. Robert O. Roswell et al., "Cultivating Empathy through Virtual Reality: Advancing Conversations about Racism, Inequity, and Climate in Medicine," *Academic Medicine* 95, no. 12 (2020): 1882–86, https://doi.org/10.1097/ACM.0000000000003615.

27. "Business Model Canvas for Medical Educators," Association of American Medical Colleges, accessed May 23, 2021, https://www.aamc.org/system/files/2019-09/profdev-gea-ugme-businessmodelcanvas.pdf.

28. Gregory W. Rouan et al., "Rewarding Teaching Faculty with a Reimbursement Plan," *Journal of General Internal Medicine* 14, no. 6 (1999): 327–32, https://doi.org/10.1046/j.1525-1497.1999.00350.x.

29. Michael M. Yeh and Daniel F. Cahill, "Quantifying Physician Teaching Productivity Using Clinical Relative Value Units," *Journal of General Internal Medicine* 14, no. 10 (1999): 617–21, https://doi.org/10.1046/j.1525-1497.1999.01029.x.

30. William T. Mallon and Robert F Jones, "How Do Medical Schools Use Measurement Systems to Track Faculty Activity and Productivity in Teaching?" *Academic Medicine* 77, no. 2 (2002): 115–23, https://doi.org/10.1097/00001888-200202000-00005.

31. Michelle Sainté, Steven L. Kanter, and David Muller, "Mission-Based Budgeting for Education: Ready for Prime Time?" *Mount Sinai Journal of Medicine* 76, no. 4 (2009): 381–86, https://doi.org/10.1002/msj.20122.

32. E. Ray Dorsey et al., "The Economics of New Faculty Hires in Basic Science," *Academic Medicine* 84, no. 1 (2009): 26–31, https://doi.org/10.1097/ACM.0b013e3181904633.

33. Stephen A. Geraci et al., "AAIM Report on Master Teachers and Clinician Educators Part 3: Finances and Resourcing." *The American Journal of Medicine* 123, no. 10 (2010): 963–67, https://doi.org/10.1016/j.amjmed.2010.06.006.

34. Steven Stites et al., "Aligning Compensation with Education: Design and Implementation of the Educational Value Unit (EVU) System in an Academic Internal Medicine Department," *Academic Medicine* 80, no. 12 (2005): 1100–106, https://doi.org/10.1097/00001888 -200512000-00006.

35. Reuben Mezrich and Paul G. Nagy, "The Academic RVU: A System for Measuring Academic Productivity," *Journal of the American College of Radiology* 4, no. 7 (2007): 471–78, https:// doi.org/10.1016/j.jacr.2007.02.009.

36. E. Benjamin Clyburn et al., "Valuing the Education Mission: Implementing an Educational Value Units System," *American Journal of Medicine* 124, no. 6 (2011): 567–72, https://doi.org /10.1016/j.amjmed.2011.01.014.

37. Joseph House et al., "Implementation of an Education Value Unit (EVU) System to Recognize Faculty Contributions," *The Western Journal of Emergency Medicine* 16, no. 6 (2015): 952– 56, https://doi.org/10.5811/westjem.2015.8.26136.

38. Linda Regan, Julianna Jung, and Gabor D. Kelen, "Educational Value Units: A Mission-Based Approach to Assigning and Monitoring Faculty Teaching Activities in an Academic Medical Department," *Academic Medicine* 91, no. 12 (2016): 1642–46, https://doi.org/10.1097 /ACM.0000000000001110.

39. Andrew Pugh et al., "Impact of a Financial Incentive on the Completion of Educational Metrics," *International Journal of Emergency Medicine* 13, no. 1 (2020): 60, https://doi.org /10.1186/s12245-020-00323-8.

40. Darcy A. Reed et al., "Association between Funding and Quality of Published Medical Education Research," *JAMA* 298, no. 9 (2007): 1002–9, https://doi.org/10.1001/jama.298.9.1002.

41. Darcy A. Reed et al., "Predictive Validity Evidence for Medical Education Research Study Quality Instrument Scores: Quality of Submissions to JGIM's Medical Education Special Issue," *Journal of General Internal Medicine* 23, no. 7 (2008): 903–7, https://doi.org/10.1007 /s11606-008-0664-3.

42. Neda Ratanawongsa et al., "Effects of a Focused Patient-Centered Care Curriculum on the Experiences of Internal Medicine Residents and Their Patients," *Journal of General Internal Medicine* 27, no. 4 (2012): 473–77, https://doi.org/10.1007/s11606-011-1881-8.

43. "Celebrating 10 Years of the Aliki Initiative," Center for Innovative Medicine, accessed May 23, 2021, https://www.hopkinscim.org/breakthrough/holiday-2017/celebrating-10-years-aliki -initiative/.

44. "Our Priorities," Josiah Macy Jr. Foundation, accessed May 23, 2021, http://macyfoundation .org/priorities.

45. Rosalyn Stewart et al., "Urban Health and Primary Care at Johns Hopkins: Urban Primary Care Medical Home Resident Training Programs," *Journal of Health Care for the Poor and Underserved* 23, no. 3 Suppl (2012): 103–13, https://doi.org/10.1353/hpu.2012.0123.

46. Malcolm S. Knowles, Elwood F. Holton III, and Richard A. Swanson, *The Adult Learner: The Definitive Classic in Adult Education and Human Resource Development*, 8th ed. (London: Routledge, 2014).

47. Stephen Brookfield, *Powerful Techniques for Teaching Adults* (San Francisco: Jossey-Bass, 2013).

48. James W. Dearing et al., "Designing for Diffusion of a Biomedical Intervention," *American Journal of Preventive Medicine* 44, no. 1 Suppl 2 (2013): S70–76, https://doi.org/10.1016/j.amepre .2012.09.038.

49. Katie W. Hsih et al., "The Student Curriculum Review Team: How We Catalyze Curricular Changes through a Student-Centered Approach," *Medical Teacher* 37, no. 11 (2015): 1008 –12, https://doi.org/10.3109/0142159X.2014.990877.

50. Priyanka Kumar et al., "Student Curriculum Review Team, 8 years Later: Where We Stand and Opportunities for Growth," *Medical Teacher* 43, no. 3 (2021): 314–19, https://doi.org /10.1080/0142159X.2020.1841891.

51. Steven C. Stoner and Sarah Billings, "Initiative to Improve Student Perceptions of Relevance and Value in a Top 200 Drugs Course through Improved Curricular Alignment and Course

Modification," *Currents in Pharmacy Teaching & Learning* 13, no. 1 (2021): 73–80, https://doi.org/10.1016/j.cptl.2020.08.006.

52. Adrienne C. Lindsey et al., "Testing a Screening, Brief Intervention, and Referral to Treatment (SBIRT) Interdisciplinary Training Program Model for Higher Education Systems," *Families, Systems & Health* (2021), https://doi.org/10.1037/fsh0000582.

53. Sarah Allen et al., "Targeting Improvements in Patient Safety at a Large Academic Center: An Institutional Handoff Curriculum for Graduate Medical Education," *Academic Medicine* 89, no. 10 (2014): 1366–69, https://doi.org/10.1097/ACM.0000000000000462.

54. Kenneth W. Thomas, *Introduction to Conflict Management: Improving Performance Using the TKI* (Mountain View, CA: CPP, 2002).

55. Kenneth W. Thomas and Ralph H. Kilmann, "An Overview of the Thomas-Kilmann Conflict Mode Instrument (TKI)," Kilmann Diagnostics, accessed May 23, 2021, http://www.kilmanndiagnostics.com/overview-thomas-kilmann-conflict-mode-instrument-tki.

56. Roger Fisher, William L. Ury, and Bruce Patton, *Getting to Yes: Negotiating Agreement without Giving In*, 3rd ed. (New York: Penguin Books, 2011).

57. Carole J. Bland et al., "Curricular Change in Medical Schools: How to Succeed," *Academic Medicine* 75, no. 6 (2000): 575–94, https://doi.org/10.1097/00001888-200006000-00006.

58. John P. Kotter, *Leading Change* (Boston: Harvard Business Review Press, 2012).

59. Westley, Frances, Brenda Zimmerman, and Michael Q. Patton, *Getting to Maybe: How the World Is Changed* (Toronto: Random House Canada, 2006).

60. William J. Rothwell, Jacqueline M. Stavros, and Roland L. Sullivan, *Practicing Organization Development: Leading Transformation and Change*, 4th ed. (Hoboken: Wiley, 2016).

61. Mica Estrada et al., "Enabling Full Representation in Science: The San Francisco BUILD Project's Agents of Change Affirm Science Skills, Belonging and Community," *BMC Proceedings* 11, Suppl 12 (2017): 25, https://doi.org/10.1186/s12919-017-0090-9.

62. Interprofessional Education Collaborative. *Core Competencies for Interprofessional Collaborative Practice: 2016 Update*, (Washington, DC: Interprofessional Education Collaborative, 2016), accessed May 23, 2021, http://www.ipecollaborative.org/ipec-core-competencies.

63. Liaison Committee on Medical Education, *Functions and Structure of a Medical School: Standards for Accreditation of Medical Education Programs Leading to the MD Degree*, March 2021, accessed May 23, 2021, https://lcme.org/publications/.

64. Laura Weiss Roberts et al., "An Invitation for Medical Educators to Focus on Ethical and Policy Issues in Research and Scholarly Practice," *Academic Medicine* 76, no. 9 (2001): 876–85, https://doi.org/10.1097/00001888-200109000-00007.

65. Jason D. Keune et al., "The Ethics of Conducting Graduate Medical Education Research on Residents," *Academic Medicine* 88, no. 4 (2013): 449–53, https://doi.org/10.1097/ACM.0b013e3182854bef.

66. William F. Miser, "Educational Research—to IRB, or Not to IRB?," *Family Medicine* 37, no. 3 (2005): 168–73.

67. Umut Sarpel et al., "Medical Students as Human Subjects in Educational Research," *Medical Education Online* 18, (2013): 1–6, https://doi.org/10.3402/meo.v18i0.19524.

68. Liselotte N. Dyrbye et al., "Medical Education Research and IRB Review: An Analysis and Comparison of the IRB Review Process at Six Institutions," *Academic Medicine* 82, no. 7 (2007): 654–60, https://doi.org/10.1097/ACM.0b013e318065be1e.

69. Rebecca C. Henry and David E. Wright, "When Do Medical Students Become Human Subjects of Research? The Case of Program Evaluation," *Academic Medicine* 76, no. 9 (2001): 871–75, https://doi.org/10.1097/00001888-200109000-00006.

70. Liselotte N. Dyrbye et al., "Clinician Educators' Experiences with Institutional Review Boards: Results of a National Survey," *Academic Medicine* 83, no. 6 (2008): 590–95, https://doi.org/10.1097/ACM.0b013e318172347a.

71. Gail M. Sullivan, "Education Research and Human Subject Protection: Crossing the IRB Quagmire," *Journal of Graduate Medical Education* 3, no. 1 (2011): 1–4, https://doi.org/10.4300/JGME-D-11-00004.1.

72. John M. Tomkowiak and Anne J. Gunderson, "To IRB or Not to IRB?" *Academic Medicine* 79, no. 7 (2004): 628–32, https://doi.org/10.1097/00001888-200407000-00004.

73. Carisa M. Cooney et al., "Comprehensive Observations of Resident Evolution: A Novel Method for Assessing Procedure-Based Residency Training," *Plastic and Reconstructive Surgery* 137, no. 2 (2016): 673–78, https://doi.org/10.1097/01.prs.0000475797.69478.0e.

74. Ricardo J. Bello et al., "The Reliability of Operative Rating Tool Evaluations: How Late Is Too Late to Provide Operative Performance Feedback?" *American Journal of Surgery* 216, no. 6 (2018): 1052–55, https://doi.org/10.1016/j.amjsurg.2018.04.005.

75. Susanne Wish-Baratz et al., "A New Supplement to Gross Anatomy Dissection: HoloAnatomy," *Medical Education* 53, no. 5 (2019): 522–23, https://doi.org/10.1111/medu.13845.

76. Example adapted with permission from the curricular project of Tahara Akmal, MA; Ty Crowe, MDiv; Patrick Hemming, MD, MPH; Tommy Rogers, MDiv; Emmanuel Saidi, PhD; Monica Sandoval, MD; and Paula Teague, DMin, MBA, for the Johns Hopkins Longitudinal Program in Faculty Development, cohort 26, 2012–2013.

77. Michael Gottlieb et al., "Applying Design Thinking Principles to Curricular Development in Medical Education," *AEM Education and Training* 1, no. 1 (2017): 21–26, https://doi.org/10.1002/aet2.10003.

78. Jacqueline E. McLaughlin et al., "A Qualitative Review of the Design Thinking Framework in Health Professions Education," *BMC Medical Education* 19, no. 1 (2019): 98, https://doi.org/10.1186/s12909-019-1528-8.

79. Michael D. Wolcott et al., "Twelve Tips to Stimulate Creative Problem-Solving with Design Thinking," *Medical Teacher*, (2020): 1–8, https://doi.org/10.1080/0142159X.2020.1807483.

80. Peter S. Cahn et al., "A Design Thinking Approach to Evaluating Interprofessional Education," *Journal of Interprofessional Care* 30, no. 3 (2016): 378–80, https://doi.org/10.3109/13561820.2015.1122582.

81. Larissa R. Thomas et al., "Designing Well-Being: Using Design Thinking to Engage Residents in Developing Well-Being Interventions," *Academic Medicine* 95, no. 7 (2020): 1038–42, https://doi.org/10.1097/ACM.0000000000003243.

82. Lauren J. Taylor et al., "Using Implementation Science to Adapt a Training Program to Assist Surgeons with High-Stakes Communication," *Journal of Surgical Education* 76, no. 1 (2019): 165–73, https://doi.org/10.1016/j.jsurg.2018.05.015.

83. Margaret L. Schwarze, "Best Case/Worst Case Training Program," UW–Madison Department of Surgery, 2016, accessed May 23, 2021, https://www.hipxchange.org/BCWC.

84. Nancy A. Hueppchen et al., "The Johns Hopkins University School of Medicine," in "A Snapshot of Medical Student Education in the United States and Canada: Reports From 145 Schools," special issue, *Academic Medicine* 95, no. 9S (2020): S206–S210, https://doi.org/10.1097/ACM.0000000000003480.

CHAPTER SEVEN

Step 6
Evaluation and Feedback

. . . assessing the achievement of objectives
and promoting continuous improvement

Brenessa M. Lindeman, MD, MEHP, David E. Kern, MD, MPH,
and Pamela A. Lipsett, MD, MHPE

DEFINITIONS

Evaluation, for the purposes of this book, is defined as the identification, clarification, and application of criteria to determine the merit or worth of what is being evaluated.[1] While often used interchangeably, *assessment* is often used to connote measurements, while *evaluation* is used to connote appraisal or judgment. In education, assessment is often of an individual, while evaluation is of a program. *Feedback* is defined as the provision of information on an individual's or curriculum's performance to learners, faculty, and other stakeholders in the curriculum.

IMPORTANCE

Step 6, Evaluation and Feedback, closes the loop in the curriculum development cycle. The evaluation process helps those who have a stake in the curriculum make a decision or judgment about the curriculum. The evaluation step helps curriculum developers ask and answer the important questions: Were the goals and objectives of the curriculum met? What outcomes were observed (both intended and unintended)? How can one explain the outcomes? What were the actual processes of the curriculum (compared to those planned)? Assessment and evaluation provide information that can be used to guide individuals and the curriculum in cycles of ongoing improvement. Evaluation results can also be used to maintain and garner support for a curriculum, to provide evidence of student achievement, to satisfy external requirements, to document the accomplishments of curriculum developers, and to serve as a basis for presentations and publications.

GENERAL CONSIDERATIONS

The assessment and evaluation methods should be feasible, transparent, and provide comprehensive information about the curriculum.[2,3] A curriculum is increasingly recognized as not an unvarying but a constantly changing process that is influenced by and alters its environmental context.[4] Therefore, multipoint and multimethod measures are preferred for understanding its processes, its learners, other stakeholders, the complex environment within which it exists, and the interactions among these[2-6] (see also Chapter 8). Such an approach lends a constant critical eye to whether there are explanations, other than the ones hypothesized, for the outcomes observed.[6]

A combination of quantitative and qualitative assessment and evaluation, termed a mixed-method approach, is generally required to achieve these goals.[7] Quantitative methods generate quantifiable/numerical data. They are used to provide descriptive or relational data and to test hypotheses through correlational, quasi-experimental, or experimental (randomized control) evaluation designs (see "Task V: Choose Evaluation Designs"), using appropriate statistics (see "Task IX: Analyze Data"). They assume an objective reality, not (or minimally) influenced by the evaluator. Qualitative methods,[8] on the other hand, focus on non-numerical data. They seek to explain, to answer "how" and "why" rather than "what" questions, to provide rich contextualized description, and to generate theory (grounded theory) and hypotheses out of data. They take a more subjective approach to data, assume the possibility of more than one reality, and recognize that results are influenced by the evaluator and qualitative method used. They are particularly helpful for formative assessment/evaluation and when it is unclear what potentially important factors and outcomes should be measured in a quantitative evaluation. While this chapter focuses primarily on quantitative approaches to evaluation, it will refer to qualitative design, methods, and data analysis when relevant.

A still-developing educational framework that needs to be considered in assessment and evaluation is the use of entrustable professional activities, or EPAs. EPAs are units of professional practice and have been defined as tasks or responsibilities that trainees are entrusted to perform without supervision, once they have attained sufficient proficiency.[9] EPAs require integration of competencies across multiple domains, such as those in the competency framework of the Accreditation Council for Graduate Medical Education (ACGME).[10,11] They are observable and measurable, often requiring both quantitative and qualitative methods, leading to a recognized output of professional practice.[12]

> **EXAMPLE:** *EPA, Evaluate and Manage a Patient with Right Lower Quadrant Pain.* The ability to evaluate and manage a patient with right lower quadrant pain without supervision involves the ACGME competency domains of medical knowledge, patient care, and interpersonal communication skills, and the achievement of multiple focused learning objectives, such as diagnostic evaluation of the presenting problem, conduct of operative management when necessary (including knowledge of the relevant anatomy and technical skills related to procedure performance), and identification of any post-procedure complications.[13]

While the EPA framework was initially formulated for the transition from residency to independent practice, this concept has been extended to develop EPAs for the transition from medical school to residency.[14] It has also been proposed that EPAs be used to create dynamic portfolios that follow physicians into practice.[15,16] EPAs, as such, are dynamic in that they are not permanent but need to be maintained within one's scope of practice.

Educators need to align the constellation of formative and summative assessments that occur within an educational program's constituent curricula with achievement of desired program outcomes, such as EPAs.[17] As the EPA framework sees rapid uptake in both the undergraduate medical education and graduate medical education environments, ongoing research is still needed to develop high-level evidence for their development, implementation, and efficacy.[18]

Whatever the conceptual framework for assessment, it is helpful to be methodical in designing the evaluation for a curriculum to ensure that important questions are answered and relevant needs met. This chapter outlines a 10-task approach that begins with consideration of the potential users and uses of an evaluation, moves to the identification of evaluation questions and methods, proceeds to the collection of data, and ends with data analysis and reporting of results.

TASK I: IDENTIFY USERS

The first step in planning the evaluation for a curriculum is to identify the likely users of the evaluation. *Participants* in the curriculum have an interest in the assessment of their own performance and the performance of the curriculum. Evaluation can provide feedback and motivation for continued improvement for *learners*, *faculty*, and *curriculum developers*.

Other stakeholders who have administrative responsibility for, allocate resources to, or are otherwise affected by the curriculum will also be interested in evaluation results. These might include individuals in the *dean's office*; *administrators*; the *department chair*; the *program director* for resident, fellow, or student education; the *division director*; *other faculty* who have contributed political support or who might be in competition for limited resources; and *individuals, granting agencies, or other organizations that have contributed funds or other resources* to the curriculum. Individuals who need to make decisions about whether to participate in the curriculum, such as *future learners or faculty*, may also be interested in evaluation results.

To the extent that a curriculum innovatively addresses an important need or tests new educational strategies, evaluation results may also be of interest to *educators from other institutions* and serve as a basis for publications/presentations. As society is often the intended beneficiary of a health care curriculum, society members are also stakeholders in this process.

Finally, evaluation results can document the achievements of *curriculum developers*. Promotion committees and department chairs assign a high degree of importance to clinician-educators' accomplishments in curriculum development.[19,20] These accomplishments can be included in the educational portfolios that are used to support applications for promotion.[21-23]

TASK II: IDENTIFY USES

Generic Uses

In designing an evaluation strategy for a curriculum, the curriculum developer should be aware of the generic uses of an evaluation. These generic uses can be classified along two axes, as shown in Table 7.1. The first axis refers to whether the evaluation is used to appraise the performance of *individuals*, the performance of the entire *program*, or both. The assessment of an individual learner usually involves determining whether the learner has achieved the cognitive, affective, psychomotor skill, behavioral, or broader competency objectives of a curriculum (see Chapter 4). Program evaluation usually determines the aggregate achievements of all individuals, clinical or other outcomes, the actual processes of a curriculum, or the perceptions of learners and faculty. The second axis in Table 7.1 refers to whether an evaluation is used for *formative* purposes (to improve performance), for *summative* purposes (to judge performance and make decisions about its future or adoption), or for both purposes.[24] From the discussion and examples below, the

Table 7.1.   Evaluation Types: Levels and Uses

Use	Level	
	Individual	Program
Formative	Assessment of an individual learner or faculty member that is used to help the individual improve performance: ■ identification of areas for improvement ■ specific suggestions for improvement	Evaluation of a program that is used to improve program performance: ■ identification of areas for improvement ■ specific suggestions for improvement
Summative	Assessment of an individual learner or faculty member that is used for judgments or decisions about the individual: ■ verification of achievement for individual ■ motivation of individual to maintain or improve performance ■ certification of performance for others ■ grades ■ promotion	Evaluation of a program that is used for judgments or decisions about the program or program developers: ■ judgments regarding success, efficacy ■ decisions regarding allocation of resources ■ motivation/recruitment of learners and faculty ■ influencing attitudes regarding value of curriculum ■ satisfying external requirements ■ prestige, power, influence, promotion ■ dissemination: presentations, publications

reader may surmise that *some evaluations can be used for both summative and formative purposes*.

Specific Uses

Having identified the likely users of the evaluation and understood the generic uses of curriculum evaluation, the curriculum developer should consider the specific needs of different users (stakeholders) and the specific ways in which they will use the evaluation.[24] Specific uses for evaluation results might include the following:

■   *Feedback on and improvement of individual performance*: Both learners and faculty can use the results of timely feedback (formative individual assessment) to direct improvements in their own performances. This type of assessment identifies areas for improvement and provides specific suggestions for improvement (feedback). It, therefore, also serves as an educational method (see Chapter 5). Guidance by mentors as to the formative nature of such assessments is critical, as studies have shown that assessments designed as formative can be perceived as summative by students.[25]

EXAMPLE: *Formative Individual Assessment.* During a women's health clerkship, students are assessed on their ability to perform the Core EPA for Entering Residency, "Provide an oral presentation of a clinical encounter,"[14] after interviewing a standardized patient, and are given specific verbal feedback about the presentation to improve their performance.

- *Judgments regarding individual performance*: The accomplishments of individual learners may need to be documented (summative individual assessment) to assign grades, to demonstrate mastery in a particular area or achievement of certain curricular objectives, or to satisfy the demands of external bodies, such as specialty boards. In these instances, it is important to clarify criteria for the achievement of objectives or competency before the evaluation. Assessment of individual faculty can be used to make decisions about their continuation as curriculum faculty, as material for their promotion portfolios, and as data for teaching awards. Used in this manner, assessments become evaluations.

EXAMPLE: *Summative Individual Assessment.* Prior to completion of postgraduate training, surgical residents must become certified in the Fundamentals of Endoscopic Surgery to be eligible for board certification. This involves a simulated technical skills test in which scores above a particular threshold must be achieved in order to obtain certification. One study identified that a train-to-proficiency curriculum can enhance preparedness for the summative exam.[26]

- *Feedback on and improvement of program performance*: Curriculum developers and coordinators can use evaluation results (formative program evaluation) to identify parts of the curriculum that are effective and parts that need improvement. This is based on the premise that both programs and their evaluations need to be developed, reexamined, and assessed at regular intervals. To accomplish this, program managers, evaluators, and stakeholders need to collaborate, and all parties must be open to change as the program design evolves.[27]

Such formative program evaluation often takes the form of surveys (see Chapter 3) of learners to obtain feedback about and suggestions for improving a curriculum. Quantitative information, such as ratings of various aspects of the curriculum, can help identify areas that need revision. Qualitative information, such as responses to open-ended questions about program strengths, program weaknesses, and suggestions for change, provides feedback in areas that may not have been anticipated and ideas for improvement. Information can also be obtained from faculty or other observers, such as nurses, other health professionals, and patients. Aggregates of formative and summative individual assessments can be used for formative program evaluation, as well, to identify specific areas of the curriculum in need of revision.

EXAMPLE: *Formative Program Evaluation.* At the end of medical students' clinical clerkships, students and their supervisors completed a workplace-based assessment utilizing 12 end-of-training EPAs. This identified gaps between students' current abilities and expectations, which allowed the students and supervisors to collectively look for opportunities to close those gaps.[28]

EXAMPLE: *Formative Program Evaluation.* After each didactic lecture of the radiology residency curriculum, residents were asked to complete a "Minute Paper" in which they briefly noted either the most important thing they had learned during the lecture or the muddiest point in the lecture, as well as an important question that remained unanswered.[29] This technique allowed the instructor to know what knowledge learners were gaining from the lecture (or not) and provided information about where to make future refinements.

- *Judgments regarding program success*: Summative program evaluation provides information on the degree to which a curriculum has met its various objectives and expectations, under what specific conditions, and at what cost. It can also document the curriculum's success in engaging, motivating, and pleasing its learners and faculty. It can identify any gaps between what the program attempted to deliver and the program's observed outcomes, including mechanisms to further elucidate and close those gaps.[30] In addition to quantitative data, summative program evaluation may include qualitative information about unintended barriers, unanticipated factors encountered in the program implementation, or unintended consequences of the curriculum. It may identify aspects of the hidden curriculum.[31,32] As mentioned above, it is important to consider the context the curriculum exists in and how the presence of the curriculum changes the context of learners' experiences.[6] The results of summative program evaluations are often reported to others to obtain or maintain curricular time, funding, and other resources.

  EXAMPLE: *Summative Program Evaluation.* At the conclusion of a psychiatry clinical clerkship, 90% of students received a passing grade in the performance of a standardized patient history and mental status examination: assessing 10 cognitive and 6 skill objectives in the areas of history, physical and mental status examination, diagnosis, management, and counseling.

  EXAMPLE: *Summative Program Evaluation Leading to Further Investigation and Change.* In an emergency medicine residency program, ratings of resident milestone achievements were based on data from faculty evaluations of resident performance. Program leadership identified that evaluation scores were missing in two areas: health advocacy and professional roles. Reasons for the missing data needed to be explored and addressed.[33]

  EXAMPLE: *Summative Program Evaluation Leading to Curricular Expansion.* Summative evaluation of all 13 Core EPAs for Entering Residency[14] among fourth-year students at one medical school revealed gaps in students' abilities to identify system failures and contribute to a culture of safety. As a result, the curriculum for intersessions between clinical clerkships was expanded to include discussions of the importance of error prevention to individual patients and to systems, a mock root cause analysis exercise, and resources for reporting of real or potential errors within the institution.

- *Justification for the allocation of resources*: Those with administrative authority can use evaluation results (summative program evaluation) to guide and justify decisions about the allocation of resources for a curriculum. They may be more likely to allocate limited resources to a curriculum if the evaluation provides evidence of success or if revisions are planned for a curriculum that demonstrates evidence of deficiency in an accreditation standard. In the above example, assessment of newly defined program outcomes identified deficiencies in student preparation, leading to expanded allocation of resources for the curriculum.
- *Motivation and recruitment*: Feedback on individual and program success and the identification of areas for future improvement (formative and summative individual assessment and program evaluation) can be motivational to faculty. Evidence of programs' responsiveness to formative program evaluation can be attractive to future learners. Evidence of programs' success through summative evaluation can also help in the recruitment of both learners and faculty.
- *Attitude change*: Evidence that significant change has occurred in learners (summative program evaluation) with the use of an unfamiliar educational method or in a previously unknown content area can significantly alter attitudes about the importance of such methods and content.

EXAMPLE: *Summative Program Evaluation Demonstrating Attitude Change.* A quality improvement project was added to the requirements for a palliative care curriculum for interprofessional learners. The pre-curriculum needs assessment revealed low ratings for participants' belief that quality improvement has a role in palliative care (2.97/5). However, after participation in the curriculum and project, this score rose to 4.32/5.[34]

- *Satisfaction of external and internal requirements*: Summative individual and program evaluation results can be used to satisfy the requirements of regulatory bodies, such as the Liaison Committee on Medical Education or Residency Review and Graduate Medical Education Committees. These evaluations, therefore, may be necessary for program accreditation and will be welcomed by those who have administrative responsibility for an overall program.
- *Demonstration of participant satisfaction*: Evidence that learners and faculty truly enjoyed and valued their experience (summative program evaluation) and evidence of other stakeholder support (patients, benefactors) may be important to educational and other administrative leaders who want to meet the needs of existing trainees, faculty, and other stakeholders and to recruit new ones. A high degree of learner, faculty, and stakeholder support provides strong political support for a curriculum.
- *Prestige, power, promotion, and influence*: A successful program (summative program evaluation) reflects positively on its institution, department chair, division chief, overall program director, curriculum developer, and faculty, thereby conveying a certain degree of prestige, power, and influence. Summative program and individual assessment data can be used as evidence of accomplishment in one's promotion portfolio.
- *Presentations, publications, and adoption of curricular components by others*: An evaluation will be of interest to educators at other institutions and to publishers if it provides evidence of success (or failure) of an innovative or insufficiently studied educational program or method (see Chapter 9).

EXAMPLE: *Summative Program Evaluation Resulting in Publication.* A quality improvement curriculum to promote administration of venous thromboembolism prophylaxis in surgical patients was implemented in a general surgery residency program. The pre-curriculum needs assessment revealed that 45% of residents prescribed appropriate prophylaxis for every patient. However, after receipt of performance scorecards and coaching, the appropriate prescription rate improved to 78%. Report of this curricular success was subsequently published in *Annals of Surgery*.[35]

TASK III: IDENTIFY RESOURCES

The most carefully planned evaluation will fail if the resources are not available to accomplish it.[36] Limits in resources may require a prioritization of evaluation questions and changes in evaluation methods. For this reason, curriculum developers should *consider resource needs early in the planning of the evaluation process*, including *time*, *personnel*, *equipment*, *facilities*, and available *funds*. Appropriate *time* should be allocated for the collection, analysis, and reporting of evaluation results. *Personnel* needs often include staff to help in the collection and collation of data and distribution of reports, as well as people with statistical or computer expertise to help verify and analyze the data. *Equipment and facilities* might include the appropriate testing environment and computer hardware and software. *Funding* from internal or external sources is required for resources that are not otherwise available, in which case a budget and budget justification may have to be developed.

> **EXAMPLE**: *Funding for a Randomized Controlled Evaluation.* For a randomized controlled evaluation of different approaches to CPR training, both external and internal funding was required. Pediatric health care providers (nurses, residents, respiratory therapists) being trained in CPR demonstrated high-quality compressions more often after ongoing practice and real-time feedback (experimental group) compared to annual training (control group).[37]

Formal funding may often be challenging to obtain, but informal networking can reveal potential assistance locally, such as computer programmers or biostatisticians interested in measurements pertinent to the curriculum or quality improvement personnel in a hospital interested in measuring patient outcomes. Survey instruments can be adopted from other residency programs or clerkships within an institution or can be shared among institutions. Health professional programs often have summative assessments in place for students and residents, in the form of subject, specialty board, and in-service training examinations. Specific information on learner performance in the knowledge areas addressed by these tests can be readily accessed through the program director, appropriate dean, or testing/examination board with little cost to the curriculum.

> **EXAMPLE**: *Use of an Existing Resource for Curricular Evaluation.* An objective of the acute neurologic event curriculum for emergency medicine residents is the appropriate administration of thrombolytic therapy within 60 minutes of hospital arrival of patients with symptoms of acute ischemic stroke. The evaluation plan included the need for a follow-up audit of this practice, but resources were not available for an independent audit. The information was then added to the comprehensive electronic medical record maintained by the emergency department staff, which provided both measures of individual resident performance and overall program success in the timely administration of thrombolytics.

An additional source of peer-reviewed assessment tools is the Association of American Medical Colleges (AAMC) MedEdPORTAL.[38]

> **EXAMPLE**: *Use of a Publicly Accessible Resource for Curricular Evaluation.* Directors of a clinical skills curriculum for preclerkship medical students added elements of the Hypothesis-Driven Physical Exam (HDPE) instrument available in MedEdPORTAL[39] to an objective structured clinical examination (OSCE) assessment of student skills and diagnostic reasoning around the physical exam.

Accommodations for testing is an increasingly important resource issue in health professions education as the professions become more inclusive of students with disability.[40–42] The prevalence of self-reported disability in US medical students is 3% to 5%, with over 97% receiving accommodations for testing.[43,44] The most frequent testing accommodations include time and half and double time, use of low-distraction or private environments, and testing breaks.[43,44] Although mobility and sensory disabilities are less common than attention-deficit/hyperactivity disorder (ADHD), learning disabilities, psychologic disorders, and chronic health conditions, assistive technology was used by over 40% of students with self-reported disability.[43] Curriculum developers planning learner assessments should be aware of the institutional or program policies and collaborate with the disability services provider to provide needed accommodations in testing.

TASK IV: IDENTIFY EVALUATION QUESTIONS

Evaluation questions direct the evaluation. They are to curriculum evaluation as research questions are to research projects. *Most evaluation questions should relate to the specific measurable learner, process, or clinical outcome objectives of a curriculum.*[45,46] As described in Chapter 4, specific measurable objectives should state <u>who will do</u> how much / how well of what <u>by when</u>. The "who" may refer to learners or instructors, or to the program itself, if one is evaluating program activities. "How much / how well of what by when" provides a standard of acceptability that is measurable. Often, in the process of writing evaluation questions and thinking through what designs and methods might be able to answer a question, it becomes clear that a curricular objective needs further clarification.

> **EXAMPLE**: *Clarifying an Objective for the Purpose of Evaluation.* The initial draft of one curricular objective stated: "By the end of the curriculum, all residents will be proficient in obtaining informed consent." In formulating the evaluation question and thinking through the evaluation methodology, it became clear to the curriculum developers that "proficient" needed to be defined operationally. Also, they determined that an increase of 25% or more of learners that demonstrated proficiency in obtaining informed consent, for a total of at least 90%, would define success for the curriculum. After appropriate revisions in the objective, the curricular evaluation questions became "By the end of the curriculum, what percent of residents have achieved a passing score on the proficiency checklist for informed consent, as assessed using standardized patients?" and "Has there been a statistically and quantitatively (>25%) significant increase in the number of proficient residents, as defined above, from the beginning to the end of the curriculum?"

The curriculum developer should also make sure that the evaluation questions are *congruent* with the related curricular objectives.

> **EXAMPLE:** *Congruence between Objectives and the Evaluation Questions.* Objectives for a curriculum teaching the 3-Act Model for goals of care discussion include that the resident would become proficient in using the model, value it, and then actually use it in practice. The evaluation questions were congruent with the objectives: "Did residents become proficient in the use of the model?"; "What approach do they use most often in practice to discuss goals of care with patients?"; and "How well do they feel the approach works for them in practice?"[47,48]

Often, resources will limit the number of objectives for which accomplishment can be assessed. In this situation, it is necessary to *prioritize and select key evaluation questions* based on the needs of the users and the feasibility of the related evaluation methodology. Sometimes, several objectives can be grouped efficiently into a single evaluation question.

> **EXAMPLE:** *Prioritizing Which Objective to Evaluate.* A curriculum on endotracheal intubation for anesthesia residents has cognitive, attitudinal, skill, and behavioral objectives. The curriculum developers decided that what mattered most was post-curricular behavior and that effective behavior required achievement of the appropriate cognitive, attitudinal, and skill objectives. Setup, placement, maintenance, and evaluation of an endotracheal intubation are all critical for success in securing a patient's airway. The curriculum developers' evaluation question and evaluation methodology, therefore, assessed post-curricular behaviors, rather than knowledge, attitudes, or technical skill mastery. If behavioral objectives were not met, the curriculum developers would need to reconsider specific assessment of cognitive, attitudinal, and/or skill objectives.

Not all evaluation questions need to relate to explicit, written learner objectives. Some curricular objectives are implicitly understood but not written down, to prevent a curriculum document from becoming unwieldy. Most curriculum developers, for example, will want to *include evaluation questions that relate to the effectiveness of specific curricular components or faculty*, even when the related objectives are implicit rather than explicit.

> **EXAMPLE:** *Evaluation Question Directed toward Curricular Processes.* What was the perceived effectiveness of the curriculum's online modules, small-group discussions, simulated patients, clinical experiences, and required case presentations?

Sometimes there are unexpected strengths and weaknesses in a curriculum. Sometimes the curriculum on paper may differ from the curriculum as delivered. Therefore, it is almost always helpful to *include some evaluation questions that do not relate to specific curricular objectives and that are open-ended in nature.*[49]

> **EXAMPLE:** *Use of Open-Ended Questions Related to Curricular Processes.* What do learners perceive as the major strengths and weaknesses of the curriculum? What did learners identify as the most important takeaway and least understood point from each session (Minute Paper/Muddiest Point technique[29])? How could the curriculum be improved?

TASK V: CHOOSE EVALUATION DESIGNS

Once the evaluation questions have been identified and prioritized, the curriculum developer should *consider which evaluation designs are most appropriate to answer the evaluation questions and most feasible in terms of resources.*[46,50–55]

An evaluation is said to possess *internal validity*[52] if it accurately assesses the impact of a specific intervention on specific subjects in a specific setting. An internally valid evaluation that is generalizable to other populations and other settings is said to possess *external validity*.[52] Usually, a curriculum's targeted learners and setting are predetermined for the curriculum developer. To the extent that the uniqueness of the targeted learners and setting can be minimized and the representativeness maximized, the external validity (or generalizability) of the evaluation will be strengthened.

The choice of evaluation design directly affects the internal validity and indirectly affects the external validity of an evaluation (an evaluation cannot have external validity if it does not have internal validity). In choosing an evaluation design, one must be aware of each design's strengths and limitations with respect to *factors that could threaten the validity of the evaluation*. These factors include attitude of subjects, history, implementation, instrumentation, location, loss of subjects (attrition), maturation, statistical regression, subject characteristics (selection bias), and testing (Table 7.2).[46,51–55] It may not be possible or feasible, in the choice of evaluation design, to prevent all of the above factors from affecting a given evaluation. However, the curriculum developer should be aware of the potential effects of these factors when choosing an evaluation design and when interpreting the results.

The most commonly used *evaluation designs* for quantitative evaluations are posttest only, pretest-posttest, nonrandomized controlled pretest-posttest, randomized controlled posttest only, and randomized controlled pretest-posttest.[50–54] *As the designs increase in methodological rigor, they also increase in the number of resources required to execute them.*

Table 7.2.   Some Factors That Can Threaten Validity

Threat	Definition	Ways to Mitigate
Attitude of subjects	The manner in which evaluation subjects view an intervention and their participation can affect the evaluation outcome. Especially true for new interventions for which expectations are high. This is also known as the Hawthorne effect.	Evaluate over several iterations of intervention. Avoid creating expectations prior to the intervention.
History	Refers to events or other interventions that affect subjects during the period of an evaluation (e.g., an unexpected weather event closes the student access to the clinical sites for a week).	Use comparison or randomized control group in evaluation design. Measure and control for events likely to influence outcome measures.
Implementation	Occurs when the results of an evaluation vary because of differences in the way the evaluation is administered that are related to the outcome (e.g., one exam proctor keeps time precisely and another allows test takers a few extra minutes).	Train evaluators. Establish standardized implementation procedures.
Instrumentation	Refers to the effects that differences in raters, changes in measurement methods, or lack of precision in the measurement instrument might have on obtained measurements (e.g., administering a survey about curriculum satisfaction with a three-point Likert scale may yield different results than the same survey given with a seven- or nine-point Likert scale).	Pilot, standardize, and test for validity of measurement instruments. Train raters. Blind raters to status of subjects. Have evaluators rate both exposed and unexposed subjects.

Table 7.2. *(continued)*

Threat	Definition	Ways to Mitigate
Location bias	Occurs when the particular place where data are collected or where an intervention has occurred may affect results. An issue to think about in multi-institutional educational research (e.g., an intervention in one intensive care unit that is modern and well-resourced with a large amount of technology may result in different outcomes than the same intervention in another intensive care unit with fewer resources).	Make sure location is similar to those to which one wants to generalize. Make sure locations in intervention group are similar to those in comparison group.
Loss of subjects (mortality/attrition)	Occurs during evaluations that span a longer period of time. When subjects who drop out are different from those who complete the evaluation, the evaluation will no longer be representative of all subjects.	Minimize dropouts. Measure differences in subjects who complete vs. dropout from evaluation to show comparability or statistically control for differences.
Maturation	Refers to changes within subjects that occur as a result of the passage of time or experience, rather than as a result of discrete external interventions.	Use comparison or randomized control group in evaluation design.
Statistical regression	Can occur when subjects have been selected on the basis of low or high pre-intervention performance. Because of temporal variations in the performance of individuals, and because of characteristics of the test itself that result in imperfect test-retest reliability (see Task VI), subsequent scores on the performance assessment are likely to be less extreme, whether or not an educational intervention takes place.	Use comparison or randomized control group in evaluation design. Be cautious about choosing subjects based on single extreme test scores.

Threat	Definition	Ways to Mitigate
Subject characteristics/selection bias	When subject characteristics are not representative of the group to which findings are being generalized or are different in the intervention vs. comparison group *and* affect the measurements of interest or the response of subjects to the intervention (e.g., studying only volunteers who are excited to learn about a particular subject may yield different results than studying all students in a cohort).	Choose representative subjects. Measure and statistically control for differences that could affect outcome measures. Use randomized controlled design.
Testing bias	Refers to the effects of an initial test on subjects' performance on subsequent tests (i.e., subjects may learn from the test the items that occur on the test but not other items felt to be important in the domain being taught). This is relevant when a test samples the material to be learned and does not cover all that is to be learned.	Develop different but equivalent tests, each of which appropriately sample items to be learned. Extend time between tests.

A *single-group, posttest-only* design can be diagrammed as follows:

$$X - - - O$$

where X represents the curriculum or educational intervention and O represents observations or measurements. This design permits assessment of what learners have achieved after the educational intervention, but the achievements could have been present before the intervention (selection bias), occurred as part of a natural maturation process during the period prior to the evaluation (maturation), or resulted from other interventions that took place prior to the evaluation (history). Because of these limitations, the conclusions of single-group, posttest-only studies are nearly always tentative. The design is acceptable when the most important evaluation question is the certification of proficiency. The design is also well suited to assess participants' perceptions of the curriculum, to solicit suggestions for improvement in the curriculum, and to solicit feedback on and ratings of student or faculty performance.

A *single-group, pretest-posttest* design can be diagrammed as

$$O_1 - - - X - - - O_2$$

where O_1 represents the first observations or measurements, in this case before the educational intervention, and O_2 the second observations or measurements, in this case after the educational intervention. This design can demonstrate that changes in proficiency have occurred in learners during the course of the curriculum. However, the changes could have occurred because of factors other than the curriculum (e.g., history, maturation, testing, and instrumentation).

The addition of a *control or comparison group* helps confirm that an observed change occurred because of the curriculum, rather than because of history, maturation, or testing, particularly if the control group was *randomized*, which also helps to eliminate selection bias. A *pretest-posttest controlled evaluation design* can be diagrammed as

$$E \qquad O_1 - - - X - - - O_2$$
$$R$$
$$C \qquad O_1 - - - - - - - O_2$$

where E represents the experimental or intervention group, C represents the control or comparison group, R (if present) indicates that subjects were randomized between the intervention and control groups, and time is represented on the x-axis. The term "control" is often used for randomized designs, and the term "comparison" for nonrandomized designs.

A *posttest-only randomized controlled design* requires fewer resources, especially when the observations or measurements are difficult and resource-intensive. It cannot, however, demonstrate changes in learners. Furthermore, the success of the randomization process in achieving comparability between the intervention and control groups before the curriculum cannot be assessed. This design can be diagrammed as follows:

$$E \qquad X - - - O_1$$
$$R$$
$$C \qquad \quad - - - O_1$$

Evaluation designs are sometimes classified as pre-experimental, quasi-experimental, and true experimental.[51–55] *Pre-experimental designs* usually lack controls. *Quasi-experimental designs* usually include comparison groups but lack random assignment. *True experimental designs* include both random assignment to experimental and control groups and concurrent observations or measurements in the experimental and control groups.

The advantages and disadvantages of each of the discussed evaluation designs are displayed in Table 7.3. Additional designs are possible (see General References).

Political or ethical considerations may prohibit withholding a curriculum from some learners. This obstacle to a controlled evaluation can sometimes be overcome by delaying administration of the curriculum to the control group until after data collection has been completed for a randomized controlled evaluation. This can be accomplished without interference when, for other reasons, the curriculum can be administered to only a portion of targeted learners at the same time.

EXAMPLE: *Controlled Evaluation without Denying the Curriculum to the Control Group.* The design for such an evaluation might be diagrammed as follows:

$$E \qquad O_1 - - -X - - - O_2 \qquad\qquad (- - - O_3)$$
$$R$$
$$C \qquad O_1 - - - - - - - O_2 - - - - - X \qquad (- - - O_3)$$

When one uses this evaluation design, a randomized controlled evaluation is accomplished without denying the curriculum to any learner. Inclusion of additional observation points, as indicated in the

Table 7.3.   Advantages and Disadvantages of Commonly Used Evaluation Designs

Design	Diagram	Advantages	Disadvantages
Single group, posttest only (pre-experimental)	$X - - - O$	Simple Economical Can document proficiency Can document process (what happened) Can ascertain learner and faculty perceptions of efficacy and value Can elicit suggestions for improvement	Accomplishments may have been preexisting Accomplishments may be due to factors other than the curriculum. Subject to history, maturation, and selection bias.
Single group, pretest-posttest (pre-experimental)	$O_1 - - - X - - - O_2$	Intermediate in complexity and cost Can demonstrate pre-post changes in cognitive, affective, psychomotor, and other outcome measures	Accomplishments may be due to factors other than the curriculum. Subject to history, maturation, and selection bias. Accomplishments could result from learning from the first test or evaluation rather than from the curriculum
Controlled pretest-posttest (quasi-experimental)	E $O_1 - - - X - - O_2$ C $O_1 - - - - - - O_2$	Controls for maturation, if control group equivalent Controls for the effects of measured factors other than the curriculum (history) Controls for learning from the test or evaluation (testing bias)	Complex Resource-intensive Comparison group may not be equivalent to the experimental group (selection bias), and changes could be due to differences in unmeasured factors Curriculum denied to some (see text)
Randomized controlled posttest only (true experimental)	EX - - - O_1 R C - - - O_1	Controls for maturation and testing bias Controls for effects of measured and unmeasured factors (history and selection bias) Less resource-intensive than a randomized controlled pretest-posttest design, while preserving the benefits of randomization	Complex Resource-intensive Does not demonstrate changes in learners Dependent on the success of the randomization process in eliminating pretest differences in independent and dependent variables Curriculum denied to some (see text)

Table 7.3.　*(continued)*

Design	Diagram	Advantages	Disadvantages
Randomized controlled pretest-posttest (true experimental)	E　O_1 - - X - - O_2 R C　O_1 - - - - - - O_2	Controls for maturation Controls for effects of measured and unmeasured factors (history) Controls for the effects of testing If randomization is successful, controls for selection bias	Most complex Most resource-intensive Curriculum denied to some (see text) Depends on success of the randomization process in eliminating pretest differences in unmeasured indepen-dent and dependent variables

Note: O = observation or measurement; X = curriculum or educational intervention; E = experimental or inter-vention group; C = control or comparison group; R = random allocation to experimental and control groups.

parentheses, is more resource-intensive but permits inclusion of all (not just half) of the learners in a noncontrolled pretest-posttest evaluation.

It is important to realize that formative assessment and feedback may occur in an ongoing fashion during a curriculum and could be diagrammed as follows:

$$O_1 - - - X - - - O_2 - - - X - - - O_3 - - - X - - - O_4$$

In this situation, a formative assessment and feedback strategy is also an educational strategy for the curriculum.

A common concern related to the efficacy of a curricular intervention is whether the desired achievements are maintained in the learners over time. This concern can be addressed by repeating post-curricular measurements after an appropriate interval:

$$O_1 - - - X - - - O_2 - - - - - - - - - - - - - - - O_3$$

Whenever publication is a goal of a curricular evaluation, it is desirable to use the strongest design for quantitative evaluation feasible (see Chapter 9, Table 9.4). Often, an evaluation plan for a curriculum or educational program with multiple constituent cur-ricula addresses multiple evaluation questions and, therefore, includes several evalua-tion designs (see "General Considerations," above, and Chapter 10, Curriculum Devel-opment for Larger Programs).

For qualitative evaluation, the design approach may be different.[7] As in quantitative evaluation, the design is predominantly determined by the evaluation question. Often qualitative data collection is embedded within quantitative designs. However, for eval-uation focused upon collecting qualitative data, sampling strategy is less likely to be random or representative and more likely to be purposive (i.e., subjects chosen inten-tionally based on their ability to elucidate all themes related to the evaluation question in order to maximize understanding). Data collection may be at one time or ongoing and sample size predetermined or expanding until data saturation is reached (i.e., no new themes related to the data emerge). Data collection and analysis may occur more or less simultaneously, with analysis being used to refine evaluation questions and sub-sequent data collection.

The use of a mixed-method (combination of quantitative and qualitative) approach can be either convergent (occurring simultaneously), where qualitative data is usually used to help interpret the meaning or deepen the understanding of quantitative data, or sequential. When qualitative follows quantitative evaluation in a sequential approach, it is usually explanatory. When it precedes quantitative, it is often used to develop hypotheses and inform quantitative approaches.

TASK VI: CHOOSE MEASUREMENT METHODS AND CONSTRUCT INSTRUMENTS

The choice of assessment or measurement methods and construction of measurement instruments are critical steps in the evaluation process because they determine the data that will be collected, determine how the data will be collected (Task VIII), and make certain implications about how the data will be analyzed (Task IX). Formal measurement methods are discussed in this section. Table 8.2 lists additional, often informal, methods for determining how a curriculum is functioning (see Chapter 8).

Choice of Measurement Methods

Measurement methods commonly used to evaluate individuals and programs include written or electronic rating forms, self-assessment forms, essays, written or computer-interactive tests, oral examinations, questionnaires (Chapter 3), individual interviews (Chapter 3), group interviews/discussions (see Chapter 3 discussion of focus groups), direct observation (real life or simulation), performance audits, and portfolios.[56-60] The uses, strengths, and limitations of each of these measurement methods are shown in Table 7.4. They can be used for either quantitative or qualitative assessment or evaluation, depending on the nature of the data collected and the analysis methods used.

As with the choice of evaluation design, it is important to *choose a measurement method that is congruent with the evaluation question*.[55-58] Multiple-choice and direct-response written tests are appropriate methods for assessing knowledge acquisition. Higher-level cognitive ability can be assessed through essay-type, case-based computer-interactive, and oral exams. Script concordance tests, in which learners' performance is compared with performance by a sample of expert clinicians, are another type of written assessment that can be used to assess higher-level reasoning abilities.[61] Direct observation (real life or simulation) using agreed-upon standards is an appropriate method for assessing skill attainment. Chart audit and unobtrusive observations are appropriate methods for assessing real-life performance.

EXAMPLE: *Script Concordance Test to Assess Clinical Reasoning.* A script concordance test (SCT) was administered to all residents and faculty at three emergency medicine training programs. The SCT inquired about how new information may or may not be useful in the clinical decision-making process across 12 different patient care scenarios. Attending physicians scored significantly higher than trainees, whose scores were similar to one another, indicating that an inflection point of clinical reasoning ability may occur around the time of beginning independent practice.[62]

EXAMPLE: *Direct Observation Patterns.* Investigators conducted focus groups of attending physicians to determine how direct observation of trainees occurs in common graduate medical education settings. Observation sessions that were preplanned were deemed important at the beginning of training and to evaluate technical skills and normalize ongoing preplanned observation sessions as part of the training relationship.[63]

Table 7.4.   Uses, Strengths, and Limitations of Commonly Used Evaluation Methods

Method	Uses	Strengths	Limitations
Global rating forms (separated in time from observation)	Cognitive, affective, or psychomotor attributes; real-life behaviors	Economical Can evaluate anything Open-ended questions can provide information for formative purposes	Subjective Rater biases Inter- and intra-rater reliability Raters frequently have insufficient data on which to base ratings
Self-assessment forms	Cognitive, affective, psychomotor attributes; real-life behaviors	Economical Can evaluate anything Promotes self-assessment Useful for formative evaluation	Subjective Rater biases Often little agreement with objective measurements Limited acceptance as method of summative evaluation
Essays on respondent's experience	Attitudes, feelings, description of respondent experiences, perceived impact	Rich in texture Provides unanticipated as well as anticipated information Respondent-centered	Subjective Rater biases Requires qualitative evaluation methods to analyze Focus varies from respondent to respondent
Written or computer-interactive tests	Knowledge; higher-level cognitive ability	Often economical Objective Multiple-choice exams can achieve high internal consistency reliability, broad sampling Good psychometric properties, low cost, low faculty time, easy to score Widely accepted Essay-type questions or computer-interactive tests can assess higher-level cognitive ability, encourage students to integrate knowledge, reflect problem-solving, and avoid cueing	Constructing tests of higher-level cognitive ability (e.g., script concordance tests), or computer-interactive tests, can be resource-intensive Reliability and validity vary with quality of test (e.g., questions that are not carefully constructed can be interpreted differently by different respondents, there may be an insufficient number of questions to validly test a domain)

Method	Uses	Strengths	Limitations
Oral examinations	Knowledge; higher-level cognitive ability; indirect measure of affective attributes	Flexible, can follow up and explore understanding Learner-centered Can be integrated into case discussions	Subjective scoring Inter- and intra-rater reliability Reliability and validity vary with quality of test (e.g., questions that are not carefully constructed can be interpreted differently by different respondents, there may be an insufficient number of questions to validly test a domain) Faculty intensive Can be costly
Questionnaires	Attitudes; perceptions; suggestions for improvement	Economical	Subjective Constructing reliable and valid measures of attitudes requires time and skill
Individual interviews	Attitudes; perceptions; suggestions for improvement	Flexible, can follow up and clarify responses Respondent-centered	Subjective Rater biases Constructing reliable and valid measures of attitudes requires time and skill Requires interviewers
Group interviews/ discussions	Attitudes; perceptions; suggestions for improvement	Flexible, can follow up and develop/explore responses Respondent-centered Efficient means of interviewing several at once Group interaction can enrich or deepen information Can be integrated into teaching sessions	Subjective Requires skilled interviewer or facilitator to control group interaction and minimize facilitator influence on responses Does not yield quantitative information Information may not be representative of all participants

Table 7.4. *(continued)*

Method	Uses	Strengths	Limitations
Direct observation using checklists or virtual reality simulators (observing real-life or simulated performance)	Skills; real-life behaviors	Firsthand data. Can provide immediate feedback to observed. Development of standards, use of observation checklists, and training of observers can increase reliability and validity; the Objective Structured Clinical Examination (OSCE)[123,124] and Objective Structured Assessment of Technical Skills (OSATS)[125] combine direct observation with structured checklists to increase reliability and validity; high-fidelity / virtual reality simulators offer the potential for automated assessment of skills[126,127]	Rater biases. Inter- and intra-rater reliability. Personnel intensive. Unless observation covert, assesses capability rather than real-life behaviors/ performance
Performance audits	Record keeping; provision of recorded care (e.g., tests ordered, provision of preventive care measures, prescribed treatments)	Objective. Reliability and accuracy can be measured and enhanced by the use of standards and the training of raters	Dependent on what is reliably recorded; much care is not documented. Dependent on available, organized records or data sources
Portfolios	Comprehensive; can assess all aspects of competence, especially practice-based learning and improvement	Unobtrusive. Actively involves learner, documents accomplishments, promotes reflection, and fosters development of learning plans	Selective, time-consuming. Requires faculty resources to provide ongoing feedback to learner

It is desirable to choose measurement methods that have *optimal accuracy (reliability and validity, as discussed below), credibility*, and *importance*. Generally speaking, patient/health care outcomes are considered most important, followed by behaviors, skills, knowledge or attitudes, and satisfaction or perceptions, in that order.[64,65] These relate to the frequently referenced Kirkpatrick's four levels of evaluation (see Chapter 4).[64] Objective measurements are usually preferred to subjective ratings. Curricular evaluations that incorporate measurement methods at the higher end of this hierarchy are more likely to be disseminated or published (see Chapter 9). However, it is more important that what is measured is congruent with the learning objectives and desired outcomes of the curriculum than to aspire to measure the "highest" level in the hierarchy.[66] Achievement of desired outcomes serves as the ultimate indicator of value to stakeholders and must be carefully considered in determining what should be measured.[67]

It is also necessary to choose measurement methods that are *feasible in terms of available resources*. Curriculum developers usually have to make difficult decisions on how to spread limited resources among problem identification, needs assessment, educational intervention, and assessment and evaluation. Global rating forms used by faculty supervisors, which assess proficiency in a number of general areas (e.g., knowledge, patient care, professionalism), and self-assessment questionnaires completed by learners can provide indirect and inexpensive measures of ability and real-life performance; however, they are subject to numerous rating biases. Direct observation (real life or simulation) and audits using trained raters and agreed-upon standards are more reliable and have more validity evidence for measuring skills and behavior in practice than global rating forms, but they also require more resources. There is little point in using the latter measurement methods, however, if their use would drain resources that are critically important for achieving a well-conceived educational intervention.

EXAMPLE: *Use of Technology to Measure and Improve Teaching Evaluation.* A residency program relied on an end-of-rotation global rating form to assess and provide feedback on teaching to residents. The evaluation methodology suffered from recall bias, and feedback was delayed. A program leader developed a smartphone-based application based upon a validated 15-question rotation evaluation tool, which delivered three randomly selected questions plus one question inviting qualitative feedback (one effective behavior and one suggestion) immediately following inpatient teaching rounds. Evaluations were automatically sent to team members three times a week using text messaging. After 10 evaluations were collected, aggregated results were sent to the resident being evaluated. Response rate was acceptable and generated a large number of completed evaluations, enabling feedback more closely juxtaposed to actual teaching behavior. Learner and teacher satisfaction with the evaluations improved.[68]

Construction of Measurement Instruments

Most evaluations will require the construction of curriculum-specific measurement instruments, such as tests, rating forms, interview schedules, or questionnaires.

The *methodological rigor* with which the instruments are constructed and administered affects the reliability and validity of the scores and, unfortunately, the cost of the evaluation. Formative individual assessments and program evaluations generally require the least rigor; summative individual assessments and program evaluations for internal use (e.g., grades, decisions about a continuation of a curriculum) an intermediate level of rigor; and summative individual assessments and program evaluations for external use (e.g., certification of mastery or publication of evaluation results) the most rigor.

When a high degree of methodological rigor is required, it is worth exploring whether there is an *already existing measurement instrument*,[69–74] which is appropriate in terms of content, reliability, validity, feasibility, and cost. When a methodologically rigorous instrument must be constructed specifically for a curriculum, it is wise to seek *advice or mentorship from individuals with expertise in designing such instruments to ensure that evidence for its validity can be maximized.*

One of the most frequent measurement instruments is the written knowledge test. Constructing knowledge tests that are supported by reliability and validity evidence requires attention to format and interpretation of statistical tests of quality. A useful reference for faculty learning to construct written knowledge tests is the online manual developed by the National Board of Medical Examiners.[75] Written tests can be used to assess both lower-level (e.g., simple knowledge) and higher-order (e.g., clinical decision-making) cognitive attributes.

A useful first step in constructing measurement instruments is to determine the desired *content*. For assessments of curricular impact, this involves the identification of independent variables and dependent variables. *Independent variables* are factors that could explain or predict the curriculum's outcomes (e.g., the curriculum itself, previous or concurrent training, environmental factors). *Dependent variables* are program outcomes (e.g., knowledge or skill attainment, real-life performance, clinical outcomes). To keep the measurement instruments from becoming unwieldy, it is prudent to focus on a few dependent variables that are most relevant to the main evaluation questions and, similarly, to focus on the independent variables that are most likely to be related to the curriculum's outcomes.

Next, attention must be devoted to the *format* of the instruments.[74,75] In determining the acceptable *length* for a measurement instrument, methodological concerns and the desire to be comprehensive must be balanced against constraints in the amount of curricular time allotted for evaluation, imposition on respondents, and concerns about response rate. Individual items should be worded and displayed in a manner that is *clear and unambiguous*. *Response scales* (e.g., true-false; strongly disagree, disagree, neither agree nor disagree, agree, strongly agree) should make sense relative to the question asked. There is no consensus about whether it is preferable for response scales to have middle points (e.g., neither agree nor disagree) or to have an even or odd number of response categories. In general, four to seven response categories permit greater flexibility in data analysis than two or three and are easier for respondents than longer scales with 7 to 10 items. It is important for the instrument as a whole to be *user-friendly* and attractive, by organizing it in a manner that facilitates quick understanding and efficient recording of responses. It is desirable for the instrument to *engage* the interest of respondents. In general, response categories should be *precoded* to facilitate data entry and analysis. *Survey software* can provide an easy mode of delivery and facilitate collation of data for different reports. Some institutions have created secure websites,[76] employ apps for real-time assessment (see example above), and have noted improved compliance in response rates, a decrease in administrative time, and an improvement in quality.[76]

Before using an instrument for evaluation purposes, it is almost always important to *pilot* it on a convenient audience.[74] Audience feedback can provide important information about the instrument: how it is likely to be perceived by respondents, acceptable length, clarity of individual items, user-friendliness of the overall format, and specific ways in which the instrument could be improved.

EXAMPLE: *Interprofessional Development of a Formative Assessment Tool.* A group of interprofessional leaders that included physicians, nurses, patients and caregivers, and other staff generated and prioritized behaviors that comprise safe and effective conduct of patient discharge from a hospital, including medication reconciliation, discharge summary, patient communication, team communication, active collaboration, and anticipation of posthospital needs. Perceptions of educators and trainees were collected prior to implementation of the instrument.[77]

Reliability, Validity, and Bias

Because measurement instruments are never perfect, the data they produce are never absolutely accurate. An understanding of potential threats to accuracy is helpful to the curriculum developer in planning the evaluation and reporting of results, and to the users of evaluation reports in interpreting results. There has been an emerging consensus in the educational literature about the meaning of the terms *validity* and *reliability*.[78–81] Validity is now considered a unitary concept that encompasses both reliability and validity. All validity relates to the construct that is being measured and is thus considered *construct validity*.

The emphasis on construct validity has emerged from the growing realization that an instrument's scores are usually meaningful only because they accurately reflect an abstract concept (or construct) such as knowledge, skill, or patient satisfaction. Validity is best viewed as a hypothesis regarding the link between the instrument's scores and the intended construct—providing evidence for a decision about the person being assessed. Evidence is collected from a variety of sources (see below) to support or refute this hypothesis. Validity can never be "proven," just as a scientific hypothesis can never be proven; it can be supported (or refuted) only as evidence accrues.

It is also important to note that validity and reliability refer to an instrument's scores and not the instrument itself. Instruments are not "validated"; they can merely have evidence to demonstrate high levels of validity (or reliability) in one context or for one purpose, but they may be ill-suited for another context (see examples in reference 81).

The construct validity of an instrument's scores can be supported by various types of evidence.[82] This evidence can take one of two forms: empirical (information acquired by observation or experimentation) or procedural (information about assessment development).[83] The *Standards for Educational and Psychological Testing* published as a joint effort from the American Educational Research Association, American Psychological Association, and National Council on Measurement in Education[78] describes five discrete sources of validity evidence identified by Messick:[81] internal structure, content, relationship to other variables, response process, and consequences. Table 7.5 provides terminology and definitions for these types of validity evidence.

Internal Structure Validity Evidence. Internal structure validity evidence relates to the psychometric characteristics of the assessment instrument and, as such, includes all forms of reliability testing, as well as other psychometrics (e.g., *item difficulty*, percentage of individuals who select the correct answer, and *item discrimination*, how well an item distinguishes between those who scored in the upper tier and those who scored in the lower tier). It includes the concepts of inter-rater and intra-rater reliability, test-retest reliability, alternate-form reliability, and internal consistency. *Reliability* refers to the consistency or reproducibility of measurements.[73,78–81] As such, it is a necessary, but not sufficient, determinant of validity evidence. There are several different methods for assessing reliability of an assessment instrument. Reliability may be calculated using a number of statistical tests but is usually reported as a coefficient between 0 and 1

Table 7.5.   Reliability and Validity Evidence: Terminology and Definitions

Construct Validity Evidence Sources	Components	Definitions	Comments/Example
Internal structure validity evidence		Psychometric characteristics of the measurement	
	Item analysis measures	Item difficulty and discrimination, other measures of item/test characteristics. Response characteristics in different settings by different populations	
	Intra-rater reliability	Consistency of measurement results when repeated by same rater	Can be assessed by statistical methods such as kappa or phi coefficient, intraclass correlation coefficient, generalizability theory analysis. See text.
	Inter-rater reliability	Consistency of measurement results when performed by different raters	
	Test-retest reliability/stability	Degree to which same test produces same results when repeated under same conditions	
	Alternate-form reliability/equivalence	Degree to which alternate forms of the same measurement instrument produce the same result	Of relevance in pretest-posttest evaluation, when each test encompasses only part of the domain being taught, and when learning, related to test taking, could be limited to the items being tested. In such situations, it is desirable to have equivalent but different tests.
	Internal consistency/homogeneity	Extent to which same items legitimately team together to measure a single characteristic	Can be assessed with statistical methods such as Cronbach's alpha. Uni- vs. multidimensionality can be assessed by factor analysis. See text.
Content validity evidence		Degree to which a measurement instrument accurately represents the skill or characteristic it is designed to measure	

Construct Validity Evidence Sources	Components	Definitions	Comments/Example
	Literature review, expert consensus	Formal methods for consensus building, including literature review and use of topic experts	Systematic reviews of the literature, focus groups, nominal group technique, Delphi techniques, etc., can contribute to expert consensus. See text.
Relationship to other variables validity evidence		How the instrument under consideration relates to other instruments or theory	
	Criterion-related validity evidence	How well the instrument under consideration compares to related measurements	Often subdivided into concurrent and predictive validity evidence.
	Concurrent validity evidence	Degree to which a measurement instrument produces the same results as another accepted or proven instrument that measures the same characteristics at the same time	E.g., comparison with a previously developed but more resource-intensive measure-ment instrument.
	Predictive validity evidence	Degree to which a measurement instrument accu-rately predicts theoretically expected outcomes	E.g., higher scores on an instrument that assesses communica-tion skills should predict higher patient satisfaction scores.
	Convergent and discriminant validity evidence	Whether an instrument performs as would theoretically be expected in groups that are known to possess or not possess the attribute being measured, or in comparison with tests that are known to measure the same attribute (high correlation) or a different attribute (low correlation)	E.g., an instrument that assesses clinical reasoning would be expected to distin-guish novice from experienced clinicians. Scores on an instru-ment designed to measure communica-tion skills would not be expected to correlate with scores on an instrument designed to measure technical proficiency in a procedure.
Response process validity evidence		Evidence of the actions and/or thought processes of test takers or observers	E.g., documentation of data collection, entry, and cleaning procedures.

Table 7.5. *(continued)*

Construct Validity Evidence Sources	Components	Definitions	Comments/Example
		Evidence of data integrity, related to test administration and data collection	
Consequences validity evidence		Degree to which the instrument has intended/useful vs. unintended/harmful consequences, the impact of its use	E.g., it would be a problem if results from a measurement method of limited reliability and validity were being used to make decisions about career advancement when the intent was to use the results as feedback to stimulate and direct trainee improvement.

(for more information, see reference 80). Regardless of the specific test used to calculate it, the reliability coefficient can also be thought of as the proportion of score variance explained by differences between subjects, with the remaining due to error (random and systematic). For high-stakes examinations (licensure), reliability should be greater than 0.9. For many testing situations a reliability of 0.7–0.8 may be acceptable. Ideally, measurement scores should be in agreement when repeated by the same rater (*intra-rater reliability*) or made by different raters (*inter-rater reliability*). Intra- or inter-rater reliability can be assessed by the percentage agreement between raters or by statistics such as kappa,[81] which corrects for chance agreement. A commonly used method of estimating inter-rater reliability is the intraclass correlation coefficient, accessible in commonly available computer software, which uses analysis of variance to estimate the variance of different factors. It permits estimation of the inter-rater reliability of the *n* raters used, as well as the reliability of a single rater. It can also manage missing data.[80] A sophisticated method for estimating inter-rater agreement often used in performance examinations uses *generalizability theory analysis*, in which variance for each of the variables in the evaluation can be estimated (i.e., subjects or true variance vs. raters and measurements or error variance). Changes can be made in the number of measurements or raters dependent on the variance seen in an individual variable.[84]

> **EXAMPLE**: *Generalizability Theory Analysis.* Medical student performance on the surgery clerkship was assessed at the end of each rotation by asking for four items to be rated by three different faculty members. Generalizability theory analysis demonstrated that the reliability (true variance / total variance) of this assessment was only 0.4; that is, that only 40% of the total variance was due to the difference between subjects (true variance), and the rest of the variance was due to differences between the raters and/or items, and/or interactions among the three sources of variation. The reliability was improved to 0.8 by adding six items, as well as requiring evaluations from three different resident raters.

Other forms of internal structure validity evidence include stability, equivalence, and internal consistency or homogeneity. *Test-retest reliability*, or *stability*, is the degree to which the same test given to the same person produces the same results when repeated under the same conditions. This is not commonly done, because of time, cost, and the possibility of contamination by intervening variables when the second test is separated in time. *Alternate-form reliability*, or *equivalence*, is the degree to which alternate forms of the same measurement instrument produce the same result. *Internal consistency*, or *homogeneity*, is the extent to which various items legitimately team together to measure a single characteristic, such as a desired attitude. Internal consistency can be assessed using the statistic Cronbach's (or coefficient) alpha,[80] which is basically the average of the correlations of each item in a scale to the total score. A complex characteristic, however, could have several dimensions. In this situation, the technique of factor analysis[85] can be used to help separate the different dimensions. When there is a need to assess the reliability of an important measure but a lack of statistical expertise among curricular faculty, statistical consultation is advisable.

EXAMPLE: *Internal Structure Validity Evidence: Internal Consistency/Homogeneity.* The group of medical student clerkship directors worked together to develop an integrative clinical reasoning assessment for chronic conditions at the completion of students' basic clerkships. Assessment of three cognitive areas was planned: (1) multidisciplinary factual knowledge for the appropriate management of diabetes mellitus and congestive heart failure in different settings; (2) clinical decision-making for diagnostic and therapeutic strategies that incorporated the use of evidence and patient preferences; and (3) cost-effectiveness of decisions in relation to outcomes. After piloting of the test, a factor analysis was able to identify separate clinical decision-making and cost-effectiveness dimensions. However, there was not a single knowledge dimension. Knowledge split into two separate factors, each of which was specific to one of the two medical disorders. Cronbach's alpha was used to assess homogeneity among items that contributed to each of the four dimensions or factors. There were a large number of items for each dimension, so those with low correlation with the overall score for each dimension were considered for elimination.

EXAMPLE: *Internal Structure Validity Evidence: Psychometrics.* All medical students must achieve a passing score on the United States Medical Licensing Examination (USMLE) to be eligible for licensure, and it is also a graduation requirement for many schools. For this high-stakes examination, the reliability coefficient determined by any means should be 0.8 or greater. That is, the reproducibility of the score must be very high. Furthermore, psychometric analysis of each item is routinely conducted, which includes an analysis of item difficulty and item discrimination, and an analysis of who answered which options.

Content Validity Evidence. Content validity evidence is the degree to which an instrument's scores accurately represent the skill or characteristic the instrument is designed to measure, based on people's experience and available knowledge. Although "face" or "surface" validity are terms that may have been considered part of this category, they are based on the appearance of an instrument rather than on a formal content analysis or empirical testing and are thus no longer appropriate for use in the literature or vocabulary of health professions educators. Content validity can be enhanced by conducting an appropriate literature review to identify the most relevant content, using topic experts, and revising the instrument until a reasonable degree of consensus about its content is achieved among knowledgeable reviewers. Formal processes, such as focus groups, nominal group technique, Delphi technique, use of daily diaries, observation by work sampling, time and motion studies, critical incident reviews, and reviews of ideal performance cases, can also contribute (see Chapter 2).

EXAMPLE: *Content Validity Evidence.* During the design of an ethics curriculum for obstetrics and gynecology residents, a group of experts in maternal-fetal medicine, genetics, neonatology, and biomedical ethics participated in a Delphi process to reach a consensus on the primary content areas to be covered during the curriculum, along with ensuring appropriate alignment of all assessment tools with the target content areas.

Relationship to Other Variables Validity Evidence. This form of validity refers to how the instrument under consideration relates to other instruments or theory. It includes the concepts of criterion-related, concurrent, and predictive validity. *Criterion-related validity evidence* encompasses concurrent validity and predictive validity evidence. *Concurrent validity evidence* demonstrates the degree to which a measurement instrument produces the same results as another accepted or proven instrument that measures the same parameters. *Predictive validity evidence* demonstrates the degree to which an instrument's scores accurately predict theoretically expected outcomes (e.g., scores from a measure of attitudes toward preventive care should correlate significantly with preventive care behaviors). Procedural evidence in this domain includes active involvement of experts in development of prediction criteria.

EXAMPLE: *Relationship to Other Variables Validity / Concurrent Validity Evidence.* Educators for a medical student psychiatry clerkship have created a computer-interactive psychiatry knowledge assessment to be given at the end of the clerkship. Scores on this examination are found to demonstrate a positive correlation with performance on the National Board of Medical Examiners Psychiatry Subject Examination, with clerkship grades, and with performance on the Clinical Knowledge examination of the USMLE, Step II.

EXAMPLE: *Relationship to Other Variables Validity / Predictive Validity Evidence.* For board certification in general surgery, the American Board of Surgery requires candidates to achieve passing scores on both a written qualifying examination (QE) and an oral certifying examination (CE). Many surgical residency programs use mock oral examinations to prepare their residents for the CE, as mock oral performance has been shown to predict performance on the CE.[86]

Concurrent and predictive validity evidence are forms of *convergent validity evidence*, in which the study measure is shown to correlate positively with another measure or construct to which it theoretically relates. *Discriminant validity evidence*, on the other hand, is a form of evidence in which the study measure is shown to not correlate or to correlate negatively with measures or constructs to which it, theoretically, is not, or is negatively, related.

EXAMPLE: *Relationship to Other Variables / Convergent and Discriminant Validity Evidence.* Scores from an instrument that measures clinical reasoning ability would be expected to distinguish between individuals rated by faculty as high or low in clinical reasoning (convergent validity evidence). Scores on the instrument would be expected to correlate significantly with grades on an evidence-based case presentation (convergent validity evidence) but not with measures of compassion (discriminate validity evidence).

Response Process Validity Evidence. Response process validity evidence includes evidence about the integrity of instrument administration and data collection so that these sources of error are controlled or eliminated. It could include information about quality control processes, use of properly trained raters, documentation of procedures used to ensure accuracy in data collection, evidence that students are familiar with test formats, or evidence that a test of clinical reasoning actually invokes higher-order thinking in test takers.

EXAMPLE: *Response Process Validity Evidence.* Use of a standardized orientation script, trained proctors at testing centers, documentation of their policies and procedures, and strict adherence to time limitations are sources of response process validity evidence for the USMLE, a high-stakes licensure exam.

Consequences Validity Evidence. This refers to the consequences of an assessment for examinees, faculty, patients, and society. It answers the question "What outcomes (good and bad) have occurred because of the assessment and related decisions?" If the consequences are intended or useful, this evidence supports the ongoing use of the instrument. If the consequences are unintended and harmful, educators may think twice before using the instrument for the same purpose in the future. Consequence validity evidence could also include the method or process to determine the cut scores, as well as the statistical properties of passing scores.

EXAMPLE: *Consequences Validity Evidence.* Medical College Admission Test (MCAT) scores have mild predictive value for medical student success, particularly in the preclinical years.[87,88] However, students with midrange scores are more diverse than students with high scores. We also know that when admissions committees admit students with midrange MCAT scores who have demonstrated the capacity and competencies needed to become physicians, those students succeed at high rates, progressing through medical school on time and passing their licensure exams on the first attempt. The consequences of relying too heavily on MCAT scores likely decreases the diversity of medical school classes and the related benefits to society.[89,90]

Scoring, Generalization, Extrapolation, and Implication. Although the above framework classifies evidence supporting the validity of an assessment in measuring a construct, it does not provide a mechanism for prioritization among the different types of validity evidence obtained. It does not analyze how they fit together into making an argument for their intended use. This was addressed by Kane in 2006 in a framework that, while incorporating the above concepts, emphasized key inferences as one progresses from measurements to decision: scoring, generalization, extrapolation, and implication.[49] Cook argues that evidence should be collected to support each of these inferences and should focus on the most questionable assumptions in the chain of inference.[49] *Scoring* (translating an observation into one or more scores) is influenced by the construction of specific items, including their response options, and fairness and standardization in assessment administration. *Generalization* (using a score as a reflection of performance in a test setting) recognizes that the items selected as part of an assessment instrument are usually a sample of potential items from a broader set of possible options. As part of testing the generalization of a single assessment observation, the question of how well the selected test items represent all of the theoretically possible relevant items is addressed. The methods utilized to ensure adequate sampling within the test domain and empiric studies to determine the reproducibility of similar scores with a new sample of items provide evidence to support this. *Extrapolation* helps the curriculum designer to understand how performance on an assessment translates to real-world performance. Evidence for this inference includes procedural methods, such as observation of—and experts thinking aloud during—task performance and empirical analyses determining the association between assessment scores and a comparable metric related to the real task, to ensure the assessment reflects key aspects of real-world performance.

EXAMPLE: *Empirical Extrapolation Evidence.* To test the ability of a laparoscopic skills trainer to increase learner readiness for intracorporeal suturing, scores of a simulated exercise were compared between medical students (novices), surgical residents (advanced beginners), and attending surgeons (experts). This analysis identified that scores improved with increasing laparoscopic experience.

Implication (using the score[s] to inform a decision or action) evaluates the consequences or impact of the assessment on the individual, stakeholders, and society more broadly, moving from thinking about the score and its interpretation to a specific use, decision, or action.

Threats to Validity. Another way to look at validity, complementary to the above perspectives, is to consider the potential threats to validity (i.e., negative validity evidence). Bias related to insufficient sampling of trainee attributes or cases, variations in the testing environment, and inadequately trained raters can threaten validity.[91] Threats to validity have been classified into two general categories: construct underrepresentation and construct-irrelevant variance.[92] These errors interfere with the interpretation of the assessment.

Construct underrepresentation connotes inadequate sampling of the domain to be assessed, biased sampling, or a mismatch of the testing sample to the domain.[92] It relates to the generalizability inference described above.

> **EXAMPLE:** *Construct Underrepresentation Variance.* An instructor has just begun to design a written examination for students at the end of their cardiopulmonary physiology module. The instructor "doesn't believe in" simple knowledge tests and plans to use questions based on one clinical scenario to assess knowledge application. A majority of students' grades will be based on this examination. Unfortunately, this exam is likely to demonstrate construct underrepresentation variance because the number of clinical scenarios is too few to represent the entire domain of cardiopulmonary knowledge expected. The problem could be addressed by increasing the number of clinical scenarios in the test and establishing content validity evidence using input from basic science and clinical experts.

Construct-irrelevant variance refers to systematic (as opposed to random) error that is introduced into the assessment and does not have a relationship to the construct being measured. It includes flawed or biased test items, inappropriately easy or difficult test items, indefensible passing scores, poorly trained standardized patients, and rater bias. Rating biases are particularly likely to occur when global rating forms are being used by untrained raters to assess learner or faculty performance. Rating biases can affect both an instrument's reliability and evidence of validity.[91] *Errors of leniency or harshness* occur when raters consistently rate higher than is accurate (e.g., rating all trainees in a health professional training program "above average") or lower than is accurate (e.g., judging junior generalist physicians against standards appropriate to senior specialist physicians). The *error of central tendency* refers to the tendency of raters to avoid extremes. The *halo effect* occurs when individuals who perform well in one area or relate particularly well to others are rated inappropriately high in other, often unobserved, areas of performance. *Attribution error* occurs when raters make inferences about why individuals behave as they do and then rate them in areas that are unobserved, based on these inferences.

> **EXAMPLE:** *Construct-Irrelevant Variance: Attribution Error.* An individual who consistently arrives late and does not contribute actively to group discussions is assumed to be lazy and unreliable. She is rated low on motivation. The individual has a problem with child care and is quiet, but she has done all of the required reading, has been active in defining her own learning needs, and has independently pursued learning resources beyond those provided in the course syllabus.

Rater biases may be reduced and inter- and intra-rater reliability improved by training those who are performing the ratings. Because not all training is effective, it is important to confirm the efficacy of training by assessing the reliability of raters and the accuracy of their ratings.

Another type of construct-irrelevant variance that has received increasing attention is *implicit bias*, often referring to age, ethnicity, gender, obesity, and race. It can affect both test items and raters. One study examined the routine use of race/ethnicity in preparatory materials for licensing examinations and found that 20% of questions in a popular question bank referred to race/ethnicity in the question stem, answer, or educational objective.[93] Because race/ethnicity is not an acceptable proxy for genetics, social class, or culture, and is associated with health care disparities, curriculum developers should be mindful that such subtle messages can contribute to the propagation of implicit bias among newly minted health care professionals. Raters can also manifest implicit bias in evaluating trainees; awareness and management of this bias may lead to its mitigation.[94]

Internal and external validity are discussed above in reference to evaluation designs (Task V). It is worth noting here that the reliability and validity of the scores for each instrument used in an evaluation affect the internal validity of the overall evaluation and, additionally, would have implications for any external validity of an evaluation.

It is also worth noting here that the reliability and validity of an instrument's scores affect the utility, feasibility, and propriety of the overall evaluation. Many of the threats to validity can be minimized once considered. Thus, open discussion of these issues should occur in the planning stages of the evaluation. Areas of validity evidence that are relatively easy to collect include internal structure and content validity evidence. Including some evidence of the validity of one's measurement methods increases the likelihood that a curriculum-related manuscript will be accepted for publication (see Chapter 9, Table 9.4).

Reliability and Validity in Qualitative Measurement. The above discussion of reliability and validity pertains to quantitative measurements. Frequently, *qualitative information* is also gathered to enrich and help explain the quantitative data that have been obtained, to describe the context of the curriculum, and to elicit suggestions for program improvement. As mentioned earlier, *qualitative evaluation methods* are also used to explore the processes and impact (such as unintended, unanticipated, or otherwise unmeasured outcomes) of a curriculum, deepen understanding, generate novel insights, and develop hypotheses about both how a curriculum works and its effects.

> **EXAMPLE:** *Qualitative Evaluation Methods.* A "boot camp" curriculum for students preparing to enter a surgical residency includes an exit interview in the form of a focus group. During this session, students are asked structured questions about the curriculum's strengths, weaknesses, processes, impact, explanations for impact, and suggestions for improvement. Their responses are recorded for further analysis and use in ongoing curriculum refinement.

When qualitative measurements are used as methods of evaluating a curriculum, those unfamiliar with this approach may have concerns about their accuracy and about the interpretation of conclusions that are drawn from the data. The methods for assessing reliability and validity described above pertain to quantitative measurements.[95] While a detailed discussion of the accuracy of qualitative measurement methods is beyond the scope of this book, it is worth noting that there are concepts in qualitative research that parallel the quantitative research concepts discussed above that relate to reliability and validity.[95-99] Collectively, these concepts address the "trustworthiness" of qualitative research, the notion of "getting it right." *Reflexivity* refers to investigators revealing their theoretical perspectives and background characteristics/experiences that may influence their interpretation of observations. It also refers to investigators reflecting on and accounting for these factors (i.e., attempting to remain as free from biases as possible when interpreting data). *Confirmability* provides assurances that the conclusions that are drawn about what is studied would be reached if another investigator undertook the same analysis of the same data or used a different measurement method. Frequently, in qualitative analysis of the same dataset, two or more investigators review and abstract themes and then have a process for reaching consensus. *Triangulation* can be used to enhance the trustworthiness of study methods (use of more than one method or source of data to study a phenomenon) or of study results (pointing out how results match or differ from those of other studies). *Dependability* refers to consistency and reproducibility of the research method over time and across research subjects and contexts. There may be quality checks on how questions are asked or the data are coded. There should be an *audit trail* or record of the study's methods and procedures, so that others can replicate what was done. *Internal validity / credibility / authenticity* refers to how much the results of the qualitative inquiry ring true. Study subjects can be asked to confirm, refute, or otherwise comment on the themes and explanations that emerge from qualitative data analysis (*respondent validation* or *member checks*). The investigators should study / account for *exceptions* to the themes that emerge from the qualitative data analysis. They should consider and discuss alternative explanations. There should be a representative, rich or *thick* description of the data, including examples, sufficient to support the investigators' interpretations. The data collection methods should be adequate to address the evaluation question. As with the quantitative research concept of *external validity*, *transferability* in qualitative research deals with the applicability of findings more broadly. Do the results apply to other cases or settings and resonate with stakeholders in those settings? Did the investigators describe their study subjects and setting in sufficient detail? Did they compare their results with those from other studies and with empirically derived theory (*triangulation* of findings)? The reader can consult this chapter's General References, "Qualitative Evaluation," for a more detailed discussion of these concepts.

As in quantitative evaluation, *implicit bias* can also affect qualitative evaluations.

EXAMPLE: *Differences in Terms Used in Letters of Recommendations.* A study of "Dean's letters" accompanying medical students' applications for residency positions revealed difference in key words used by race/ethnicity and gender. This persisted despite controlling for USMLE Step 1 scores and was thought to represent implicit bias.[100]

Conclusions

Because all measurement instruments are subject to threats to their reliability and validity, the ideal evaluation strategy will employ *multiple measurements using several different measurement methods and several different raters*. When all results are similar, the findings are said to be *robust*. One can feel even more comfortable when a variety of validity evidence supports their use. This point cannot be overemphasized, as multiple concordant pieces of evidence, each individually weak, can collectively provide strong evidence to support judgments based on evaluation.

TASK VII: ADDRESS ETHICAL CONCERNS

Propriety Standards

More than any other step in the curriculum development process, evaluation is likely to raise ethical and what are formally called propriety concerns.[46,101] This can be broken down into seven categories[46] (Table 7.6). Major concerns relate to concern for human rights and human interactions, which usually involves issues of confidentiality, access, student rights, and consent; resource allocation; and potential impact of the evaluation. It is wise for curriculum developers to anticipate these ethical concerns and address them in planning the evaluation. In addressing important ethical concerns, it can be helpful to obtain input both from the involved parties, such as learners and faculty, and from those with administrative oversight for the overall program. Institutional policies and

Table 7.6.   Ethical-Propriety Concerns Related to Evaluation

Issue	Recommendation
Responsive and inclusive orientation	Place the needs of program participants and stakeholders in the center. Elicit suggestions for program improvement.
Formal policy / agreements	Have a formal policy or agreement regarding the purpose and questions of the evaluation, the release of reports, and confidentiality and anonymity of data.
Rights of human subjects	Clearly establish the protection of the rights of human subjects. Clarify intended uses of the evaluation. Ensure informed consent. Follow due process. Respect diversity; avoid implicit bias. Keep stakeholders informed. Understand participant values. Follow stated protocol. Honor confidentiality and anonymity agreements. Do no harm.
Clarity and fairness	Assess and report a balance of the strengths and weaknesses and unintended outcomes. Acknowledge limitations of the evaluation.
Transparency and disclosure	Define right-to-know audiences (i.e., stakeholders). Clearly report the findings and the basis for conclusions. Disclose limitations. Assure that reports reach their intended audiences.
Conflict of interest	Identify real and perceived conflicts of interest. Assure protection against conflicts of interest. Use independent parties or reporting agencies as needed to avoid conflicts of interest.
Fiscal responsibility	Consider and specify budgetary needs. Keep some flexibility. Be frugal. Include a statement of use of funds. Consider evaluation process in the context of entire program budget.

Source: Adapted from Yarbrough et al.[46]

procedures, external guidelines, and consultation with uninvolved parties, including those in the community, can also provide assistance.

Confidentiality, Access, Student Rights, and Consent

Concerns about confidentiality, access, and consent usually relate to those being evaluated, and their rights. Decisions about confidentiality must be made regarding who should have access to an individual's assessments. Concerns are magnified when feasibility considerations have resulted in the use of measurement methods of limited reliability and validity, and when there is a need for those reviewing the assessments to understand these limitations. Curriculum developers should also be aware of relevant law (e.g., the Family Educational Rights and Privacy Act, or FERPA) and other regulations regarding the use of learner and health care data in evaluations pertinent to their program and location.

The curriculum developer must decide whether any evaluators should be granted confidentiality (the evaluator is unknown to the evaluated but can be identified by someone else) or anonymity (the evaluator is known to no one). This concern usually pertains to individuals in subordinate positions (e.g., students, employees) who have been asked to evaluate those in authority over them, and who might be subject to retaliation for an unflattering assessment. Anonymous raters may be more open and honest, but they may also be less responsible in criticizing the person being rated.

Finally, it is necessary to decide whether those being assessed need to provide informed consent for the assessment process. Even if a separate formal consent for the evaluation is not required, decisions need to be made regarding the extent to which those being assessed will be informed about the following: the assessment methods being used; the strengths and limitations of the assessment methods; the potential users of the assessments (e.g., deans, program directors, board review committees); the uses to which assessment results will be put (e.g., formative purposes, grades, certification of proficiency for external bodies); the location of assessment results, their confidentiality, and methods for ensuring confidentiality; and, finally, the assessment results themselves. Which assessment results will be shared with whom, and how will that sharing take place? Will collated or individual results be shared? Will individual results be shared with those being assessed? If so, how? Do students have a right to contest a test result? Is there an institutional policy on student appeals? Each of these issues should be addressed and answered during the planning stage of the evaluation process. The "need to know" principle should be widely applied. Publication of evaluation results beyond one's institution constitutes educational research. When publication or other forms of dissemination are contemplated (see Chapter 9), curriculum developers should consult their institutional review board or relevant research ethics committee in the planning stages of the evaluation, before data are collected (see Chapters 6 and 9).

Resource Allocation

The use of resources for one purpose may mean that fewer resources are available for other purposes. The curriculum developer may need to ask whether the allocation of resources for a curriculum is fair and whether the allocation is likely to result in the most overall good. A strong evaluation could drain resources from other curriculum development steps. Therefore, it is appropriate to think about the impact of resource allocation on learners, faculty, curriculum coordinators, and other stakeholders in the curriculum.

A controlled evaluation design, for example, may deny an educational intervention to some learners. This consequence may be justified if the efficacy of the intervention is widely perceived as questionable and if there is consensus about the need to resolve the question through a controlled evaluation.

On the other hand, allocation of resources to an evaluation effort that is important for a faculty member's academic advancement, but that diverts needed resources from learners or other faculty, is ethically problematic.

There may also be concerns about the allocation of resources for different evaluation purposes. How much should be allocated for formative purposes, to help learners and the curriculum improve, and how much for summative purposes, to ensure trainees' competence for the public or to develop evidence of programmatic success for the curriculum developers, one's institution, or those beyond one's institution? It is important to plan for these considerations during the development process, before implementation of the curriculum (Chapter 6).

Potential Impact/Consequences

The evaluation may have an impact on learners, faculty, curriculum developers, other stakeholders, and the curriculum itself. It is helpful to consider the way evaluation results might be used, and whether the evaluation is likely to result in more good than harm. An evaluation that lacks methodological rigor due to resource limitations could lead to false conclusions, improper interpretation, and harmful use. It is therefore important to ensure that the uses to which an evaluation is put are appropriate for its degree of methodological rigor, to ensure that the necessary degree of methodological rigor is maintained over time, and to inform users of an evaluation's methodological limitations as well as its strengths.

EXAMPLE: *Inability to Conduct Sufficiently Accurate Individual Summative Assessments.* The director for the internal medicine clerkship wants to evaluate the overall progress of students in the competencies of medical knowledge and patient care at the midpoint of the clerkship; however, there are not sufficient resources to develop individual summative assessments of high accuracy. The director instead elects to obtain individual observational assessments from one faculty member and one resident for each student. Because the assessments lack sufficient inter-rater reliability and validity evidence, they are used for formative purposes and discussed in an interactive way with learners, with suggestions for how to improve their skills. The results of these assessments are kept only until the end of the clerkship to evaluate longitudinal progress, and they are not used for summative assessment purposes or entered into the student's record where others could have access to them.

EXAMPLE: *Inability to Conduct a Sufficiently Accurate Summative Program Evaluation.* As a pilot program, a medical school designed and implemented a longitudinal third- and fourth-year curriculum around the core EPAs for entering residency.[14] After four months, the curriculum committee requested a report about whether the third-year students demonstrated "entrustability" yet, as proof of measurable benefits of the new curriculum. Curriculum developers had planned an evaluation at the end of one year, based on sample size, cost of the simulation-heavy evaluation, and reliability and validity evidence of the assessment tools. Given the possibility that a false conclusion could be drawn on the outcome of the curriculum after four months, and that more harm than good could result from the evaluation, the curriculum developers instead reported formative evaluation results of student and faculty satisfaction and engagement with the curriculum.

EXAMPLE: *Informing Users of Methodological Limitations of an Evaluation Method.* In a surgery residency program, multiple types of assessment data are used to rate residents' performance against the milestones that have been mapped to each of the ACGME Core Competencies to satisfy requirements for the Next Accreditation System.[102] A listing of the limitations of and validity evidence for each instrument used in milestone assessment is included in each resident's record, along with advice about how to interpret each of the measures.

Equity in evaluation is an increasingly recognized concern related to the impact/consequences of evaluation. As discussed above under construct-irrelevant variance and consequences validity evidence, implicit bias[93,94] and structural aspects of assessment[89,90] can adversely affect students underrepresented in medicine. Structural aspects include overemphasis on certain measurements, failure to measure important attributes, insufficient transparency and criteria in assessment, and making major decisions based upon small differences.[89,90,103,104]

TASK VIII: COLLECT DATA

Sufficient data must be collected to ensure a useful analysis. Failure to collect important evaluation data that match the evaluation questions or low response rates can seriously compromise the value of an evaluation. While it may be tempting to cast a wide net in data collection, doing so excessively or inefficiently can consume valuable resources and lead to fatigue in respondents.

Response Rates and Efficiency

While the evaluation data design dictates when data should be collected relative to an intervention, curriculum coordinators usually have flexibility with respect to the precise time, place, and manner of data collection. Data collection can therefore be planned to maximize response rates, feasibility, and efficiency. Today, secure web-based assessment and evaluation tools may allow efficiency in the collection and analysis of data.[76]

Response rates can be boosted and the need for follow-up reduced when data collection is built into scheduled learner and faculty activities. This may be further facilitated using asynchronous and online learning activities, for which electronic platforms may offer mechanisms for built-in evaluation. Response rates can also be increased if a learner's completion of an evaluation is required to achieve needed credit.

> **EXAMPLE**: *Integrating Data Collection into the Curriculum.* A 15-question evaluation was embedded on the last page of an interactive online learning module on the pediatrics clerkship. Students were required to complete both the module and its evaluation to receive credit, and all students completed the evaluation without need for follow-up.

Sometimes an evaluation method can be designed to serve simultaneously as an educational method. This strategy reduces imposition on the learner and uses curriculum personnel efficiently.

> **EXAMPLE**: *A Method Used for Both Teaching and Evaluation.* Test-enhanced learning, a method for increasing knowledge retention through repeated testing without interval studying as a type of "retrieval practice," was utilized at a continuing professional development conference among pediatricians in Canada. Participants were randomized to no testing and pre- and post-session multiple-choice testing groups. Participants in the testing group showed a moderate effect size (measure of the size of change, see below, Task IX) from testing (0.46, 95% CI 0.26–0.67), and the majority (65%) reported improved learning from the tests.[105]

Occasionally, data collection can be incorporated into already scheduled evaluation activities.

EXAMPLE: *Use of an Existing Evaluation Activity.* A multistation examination was used to assess students' accomplishments at the end of a clinical clerkship in neurology. Curriculum developers for a procedural curriculum on lumbar puncture were granted a station for a simulated patient assessment during the examination.

EXAMPLE: *Use of an Existing Evaluation Activity.* Evaluation of a new competency-based evaluation method (observable practice activities) was embedded into the existing evaluation workflow within an internal medicine residency program, with assessments at the midpoint and end of each rotation. Over a three-year period, over 300,000 data points were collected and demonstrated increasing proficiency with increasing level of training.[106]

Finally, curriculum developers may be able to use existing data sources, such as electronic medical records, to collect data automatically for evaluation purposes.

EXAMPLE: *Use of Available Data.* Developers of an ambulatory primary care curriculum were able to obtain reports from electronic medical records to assess pre-post curriculum delivery of targeted preventive care measures, such as immunizations, cholesterol profiles, and breast and colon cancer screening. They were also able to track these measures longitudinally to assess post-curricular maintenance versus decay of preventive care measures.

Interaction between Data Collection and Instrument Design

What data are collected is determined by the choice of measurement instruments (see Task VI). However, the design of measurement instruments needs to be tempered by the process of data collection. Response rates for questionnaires will fall as their length and complexity increase. The amount of time and resources that have been allocated for data collection cannot be exceeded without affecting learners, faculty, or other priorities.

EXAMPLE: *Impact of Instrument Length.* In a study where paramedic educators were asked to either rate four clinical observations in all six performance dimensions or sequentially rate three performances on two of the six performance dimensions, the authors found that the amount and quality of unique feedback was decreased when raters were asked about more performance dimensions. They posited that this may be due either to time constraints or limits of raters' attention.[107]

Assignment of Responsibility

Measurement instruments must be distributed, collected, and safely stored. Non-respondents require follow-up. While different individuals may distribute or administer measurement instruments within scheduled sessions, it is usually wise to delegate overall responsibility for data collection to one person.

EXAMPLE: *Assignment of Responsibility.* A multicenter study of a medical student simulation curriculum recruited a site director for each participating institution. These individuals oversaw all training, collected data, and tracked students' completion of surveys.[108]

TASK IX: ANALYZE DATA

After the data have been collected, they need to be analyzed.[109–115] *Data analysis, however, should be planned at the same time that evaluation questions are being identified and measurement instruments developed.* Tools previously utilized in business or in the delivery of clinical care are now being made available within health professional education. Termed *learning analytics*, these tools can be thought of as a compendium of data analysis techniques that describe, characterize, and predict the learning behaviors of individuals,[116] and they can be deployed to gather information about learner- or system-level performance. Congruent with the repeated theme in this chapter that advance planning lies at the heart of useful assessment, optimal deployment of learning analytics can only occur when the data that are inputted have sufficient validity evidence and are placed in a database constructed with analysis in mind.

> **EXAMPLE:** *Learning Analytics Using Resident Dashboards.* Aggregated workplace-based assessment data from three Canadian emergency medicine residency programs generated a dataset of nearly 1,500 unique ratings about 23 residents. With computational modeling, study authors were able to visually display that residents begin at different points and progress at different rates, but that rating scores tended to increase with each additional assessment, indicating progress over time.[117]

Relation to Evaluation Questions

The nature of evaluation questions will determine, in part, the type of statistical approach required to answer them. Questions related to participants' perceptions of a curriculum, or to the percentage of learners who achieved a specific objective, generally require only descriptive statistics. Questions about changes in learners generally require more sophisticated tests of statistical significance.

Statistical considerations may also influence the choice of evaluation questions. A *power analysis*[109–111] is a statistical method for estimating the ability of an evaluation to detect a statistically significant relationship between an outcome measure (dependent variable) and a potential determinant of the outcome (independent variable, such as exposure to a curriculum). The power analysis can be used to determine whether a curriculum has a sufficient number of learners over a given period of time to justify a determination of the statistical significance of its impact. Sometimes there are limitations in the evaluator's statistical expertise and in the resources available for statistical consultation. Evaluation questions can then be worded in a way that at least ensures *congruence* between the questions and the analytic methods that will be employed.

> **EXAMPLE:** *Congruence between the Evaluation Question and the Analytic Methods Required.* A curriculum developer has a rudimentary knowledge of statistics and few resources for consultation. After designing the assessment instruments, an evaluation question was changed. "Does the curriculum result in a statistically significant improvement in the proficiency of its learners in skill X?" was changed to "What percentage of learners improve or achieve proficiency in skill X by the end of the curriculum?" so that application of tests of statistical significance could be avoided.

When the curriculum evaluation involves a large number of learners, analysis could reveal a statistically significant but an educationally meaningless impact on learners. The latter consideration might prompt curriculum evaluators to develop an evaluation question that addresses the magnitude as well as the statistical significance of any impact. *Effect size* is increasingly used to provide a measure of the size of a change, or the degree to which sample results diverge from the null hypothesis.[112] Several measurements have been used to give an estimate of effect size: *correlation coefficient, r,* which is the measure of the relationship between variables, with the value of r^2 indicating the percentage of variance explained by the measured variables; *eta-square (η^2)*, which is reported in analysis of variance and is interpreted as the proportion of the variance of an outcome variable explained by the independent variable; odds ratios; risk ratios; absolute risk reduction; and *Cohen's d*, which is the difference between two means (e.g., pre-post scores or experimental vs. control groups) divided by the pooled standard deviation associated with that measurement. The effect size is said to be small if Cohen's $d = 0.20$, medium if 0.50, and large if ≥ 0.80.[111] However, measures of effect size are probably more meaningful when judging the results of several studies with similar designs and directly comparable interventions, rather than using these thresholds in absolute terms. For example, it would not be surprising to see a large Cohen's *d* when comparing a multimodal curriculum against no intervention, whereas the expected Cohen's *d* for a study comparing two active educational interventions would be much smaller. It is important to remember that educational meaningfulness is still an interpretation that rests not only on the statistical significance and size of a change but also on the nature of the change and its relation to other outcomes deemed important. Examples of such outcomes might be improvements in adherence to management plans or a reduction in risk behaviors, morbidity, or mortality.

Relation to Measurement Instruments: Data Type and Entry

The measurement instrument determines the type of data collected. The *type of data*, in turn, *helps determine the type of statistical test that is appropriate to analyze the data*[113–115] (Table 7.7). Data are first divided into one of two types: numerical or categorical. *Numerical* data are data that have meaning on a numerical scale. Numerical data can be continuous (e.g., age, weight, height) or discrete, such as count data (no fractions, only non-negative integer values—e.g., number of procedures performed or the number of sessions attended). Numerical data can also be subdivided into interval and ratio data. *Interval data* are numerical data with equal intervals, distances, or differences between categories but no zero point (e.g., year, dates on a calendar). *Ratio data* are numerical data with equal intervals and a meaningful zero point (e.g., weight, age, number of procedures completed appropriately without assistance). *Categorical* data are data that fit into discrete categories. *Within the categorical domain, data can additionally be described as either nominal or ordinal. Nominal* data are categorical data that fit into discrete, nonordered categories (e.g., sex, race, eye color, exposure or not to an intervention). *Ordinal data* are categorical data that fit into discrete but inherently ordered or hierarchical categories (e.g., grades: A, B, C, D, and F; highest educational level completed: grade school, high school, college, postcollege degree program; condition: worse, same, better).

Data analysis considerations affect the design of the measurement instrument. When a computer is being used, the first step in data analysis is *data entry*. In this situation, it is helpful to construct one's measurement instruments in a way that facilitates data entry, such as the precoding of responses or using electronic evaluation software that can download data into a usable spreadsheet format. *Technology* can also be utilized for other aspects of the assessment and evaluation process—for example, participant registration, tracking, and retention; process evaluation including assignment completion; and outcomes evaluation including changes in knowledge and behavior.[118]

Choice of Statistical Methods

The choice of statistical method depends on several factors, including the evaluation question, evaluation design, sample size, number of study groups, whether groups

Table 7.7. Commonly Used Statistical Methods

Type of Measurement (Dependent Variable)	Tests/Methods Used for Evaluating Statistically Significant Differences or Associations						
	One Sample (Observed vs. Expected)	Two Samples		N Samples			
		Independent	Related (pre-post)	Independent	Related (pre-post)	Correlation	Multivariate Analysis*
Nominal	Binomial test Chi-square	Fisher exact test Chi-square	McNemar's test	Chi-square	Cochran's Q test	Contingency coefficient	Cumulative logistic regression Discriminant function analysis
Dichotomous	Binomial test Chi-square	Chi-square Odds ratio Relative risk Prevalence ratio	McNemar's test	Chi-square Logistic regression (odds ratios)	Logistic regression (odds ratios)		Logistic regression (odds ratios) Generalized estimating equations (GEE) Discriminant functional analysis
Ordinal or ordered	Kolmogorov-Smirnov one-sample test One-sample runs test	Median test Mann-Whitney U Kolmogorov-Smirnov test Wald-Wolfowitz runs test	Sign test Wilcoxon matched pairs signed rank test	Kruskal-Wallis ANOVA† (one-way ANOVA)	Friedman's two-way ANOVA	Spearman's r Kendall's τ (tau) Kendall's w	Multiple regression Polychotomous logistic regression Generalized estimating equations (GEE) Hierarchical regression models (mixed regression)

	Mean, SD,‡ confidence interval	t-test	Paired t-test Wilcoxon matched pairs signed rank test	ANOVA	Repeated-measures ANOVA Generalized estimating equations (GEE) Hierarchical regression models (mixed regression)	Pearson r	Linear regression Partial correlation Multiple correlation Multiple regression ANCOVA§ Generalized estimating equations (GEE) Hierarchical regression models (mixed regression) Canonical correlation
Interval and ratio	Mean, SD,‡ confidence interval	t-test	Paired t-test Wilcoxon matched pairs signed rank test	ANOVA	Repeated-measures ANOVA Generalized estimating equations (GEE) Hierarchical regression models (mixed regression)	Pearson r	Linear regression Partial correlation Multiple correlation Multiple regression ANCOVA§ Generalized estimating equations (GEE) Hierarchical regression models (mixed regression) Canonical correlation
Count data	Confidence interval using Poisson distribution	Poisson, negative binomial, or zero-inflated Poisson models	Poisson, negative binomial, or zero-inflated Poisson models Paired t-test Wilcoxon matched pairs signed rank test	Poisson, negative binomial. or zero-inflated Poisson models	Poisson, negative binomial, or zero-inflated Poisson models	Spearman's r, if well enough distributed	Poisson, negative binomial, or zero-inflated Poisson models
Time to event—survival analysis	Kaplan-Meier survival curves (survival function)	Kaplan-Meier survival curves Log-rank test Proportional hazards regression Hazard ratios		Kaplan-Meier survival curves Log-rank test Proportional hazards regression Hazard ratios	Kaplan-Meier survival curves Log-rank test Proportional hazards regression Adjusted hazard ratios		Kaplan-Meier survival curves Log-rank test Proportional hazards regression Adjusted hazard ratios

*Multivariate analysis involves analysis of more than one variable at a time and permits analysis of the relationship between one independent variable (e.g., the curriculum) and a dependent variable of interest (e.g., learner skill or behavior) while controlling for other independent variables (e.g., age, gender, level of training, previous or concurrent experiences).

† ANOVA = analysis of variance.

‡ SD = standard deviation.

§ ANCOVA = analysis of covariance.

are matched or paired for certain characteristics, number of measures, data distribution, and the type of data collected. *Descriptive statistics* are often sufficient to answer questions about participant perceptions, distribution of characteristics and responses, and percentage change or achievement. For all types of data, a display of the percentages or proportions in each response category is an important first step in analysis. Medians and ranges are sometimes useful in characterizing ordinal as well as numerical data. Means and standard deviations are reserved for describing numerical data. Ordinal data (e.g., from Likert scales) can sometimes be treated as numerical data so that means and standard deviations (or other measures of variance) can be applied.

> **EXAMPLE:** *Conversion of Ordinal to Numerical Data for the Purpose of Statistical Analysis.* Questions from one institution's 360° resident evaluations use a Likert scale with the following categories: strongly disagree, disagree, neutral, agree, and strongly agree. For analysis, these data were converted to numerical data so that responses could be summarized by means: strongly disagree [1], disagree [2], neutral [3], agree [4], strongly agree [5].

Statistical tests of significance are required to answer questions about the statistical significance of changes in individual learners or groups of learners, and of associations between various characteristics. *Bivariate analysis* explores the relationship between two variables at a time. Most often, the curriculum developer is interested in establishing the relationship between an outcome (the *dependent* variable) and the intervention (the primary *independent* variable), along with additional characteristics. Bivariate analysis is usually not sufficient. *Multivariate analysis* attempts to tease out the independent effects of multiple characteristics (including potentially confounding variables).

> **EXAMPLE:** *Use of Multivariate Analysis.* In the example above of test-enhanced learning, multivariate analysis was used to control for covariates (e.g., number of workshops attended) during the continuing education conference. The covariates could not account for the differences in knowledge retention observed between the experimental and control groups.[105]

Parametric statistics, such as *t*-tests, analysis of variance, regression, and Pearson correlation analysis, are often appropriate for numerical data. In choosing an appropriate statistical method for analysis, careful consideration must be given to the distribution of the data. Table 7.7 is intended as a general guide. Parametric tests assume that the sample has been randomly selected from the population it represents and that the distribution of data in the population has a known underlying distribution. However, these tests are often robust enough to tolerate some deviation from this assumption. The most common distribution assumption is that the distribution is normal. Other common distributions include the binomial distribution (used for binary outcomes) and the Poisson distribution (used for count data). Sometimes ordinal data can be treated as numerical data (see example above) to permit the use of parametric statistics.

Nonparametric tests, such as chi-square, Wilcoxon rank-sum test, Spearman's correlation statistic, and nonparametric versions of analysis of variance, do not make, or make few, assumptions about the distribution of data in a population. They are often appropriate for small sample sizes, categorical data, and non-normally distributed data.

Statistical software packages are available that can perform parametric and nonparametric tests on the same data. This approach can provide a check of the statistical results when numerical data do not satisfy all of the assumptions for parametric tests. One can be confident about using parametric statistics on ordinal level data when nonparametric statistics confirm decisions regarding statistical significance obtained using parametric statistics. For non-normally distributed data, it may be possible to normalize the data through transformation (e.g., log transformation) in order to use parametric rather than nonparametric statistics (which tend to have lower power).

The most common multivariate statistical methods include multiple regression (used for a continuous outcome variable), logistic regression (used for a binary outcome), Poisson regression (used for count data), and Cox regression (used for time-to-event outcomes). Each of these methods has the capacity of controlling for multiple variables at a time. With each method, the goal is to parse the statistical contributions of independent relationships of various characteristics (the independent variables) with an outcome.

Curriculum developers have varying degrees of statistical expertise. Those with modest levels of expertise and limited resources (the majority) may choose to keep data analysis simple. They can consult textbooks (see below, General References, "Statistics") on how to perform simple statistical tests, such as *t*-tests, chi-squares, and the Wilcoxon rank-sum test. These tests, especially for small sample sizes, can be performed by hand or with a calculator (online calculators are now available) and do not require access to computer programs. Sometimes, however, the needs of users will require more sophisticated approaches. Often there are individuals within or beyond one's institution who can provide statistical consultation. The curriculum developer will use the statistician's time most efficiently when the evaluation questions are clearly stated and the key independent and dependent variables are clearly defined. Some familiarity with the range and purposes of commonly used statistical methods can also facilitate communication. Table 7.7 displays the situations in which statistical methods are appropriately used, based on the type of data being analyzed, the number and type of samples, and whether correlational or multivariate analysis is desired. As indicated toward the bottom of the table, count data require special consideration. Another type of situation that is captured at the bottom of the table is statistical analysis of time to a desired educational outcome or event, which can be analyzed using various survival analysis techniques, such as the log-rank test or Cox regression. Cox (or proportional hazards) regression has the advantage of providing hazard ratios (akin to odds ratios).

Analysis of Qualitative Data

Analysis of qualitative data may involve counts but does not employ tests of statistical significance. It usually starts with reduction, or extracting the essence, of data, often through thematic analysis.[7,119] It then proceeds to organizing the reduced data or themes in ways that enhance meaning[7] Finally, the analysis leads to conclusions or proposed explanations for the findings.[7] Throughout, attention should be paid to the integrity and rigor of the analysis, as described above (see "Reliability and Validity in Qualitative Measurement").

TASK X: REPORT RESULTS

The final step in evaluation is the reporting and distribution of results.[120] In planning evaluation reports, it is helpful to think of the *needs of users*.

The *timeliness* of reports can be critical. Individual learners benefit from the immediate feedback of formative assessment results, so that the information can be processed while the learning experience is still fresh and can be used to enhance subsequent learning within the curriculum. Evaluation results are helpful to faculty and curriculum planners when they are received in time to prepare for the next curricular cycle. Important decisions, such as the allocation of educational resources for the coming year, may be influenced by the timely reporting of evaluation results to administrators in concert with budget cycles. External bodies, such as funding agencies or specialty boards, may also impose deadlines for the receipt of reports.

The *format* of a report should match the needs of its users in content, language, and length. Individual learners, faculty members, and curriculum developers may want detailed evaluation reports pertaining to their particular (or the curriculum's) performance that include all relevant quantitative and qualitative data provided by the measurement instruments. Administrators, deans, and department chairs may prefer brief reports that provide background information on the curriculum and that synthesize the evaluation information relevant to their respective needs. External bodies and publishers (see Chapter 10) may specify the format they expect for a report.

It is always desirable to *display results in a succinct and clear manner and to use plain language*. An *Executive Summary* can be helpful to the reader, particularly when it precedes detailed and/or lengthy reports. Specific examples can help explain and bring to life summaries of qualitative data. Collated results can be enhanced by the addition of descriptive statistics, such as percentage distributions, means, medians, and standard deviations. Other results can be displayed in a clear and efficient manner in tables, graphs, or figures.

> **EXAMPLE:** *Use of Figures to Communicate Educational Outcomes.* Construction of learning curves (effort on x-axis, learning on y-axis) to demonstrate the relationship between learning effort and outcome achievement have been noted to be useful at several levels: at an individual learner level for self and teacher-directed instruction; at the level of curriculum developers and administrators for educational management and outcomes tracking. Learning curves can be used to visually demonstrate the rate of learning (slope of the line), times when learning is more effortful (an inflection point), and when mastery is achieved (upper asymptote).[121]

Dashboards, which incorporate the use of figures and tables, are being increasingly used to meet the needs of users, such as Clinical Competency Committees, and the requirements of regulatory bodies, such as the ACGME.[122]

CONCLUSION

Evaluation is not the final step in curriculum planning, but one that directly affects and should evolve in concert with other steps in the curriculum development process (see also Chapter 1). It provides important information that can help both individuals and programs improve their performance. It provides information that facilitates judgments and decisions about individuals and the curriculum. A stepwise approach can help ensure an evaluation that meets the needs of its users and that balances methodological rigor with feasibility.

Congratulations! You have read and thought about six steps critical to curriculum development. At this point, rereading Chapter 1 may be worthwhile, to review briefly the six steps and reflect on how they interact.

ACKNOWLEDGMENTS

We thank Joseph Carrese, MD, MPH, for his review of all parts of this chapter related to qualitative evaluation. We thank Ken Kolodner, ScD, for his review of and input to the section "Task IX: Analyze Data," Table 7.7, our mention of specific statistical tests throughout the chapter, and "Statistics" under General References.

QUESTIONS

For the curriculum you are coordinating, planning, or would like to be planning, please answer or think about the following questions and prompts:

1. Who will be the *users* of your curriculum?

2. What are their needs? *How will evaluation results be used?*

3. What *resources* are available for evaluation, in terms of *time*, *personnel*, *equipment*, *facilities*, *funds*, and *existing data*?

4. Identify one to three critical *evaluation questions*. Are they *congruent* with the objectives of your curriculum? Do either the objectives or the evaluation questions need to be changed?

5. Name and diagram the most appropriate *evaluation design* for each evaluation question, considering both methodological rigor and feasibility (see Table 7.3 and text). What issues related to validity are pertinent for your evaluation design (see Table 7.2)?

6. Choose the most appropriate *measurement methods* for the evaluation you are designing (see Table 7.4). Are the measurement methods *congruent* with the evaluation questions (i.e., are you measuring the correct items)? Would it be *feasible* for you, given available resources, to construct and administer the required measurement instruments? If not, do you need to revise the evaluation questions or choose other evaluation methods? What issues related to reliability and validity are pertinent for your measurement instrument (see Table 7.5)?

7. What *ethical issues* are likely to be raised by your evaluation in terms of confidentiality, access, consent, resource allocation, potential impact, or other concerns? Should you consult your institutional review board?

8. Consider the *data collection* process. *Who will be responsible* for data collection? How can the data be collected so that *resource use* is minimized and *response rate* is maximized? Are data collection considerations likely to influence the *design of your measurement instruments*?

9. How will the data that are collected be *analyzed*? Given your evaluation questions, are *descriptive statistics* sufficient or are *tests of statistical significance* required? Is a *power analysis* desirable? Will statistical consultation be required?

10. List the goals, content, format, and time frame of the various *evaluation reports* you envision, given the needs of the users (refer to Questions 1 and 2). How will you ensure that the reports are completed?

GENERAL REFERENCES

Comprehensive

Fink, Arlene. *Evaluation Fundamentals: Insights into the Outcomes, Effectiveness, and Quality of Health Programs*. 3rd ed. Thousand Oaks, CA: SAGE Publications, 2014.
Reader-friendly, basic comprehensive reference on program evaluation, with examples from the health and social science fields. 273 pages.

Fitzpatrick, Jody L., James R. Sanders, and Blaine R. Worthen. *Program Evaluation: Alternative Approaches and Practical Guidelines*. 4th ed. Upper Saddle River, NJ: Pearson Education, 2011.
Comprehensive text on evaluation methods and a systematic, detailed approach to design, implementation, and reporting of an evaluation. Excellent use of a longitudinal evaluation problem throughout the text. 560 pages.

Green, Lawrence W., and Frances M. Lewis. *Measurement and Evaluation in Health Education and Health Promotion*. Palo Alto, CA: Mayfield Publications, 1986.
Clearly written, comprehensive text with examples from community health and patient education programs with easy applicability to medical education programs. Both quantitative and qualitative methods are included. 411 pages.

Kalet, Adina, and Calvin L. Chou, eds. *Remediation in Medical Education: A Mid-course Correction*. New York: Springer Publishing Co., 2014.
This multiauthored and pithy text brings together the array of potential learner assessment methods in the new era of competency-based education, current understanding of root causes of learner failures, and potential approaches to remediation. There are numerous examples and models that can be transferred to other institutions. 367 pages.

McGaghie, William C., ed. *International Best Practices for Evaluation in the Health Professions*. London, New York: Radcliffe Publishing, 2013.
Multiauthored text encompassing an international group of 69 educational experts. Sixteen chapters cover topics including the need for and methodology of evaluation and specific foci of evaluation, such as clinical competence, knowledge acquisition, professionalism, team performance, continuing education, outcomes, workplace performance, leadership/management, recertification, and accreditation. The final chapter describes a new educational framework of mastery learning and deliberative practice. 377 pages.

Windsor, Richard A. *Evaluation of Health Promotion, Health Education, and Disease Prevention Programs*. 3rd ed. Boston: McGraw-Hill, 2004.
Written for health professionals who are responsible for planning, implementing, and evaluating health education or health promotion programs, with direct applicability to medical education. Especially useful are the chapters on process evaluations and cost evaluation. 292 pages.

Measurement

DeVellis, Robert F. *Scale Development: Theory and Applications*. 4th ed. Thousand Oaks, CA: SAGE Publications, 2016.
Authoritative text in the Applied Social Research Methods series that provides an eight-step framework for creation and refinement of surveys and scales for use in social sciences research. 280 pages.

Fink, Arlene, ed. *The Survey Kit*. 2nd ed. Thousand Oaks, CA: SAGE Publications, 2002.
Ten user-friendly, practical handbooks about various aspects of surveys, both for the novice and for those who are more experienced but want a refresher reference. The first book is an overview of the survey method. The other handbooks are "how-to" books on asking survey questions; conducting self-administered and mail surveys; conducting interviews by telephone; conducting interviews in person; designing surveys; sampling for surveys; assessing and interpreting survey psychometrics; managing, analyzing, and interpreting survey data; and reporting on surveys. Ten books, ranging from 75 to 325 pages in length.

Lane, Suzanne, Mark R. Raymond, and Thomas M. Halayna. *Handbook of Test Development*. 2nd ed. Philadelphia, PA: Routledge, 2015.
Up-to-date, research-oriented guide to the latest developments in the field. Thirty-two chapters, divided into five sections, covering the foundations of test development, content definition, item development, test design and form assembly, and the processes of test administration, documentation, and evaluation. 692 pages.

Miller, Delbert Charles, and Neil J. Salkind. *Handbook of Research Design and Social Measurement*. 6th ed. Thousand Oaks, CA: SAGE Publications, 2002.
The most useful part of this textbook is Part 7 (209 pages), selected sociometric scales and indices to measure social variables. Scales in the following areas are discussed: social status; group structure and dynamics; social indicators; measures of organizational structure; community; social participation; leadership in the work organization; morale and job satisfaction; scales of attitudes, values, and norms; personality measurements; and others. 808 pages.

Paniagua, Miguel A., and Kimberly A. Swygert, eds. *Constructing Written Test Questions for the Basic and Clinical Sciences*. 4th ed. Philadelphia: National Board of Medical Examiners, 2016. Accessed September 20, 2021. https://www.bumc.bu.edu/busm/files/2018/10/NBME -Constructing-Written-Test-Questions.pdf.
Written for medical school educators who need to construct and interpret flawlessly written test questions. Frequent examples. 94 pages.

Waugh, C. Keith, and Norman Gronlund. *Assessment of Student Achievement*. 10th ed. Upper Saddle River, NJ: Pearson Education, 2012.
Basic text with review of assessment methods, validity and reliability in planning, preparing and using achievement tests, performance assessments, grading and reporting, and interpretation of scores. 288 pages.

Evaluation Designs

Campbell, Donald T., N. L. Gage, and Julian C Stanley. *Experimental and Quasi-experimental Designs for Research*. Boston: Houghton Mifflin, 1963.
Succinct, classic text on research/evaluation designs for educational programs. More concise than the later edition, and tables more complete. Table 1 (p. 8), Table 2 (p. 40), and Table 3 (p. 56) diagram different experimental designs and the degree to which they control or do not control for threats to internal and external validity; pages 5–6 concisely summarize threats to internal validity; pages 16–22 discuss external validity. 84 pages.

Fraenkel, Jack R., Norman E. Wallen, and Helen H. Hyun. *How to Design and Evaluate Research in Education*. 10th ed. New York, NY: McGraw-Hill Education, 2018.
Comprehensive and straightforward review of educational research methods, with step-by-step analysis of research and real case studies. 640 pages.

Qualitative Evaluation

Crabtree, Benjamin F., and William L. Miller. *Doing Qualitative Research*. 2nd ed. Thousand Oaks, CA: SAGE Publications, 1999.
Practical, user-friendly text with an emphasis on using qualitative methods in primary care research. 424 pages.

Denzin, Norman K., and Yvonna S. Lincoln. *Handbook of Qualitative Research*. 5th ed. Thousand Oaks, CA: SAGE Publications, 2017.
Comprehensive text that is useful as a reference to look up particular topics. 992 pages.

Miles, Matthew B., A. Michael Huberman, and Johnny Saldaña. *Qualitative Data Analysis: A Methods Sourcebook*. 4th ed. Thousand Oaks, CA: SAGE Publications, 2019.
Practical text and useful resource on qualitative data analysis. Chapter 11 focuses on drawing and verifying conclusions, as well as issues of reliability and validity. 408 pages.

Patton, Michael Q. *Qualitative Research & Evaluation Methods*. 4th ed. Thousand Oaks, CA: SAGE Publications, 2014.
Readable, example-filled text emphasizing strategies for generating useful and credible qualitative information for decision-making. The three sections of the book cover conceptual issues in the use of qualitative methods; qualitative designs and data collection; and analysis, interpretation, and reporting of such studies. 832 pages.

Richards, Lyn, and Janice M. Morse. *README FIRST for a User's Guide to Qualitative Methods*. 3rd ed. Thousand Oaks, CA: SAGE Publications, 2012.
Readable, introductory book to qualitative research methods. 336 pages.

Statistics

Kanji, Gopal K. *100 Statistical Tests*. 3rd ed. Thousand Oaks, CA: SAGE Publications, 2006.
A handy reference for the applied statistician and everyday user of statistics. An elementary knowledge of statistics is sufficient to allow the reader to follow the formulae given and to carry out the tests. All 100 tests are cross-referenced to several headings. Examples also included. 256 pages.

Norman, Geoffrey R., and David L. Streiner. *Biostatistics: The Bare Essentials*. 4th ed. Shelton, CT: People's Medical Publishing House–USA, 2014.
Practical, irreverent guide to statistical tests that explains them with clarity and humor. 438 pages.

Norman, Geoffrey R., and David L. Streiner. *PDQ Statistics*. 3rd ed. Hamilton, ON: B. C. Decker, 2003.
This short, well-written book covers types of variables, descriptive statistics, parametric and nonparametric statistics, multivariate methods, and research designs. The authors assume that the reader has had some introductory exposure to statistics. The intent of the book is to help the reader understand the various approaches to analysis when reading/critiquing the results section of research articles. Useful also for planning an analysis, in order to avoid misuse and misinterpretation of statistical tests. 218 pages.

Shott, Susan. *Statistics for Health Professionals*. Philadelphia: W. B. Saunders Co., 1990.
The author states that after studying this text and working the problems, the reader should be able to select appropriate statistics for most datasets, interpret results, evaluate analyses reported in the literature, and interpret SPSS and SPS output for the common statistical procedures. 418 pages.

Assessment Frameworks and Instruments

Association of American Medical Colleges (AAMC). MedEdPORTAL. Available at www.mededportal .org. Search "Directory and Repository for Educational Assessment Measures."
Provides easy to locate, publicly accessible information about assessment instruments.

Pangaro, Louis, and Olle ten Cate. "Frameworks for Learner Assessment in Medicine: AMEE Guide No. 78," *Medical Teacher* 35 (2013): e1197-200. https://doi.org/10.3109/0142159X.2013 .788789.

REFERENCES CITED

1. Jody L. Fitzpatrick, James R. Sanders, and Blaine R. Worthen, "Evaluation's Basic Purpose, Uses, and Conceptual Distinctions," in *Program Evaluation: Alternative Approaches and Practical Guidelines*, 4th ed. (Upper Saddle River, NJ: Pearson Education, 2011), 3–38.
2. John Norcini et al., "2018 Consensus Framework for Good Assessment," *Medical Teacher* 40, no. 11 (2018): 1102–9, https://doi.org/10.1080/0142159x.2018.1500016.
3. C. P. M. Van Der Vleuten et al., "Twelve Tips for Programmatic Assessment," *Medical Teacher* 37, no. 7 (2015): 641–46, https://doi.org/10.3109/0142159x.2014.973388.

4. Dario M. Torre, L. W. T. Schuwirth, and C. P. M. Van der Vleuten, "Theoretical Considerations on Programmatic Assessment," *Medical Teacher* 42, no. 2 (2020): 213–20, https://doi.org/10.1080/0142159x.2019.1672863.

5. Ann W. Frye and Paul A. Hemmer, "Program Evaluation Models and Related Theories: AMEE Guide No. 67," *Medical Teacher* 34, no. 5 (2012): e288–99, https://doi.org/10.3109/0142159x.2012.668637.

6. Faizal Haji, Marie-Paul Morin, and Kathryn Parker, "Rethinking Programme Evaluation in Health Professions Education: Beyond 'Did It Work?,'" *Medical Education* 47, no. 4 (2013): 342–51, https://doi.org/10.1111/medu.12091.

7. Jennifer Cleland. "Exploring versus Measuring: Considering the Fundamental Differences between Qualitative and Quantitative Research," in *Researching Medical Education*, ed. Jennifer Cleland and Steven J. Durning (Oxford: Wiley Blackwell, 2015), 1–14.

8. Ayelet Kuper, Scott Reeves, and Wendy Levinson. "An Introduction to Reading and Appraising Qualitative Research," *BMJ* 337 (2008): a288, https://www.doi.org/10.1136/bmj.a288.

9. Olle ten Cate, "Nuts and Bolts of Entrustable Professional Activities," *Journal of Graduate Medical Education* 5, no. 1 (2013): 157–58, https://doi.org/10.4300/JGME-D-12-00380.1.

10. Susan R. Swing, "The ACGME Outcome Project: Retrospective and Prospective," *Medical Teacher* 29, no. 7 (2007): 648–54, https://doi.org/10.1080/01421590701392903.

11. Olle ten Cate and Fedde Scheele, "Competency-Based Postgraduate Training: Can We Bridge the Gap between Theory and Clinical Practice?" *Academic Medicine* 82, no. 6 (2007): 542–47, https://doi.org/10.1097/ACM.0b013e31805559c7.

12. Olle ten Cate, "Entrustability of Professional Activities and Competency-Based Training," *Medical Education* 39, no. 12 (2005): 1176–77, https://doi.org/10.1111/j.1365-2929.2005.02341.x.

13. Karen J. Brasel et al. "Entrustable Professional Activities in General Surgery: Development and Implementation," *Journal of Surgical Education* 76, no. 5 (2019): 1174–86, https://doi.org/10.1016/j.jsurg.2019.04.003.

14. "Core Entrustable Professional Activities for Entering Residency (CEPAER)," Association of American Medical Colleges, March 2014, accessed September 16, 2021, https://www.aamc.org/system/files/c/2/484778-epa13toolkit.pdf.

15. David P. Sklar, "Creating a Medical Education Continuum with Competencies and Entrustable Professional Activities," *Academic Medicine* 94, no. 9 (2019): 1257–60, https://doi.org/10.1097/acm.0000000000002805.

16. Olle ten Cate and Carol Carraccio, "Envisioning a True Continuum of Competency-Based Medical Education, Training, and Practice," *Academic Medicine* 94, no. 9 (2019): 1283–88, https://doi.org/10.1097/acm.0000000000002687.

17. Brandon David Moore, *Designing and Aligning Learning Outcome Assessments for Academic Programs: Proficiencies That Students Are Expected to Demonstrate — Learning Institutions Are Expected to Authenticate* (Urbana: University of Illinois and Indiana University), National Institute for Learning Outcomes Assessment, 2020, accessed September 16, 2021, www.learningoutcomesassessment.org/wp-content/uploads/2020/02/AiP-Moore.pdf.

18. Shefaly Shorey et al., "Entrustable Professional Activities in Health Care Education: A Scoping Review," *Medical Education* 53, no. 8 (2019): 766–77, https://doi.org/10.1111/medu.13879.

19. Ayse Atasoylu et al., "Promotion Criteria for Clinician-Educators." *Journal of General Internal Medicine* 18, no. 9 (2003): 711–16, https://doi.org/10.1046/j.1525-1497.2003.10425.x.

20. Brent W. Beasley et al., "Promotion Criteria for Clinician-Educators in the United States and Canada. A Survey of Promotion Committee Chairpersons," *JAMA* 278, no. 9 (1997): 723–28.

21. Victoria M. Fleming et al., "Separate and Equitable Promotion Tracks for Clinician-Educators," *JAMA* 294, no. 9 (2005): 1101–4, https://doi.org/10.1001/jama.294.9.1101.

22. Deborah Simpson et al., "Advancing Educators and Education by Defining the Components and Evidence Associated with Educational Scholarship," *Medical Education* 41, no. 10 (2007): 1002–9, https://doi.org/10.1111/j.1365-2923.2007.02844.x.

23. Jorge G. Ruiz et al., "E-learning as Evidence of Educational Scholarship: A Survey of Chairs of Promotion and Tenure Committees at U.S. Medical Schools," *Academic Medicine* 84, no. 1 (2009): 47–57, https://doi.org/10.1097/ACM.0b013e3181901004.

24. John Norcini et al., "Criteria for Good Assessment: Consensus Statement and Recommendations from the Ottawa 2010 Conference," *Medical Teacher* 33, no. 3 (2011): 206–14, https://doi.org/10.3109/0142159x.2011.551559.

25. Harold G. J. Bok et al., "Programmatic Assessment of Competency-Based Workplace Learning: When Theory Meets Practice," *BMC Medical Education* 13 (2013): 123, https://doi.org/10.1186/1472-6920-13-123.

26. Susan Gearhart et al., "Development of a Train-to-Proficiency Curriculum for the Technical Skills Component of the Fundamentals of Endoscopic Surgery Exam," *Surgical Endoscopy* 32, no. 7 (2018): 3070–75, https://doi.org/10.1007/s00464-017-6018-7.

27. Jori Hall, Melissa Freeman, and Kathy Roulston, "Right Timing in Formative Program Evaluation," *Evaluation and Program Planning* 45 (2014): 151–56, https://doi.org/10.1016/j.evalprogplan.2014.04.007.

28. Harm Peters et al., "Introducing an Assessment Tool Based on a Full Set of End-of-Training EPAs to Capture the Workplace Performance of Final-Year Medical Students," *BMC Medical Education* 19, no. 1 (2019): 207, https://doi.org/10.1186/s12909-019-1600-4.

29. David R. Stead, "A Review of the One-Minute Paper," *Active Learning in Higher Education* 6, no. 2 (2005): 118–31, https://doi.org/10.1177/1469787405054237.

30. Barbara G. Lubejko, "Developing a Program Evaluation Plan: Options and Opportunities," *Journal of Continuing Education in Nursing* 47, no. 9 (2016): 388–89, https://doi.org/10.3928/00220124-20160817-02.

31. Frederic W. Hafferty and Ronald Franks, "The Hidden Curriculum, Ethics Teaching, and the Structure of Medical Education," *Academic Medicine* 69, no. 11 (1994): 861–71, https://doi.org/10.1097/00001888-199411000-00001.

32. Janet P. Hafler et al., "Decoding the Learning Environment of Medical Education: A Hidden Curriculum Perspective for Faculty Development," *Academic Medicine* 86, no. 4 (2011): 440–44, https://doi.org/10.1097/ACM.0b013e31820df8e2.

33. Meghan McConnell, Jonathan Sherbino, and Teresa M. Chan, "Mind the Gap: The Prospects of Missing Data," *Journal of Graduate Medical Education* 8, no. 5 (2016): 708–12, https://doi.org/10.4300/JGME-D-16-00142.1.

34. Joshua R. Lakin et al. "A Curriculum in Quality Improvement for Interprofessional Palliative Care Trainees," *American Journal of Hospice and Palliative Medicine* 37, no. 1 (2020): 41–45, https://doi.org/10.1177/1049909119850794.

35. Brandyn Lau et al., "Individualized Performance Feedback to Surgical Residents Improves Appropriate Venous Thromboembolism Prophylaxis Prescription and Reduces Potentially Preventable VTE: A Prospective Cohort Study," *Annals of Surgery* 264, no. 6 (2016): 1181–87, https://doi.org/10.1097/sla.0000000000001512.

36. Linda Suskie, "Supporting Assessment Efforts with Time, Infrastructure, and Resources," in *Assessing Student Learning: A Common Sense Guide*, 2nd ed., ed. Linda Suskie (San Francisco: Jossey-Bass, 2009), 86–97.

37. Yiqun Lin et al., "Improving CPR Quality with Distributed Practice and Real-Time Feedback in Pediatric Healthcare Providers—a Randomized Controlled Trial," *Resuscitation* 130 (2018): 6–12, https://doi.org/10.1016/j.resuscitation.2018.06.025.

38. Association of American Medical Colleges (AAMC), *MedEdPORTAL*, accessed October 6, 2021, https://www.mededportal.org. Search "critical synthesis package."

39. Toshiko Uchida and Heather L. Heiman, "Critical Synthesis Package: Hypothesis-Driven Physical Examination (HDPE)," *MedEdPORTAL* 9 (2013), https://doi.org/10.15766/mep_2374-8265.9435.

40. Sarah H. Ailey and Beth Marks, "Technical Standards for Nursing Education Programs in the 21st Century," *Rehabilitation Nursing* 45, no. 6 (2020): 311–20, https://doi.org/10.1097/rnj.0000000000000297.

41. Constance Burke, "Diversity and Inclusion: Addressing Underrepresentation of Students with Disabilities in Health Care Education," *Journal of Physician Assistant Education* 30, no. 1 (2019): 61–63, https://doi.org/10.1097/JPA.0000000000000244.

42. Philip Zazove et al., "U.S. Medical Schools' Compliance with the Americans with Disabilities Act: Findings from a National Study," *Academic Medicine* 91, no. 7 (2016): 979–986, https://doi.org/10.1097/ACM.0000000000001087.

43. Lisa M. Meeks and Kurt R. Herzer, "Prevalence of Self-Disclosed Disability among Medical Students in US Allopathic Medical Schools," *JAMA* 316, no. 21 (2016): 2271–72, https://doi.org/10.1001/jama.2016.10544.

44. Lisa M. Meeks et al., "National Prevalence of Disability and Clinical Accommodations in Medical Education," *Journal of Medical Education and Curricular Development* 7 (2020): 1–4, https://doi.org/10.1177/2382120520965249.

45. C. Keith Waugh and Norman E. Gronlund, "Planning for Assessment," in *Assessment of Student Achievement*, 10th ed. (Upper Saddle River, NJ: Pearson Education, 2012), 31–47.

46. Donald B. Yarbrough et al. (Joint Committee on Standards for Educational Evaluation), *The Program Evaluation Standards: A Guide for Evaluators and Evaluation Users, 3rd ed.* (Thousand Oaks, CA: SAGE Publications, 2011), accessed September 18, 2021, www.jcsee.org.

47. David Shih Wu et al., "Narrative Approach to Goals of Care Discussions: A Novel Curriculum," *Journal of Pain and Symptom Management* 58, no. 6 (2019): 1033–39.e1, https://doi.org/10.1016/j.jpainsymman.2019.08.023.

48. Benjamin Roberts et al., "Narrative Approach to Goals of Care Discussions: Adapting the 3-Act Model Training to an Online Format," *Journal of Pain and Symptom Management* 60 (2021): 874–78, https://doi.org/10.1016/j.jpainsymman.2021.02.009.

49. David A. Cook et al., "A Contemporary Approach to Validity Arguments: A Practical Guide to Kane's Framework," *Medical Education* 49, no. 6 (2015): 560–75, https://doi.org/10.1111/medu.12678.

50. Arlene Fink, "Designing Program Evaluations," in *Evaluation Fundamentals: Insights into the Outcomes, Effectiveness, and Quality of Health Programs*, 3rd ed. (Thousand Oaks, CA: SAGE Publications, 2014), 67–100.

51. Jody L. Fitzpatrick, James R. Sanders, and Blaine R. Worthen, "Collecting Evaluative Information: Design, Sampling, and Cost Choices," in Fitzpatrick et al., *Program Evaluation,* 380–417.

52. Jack R. Fraenkel, Norman E. Wallen, and Helen Hyun, "Internal Validity," and "Experimental Research," in *How to Design and Evaluate Research in Education*, 10th ed. (New York: McGraw-Hill Publishing, 2018).

53. Matthew Lineberry, "Validity and Quality" and "Assessment Affecting Learning," in *Assessment in Health Professions Education*, 2nd ed., ed. Rachel Yudowsky, Yoo Soon Park, and Steven M. Downing (New York: Taylor & Francis; 2019), 21–56, 257–71.

54. C. Keith Waugh and Norman E. Gronlund, "Validity and Reliability," in Waugh and Gronlund, *Assessment of Student Achievement*, 48–70.

55. Richard Windsor et al., "Formative and Impact Evaluations," in *Evaluation of Health Promotion, Health Education, and Disease Prevention Programs*, ed. Richard A. Windsor et al. (New York: McGraw-Hill Publishing, 2004), 215–63.

56. Ronald M. Epstein, "Assessment in Medical Education," *New England Journal of Medicine* 356, no. 4 (2007): 387–96, https://doi.org/10.1056/NEJMra054784.

57. "Evaluating Student Learning," in *Student Learning Assessment: Options and Resources* (Philadelphia: Middle States Commission on Higher Education, 2007), 27–53.

58. Donald G. Kassebaum, "The Measurement of Outcomes in the Assessment of Educational Program Effectiveness," *Academic Medicine* 65, no. 5 (1990): 293–96, https://doi.org/10.1097/00001888-199005000-00003.

59. C. Keith Waugh and Norman E. Gronlund, "Performance Assessments," in Waugh and Gronlund, *Assessment of Student Achievement*, 144–74.

60. Eric S. Holmboe, Steven J. Durning, and Richard E. Hawkins, eds., *Practical Guide to the Evaluation of Clinical Competence*, 2nd ed. (Philadelphia: Elsevier, 2018).

61. Bernard Charlin et al., "The Script Concordance Test: A Tool to Assess the Reflective Clinician," *Teaching and Learning in Medicine* 12, no. 4 (2000): 189–95, https://doi.org/10.1207/s15328015tlm1204_5.

62. Eric Steinberg et al., "Assessment of Emergency Medicine Residents' Clinical Reasoning: Validation of a Script Concordance Test," *Western Journal of Emergency Medicine* 21, no. 4 (2020): 978–84, https://doi.org/10.5811/westjem.2020.3.46035.

63. Chris B. T. Rietmeijer et al., "Patterns of Direct Observation and Their Impact During Residency: General Practice Supervisors' Views," *Medical Education* 52, no. 9 (2018): 981–91, https://doi.org/10.1111/medu.13631.

64. Donald I. Kirkpatrick and James D. Kirkpatrick, *Evaluating Training Programs: The Four Levels*, 3rd ed. (San Francisco: Berrett-Koehler, 2006).

65. Clive Belfield et al., "Measuring Effectiveness for Best Evidence Medical Education: A Discussion," *Medical Teacher* 23, no. 2 (2001): 164–70, https://doi.org/10.1080/0142150020031084.

66. Sarah Yardley and Tim Dornan, "Kirkpatrick's Levels and Education 'Evidence,'" *Medical Education* 46, no. 1 (2012): 97–106, https://doi.org/10.1111/j.1365-2923.2011.04076.x.

67. Lynore DeSilets, "An Update on Kirkpatrick's Model of Evaluation: Part Two." *Journal of Continuing Education in Nursing* 49, no. 7 (2018): 292–93, https://doi.org/10.3928/00220124-20180613-02.

68. Example adapted with permission from the curricular project of Michael Melia, MD, Johns Hopkins University School of Medicine, 2016.

69. Ian McDowell, *Measuring Health: A Guide to Rating Scales and Questionnaires*, 3rd ed. (New York: Oxford University Press, 2006).

70. Delbert Charles Miller, "Assessing Social Variables: Scales and Indexes," in *Handbook of Research Design and Social Measurement,* ed. Delbert C. Miller and Neil J. Salkind (Thousand Oaks, CA: SAGE Publications, 2002), 453–660.

71. Carolyn F. Waltz et al., eds., *Measurement of Nursing Outcomes*, 2nd ed., 3 vols. (New York: Springer Publishing Co., 2001–2003).

72. Association of American Medical Colleges (AAMC), MedEdPORTAL, accessed September 20, 2021, www.mededportal.org. Search "Directory and for Educational Assessment Measures Repository."

73. Arlene Fink, "Collecting Information: The Right Data Sources," and "Evaluation Measures," in Fink, *Evaluation Fundamentals*, 119–64.

74. C. Keith Waugh and Norman E. Gronlund, "Writing Selection Items: Multiple Choice," "Writing Selection Items: True-False, Matching, and Interpretive Exercise," "Writing Selection items: Short Answer and Essay," in Waugh and Gronlund, *Assessment of Student Achievement*, 91–143.

75. National Board of Medical Examiners. *NBME Item Writing Guide* (Philadelphia: National Board of Medical Examiners, 2021), accessed September 20, 2021, https://www.nbme.org/item-writing-guide.

76. Lawrence B. Afrin et al., "Improving Oversight of the Graduate Medical Education Enterprise: One Institution's Strategies and Tools," *Academic Medicine* 81, no. 5 (2006): 419–25, https://doi.org/10.1097/01.ACM.0000222258.55266.6a.

77. Lauren B. Meade et al., "Patients, Nurses, and Physicians Working Together to Develop a Discharge Entrustable Professional Activity Assessment Tool," *Academic Medicine* 91, no. 10 (2016): 1388–91, https://doi.org/10.1097/ACM.0000000000001189.

78. American Educational Research Association, American Psychological Association, National Council on Measurement in Education, *Standards for Educational and Psychological Testing* (Washington, DC: American Educational Research Association, 2014).

79. Steven M. Downing, "Validity: On Meaningful Interpretation of Assessment Data." *Medical Education* 37, no. 9 (2003): 830–37, https://doi.org/10.1046/j.1365-2923.2003.01594.x.

80. Steven M. Downing, "Reliability: On the Reproducibility of Assessment Data." *Medical Education* 38, no. 9 (2004): 1006–12, https://doi.org/10.1111/j.1365-2929.2004.01932.x.
81. David A. Cook and Thomas J. Beckman, "Current Concepts in Validity and Reliability for Psychometric Instruments: Theory and Application," *American Journal of Medicine* 119, no. 2 (2006): 166.e7–16, https://doi.org/10.1016/j.amjmed.2005.10.036.
82. Mitchell Goldenberg and Jason Y. Lee, "Surgical Education, Simulation, and Simulators-Updating the Concept of Validity." *Current Urology Reports* 19, no. 7 (2018): 52, https://doi.org/10.1007/s11934-018-0799-7.
83. Thomas M. Haladyna, "Roles and Importance of Validity Studies in Test Development," in *Handbook of Test Development*, ed. Steven M. Downing and Thomas M. Haladyna (Mahwah, NJ: Lawrence Erlbaum Associates, 2006), 739–58.
84. Jim Crossley et al., "Generalisability: A Key to Unlock Professional Assessment," *Medical Education* 36, no. 10 (2002): 972–78, https://doi.org/10.1046/j.1365-2923.2002.01320.x.
85. Geoffrey R. Norman and David L. Streiner, "Principal Components and Factor Analysis: Fooling Around with Factors," in *Biostatistics: The Bare Essentials*, ed. Geoffrey R. Norman and David L. Streiner (Lewiston, NY: B. C. Decker, 2008), 194–209.
86. Armen Aboulian et al., "The Public Mock Oral: A Useful Tool for Examinees and the Audience in Preparation for the American Board of Surgery Certifying Examination," *Journal of Surgical Education* 67, no. 1 (2010): 33–36, https://doi.org/10.1016/j.jsurg.2009.10.007.
87. Tyronne Donnon, Elizabeth O. Paolucci, and Claudio Violato, "The Predictive Validity of the MCAT for Medical School Performance and Medical Board Licensing Examinations: A Meta-analysis of the Published Research," *Academic Medicine* 82, no. 1 (2007): 100–106, https://doi.org/10.1097/01.ACM.0000249878.25186.b7.
88. Kevin Busche et al., "The Validity of Scores from the New MCAT Exam in Predicting Student Performance: Results from a Multisite Study," *Academic Medicine* 95, no. 3 (2020): 387–95, https://doi.org/10.1097/acm.0000000000002942.
89. Carol A. Terregino et al., "The Diversity and Success of Medical School Applicants with Scores in the Middle Third of the MCAT Score Scale," *Academic Medicine* 95, no. 3 (2020): 344–50, https://doi.org/10.1097/acm.0000000000002941.
90. Catherine Reinis Lucey and Aaron Saguil, "The Consequences of Structural Racism on MCAT Scores and Medical School Admissions: The Past Is Prologue," *Academic Medicine* 95, no. 3 (2020): 351–56, https://doi.org/10.1097/ACM.0000000000002939.
91. Reed G. Williams, Debra A. Klamen, and William C. McGaghie. "Cognitive, Social and Environmental Sources of Bias in Clinical Performance Ratings," *Teaching and Learning in Medicine* 15, no. 4 (2003): 270–92, https://doi.org/10.1207/s15328015tlm1504_11.
92. Steven M. Downing and Thomas M. Haladyna, "Validity Threats: Overcoming Interference with Proposed Interpretations of Assessment Data," *Medical Education* 38, no. 3 (2004): 327–33, https://doi.org/10.1046/j.1365-2923.2004.01777.x.
93. Kelsey Ripp and Lundy Braun, "Race/Ethnicity in Medical Education: An Analysis of a Question Bank for Step 1 of the United States Medical Licensing Examination," *Teaching and Learning in Medicine* 29, no. 2 (2017): 115–22, https://doi.org/10.1080/10401334.2016.1268056.
94. Charles M. Maxfield et al., "Awareness of Implicit Bias Mitigates Discrimination in Radiology Resident Selection," *Medical Education* 54, no. 7 (2020): 637–42, https://doi.org/10.1111/medu.14146.
95. David A. Cook et al., "When Assessment Data Are Words: Validity Evidence for Qualitative Educational Assessment." *Academic Medicine* 91, no. 10 (2016): 1359–69, https://doi.org/10.1097/ACM.0000000000001175.
96. Nicholas Mays and Catherine Pope, "Assessing Quality in Qualitative Research," *BMJ* 320, no. 7226 (2000): 50–52, https://doi.org/10.1136/bmj.320.7226.50.
97. Rosaline S. Barbour, "Checklists for Improving Rigour in Qualitative Research: A Case of the Tail Wagging the Dog?" *BMJ* 322, no. 7294 (2001): 1115–17, https://doi.org/10.1136/bmj.322.7294.1115.

98. Mita K. Giacomini and Debra J. Cook, "Users' Guides to the Medical Literature: XXIII. Qualitative Research in Health Care: A. Are the Results of the Study Valid?," *JAMA* 284, no. 3 (2000): 357–62, https://doi.org/10.1001/jama.284.3.357.

99. Mita K. Giacomini and Debra J. Cook, "Users' Guides to the Medical Literature: XXIII. Qualitative Research in Health Care: B. What Are the Results and How Do They Help Me Care for My Patients?," *JAMA* 284, no. 4 (2000): 478–82, https://doi.org/10.1001/jama.284.4.478.

100. David A. Ross et al., "Differences in Words Used to Describe Racial and Gender Groups in Medical Student Performance Evaluations." *PLOS One* 12, no. 8 (2017): e0181659, https://doi.org/10.1371/journal.pone.0181659.

101. "Guiding Principles for Evaluators," American Evaluation Association, accessed September 20, 2021, https://www.eval.org/About/Guiding-Principles.

102. Thomas J. Nasca et al., "The Next GME Accreditation System—Rationale and Benefits," *New England Journal of Medicine* 366, no. 11 (2012): 1051–56, https://doi.org/10.1056/NEJMsr1200117.

103. Arianne Teherani et al. "How Small Differences in Assessed Clinical Performance Amplify to Large Differences in Grades and Awards: A Cascade with Serious Consequences for Students Underrepresented in Medicine," *Academic Medicine* 93, no. 9 (2018): 1286–92, https://doi.org/10.1097/ACM.0000000000002323.

104. Catherine R. Lucey et al., "Medical Education's Wicked Problem: Achieving Equity in Assessment for Medical Learners," *Academic Medicine* 95, no. 12S (2020): S98–S108, https://doi.org/10.1097/ACM.0000000000003717.

105. Mark Feldman et al., "Testing Test-Enhanced Continuing Medical Education: A Randomized Controlled Trial," *Academic Medicine* 93, no. 11S (2018): S30–S36, https://doi.org/10.1097/acm.0000000000002377.

106. Eric J. Warm et al., "Entrusting Observable Practice Activities and Milestones over the 36 Months of an Internal Medicine Residency," *Academic Medicine* 91, no. 10 (2016): 1398–405, https://doi.org/10.1097/acm.0000000000001292.

107. Walter Tavares et al., "Asking for Less and Getting More: The Impact of Broadening a Rater's Focus in Formative Assessment," *Academic Medicine* 93, no. 10 (2018): 1584–90, https://doi.org/10.1097/acm.0000000000002294.

108. Chad S. Kessler et al., "The 5Cs of Consultation: Training Medical Students to Communicate Effectively in the Emergency Department," *Journal of Emergency Medicine* 49, no. 5 (2015): 713–21, https://doi.org/10.1016/j.jemermed.2015.05.012.

109. Ronald J. Markert, "Enhancing Medical Education by Improving Statistical Methodology in Journal Articles," *Teaching and Learning in Medicine* 25, no. 2 (2013): 159–64, https://doi.org/10.1080/10401334.2013.770746.

110. Fink, "Sampling," in Fink, *Evaluation Fundamentals*, 101–18.

111. Jacob Cohen, *Statistical Power Analysis for the Behavioral Sciences* (Hillsdale, NJ: Lawrence Erlbaum Associates, 1988).

112. Heibatollah Baghi, Siamak Noorbaloochi, and Jean B. Moore, "Statistical and Nonstatistical Significance: Implications for Health Care Researchers," *Quality Management in Health Care* 16, no. 2 (2007): 104–12, https://doi.org/10.1097/01.Qmh.0000267447.55500.57.

113. Jack R. Fraenkel, Norman E. Wallen, and Helen Hyun, *How to Design and Evaluate Research in Education*, 10th ed. (New York: McGraw-Hill Publishing, 2018).

114. Fink, "Analyzing Evaluation Data," in Fink, *Evaluation Fundamentals*, 187–216.

115. Donna M. Windish and Marie Diener-West, "A Clinician-Educator's Roadmap to Choosing and Interpreting Statistical Tests," *Journal of General Internal Medicine* 21, no. 6 (2006): 656–60, https://doi.org/10.1111/j.1525-1497.2006.00390.x.

116. Teresa Chan et. al., "Learning Analytics in Medical Education Assessment: The Past, the Present, and the Future," *Academic Emergency Medicine Education and Training* 2, no. 2 (2018): 178–87, https://doi.org/10.1002/aet2.10087.

117. Teresa M. Chan, Jonathan Sherbino, and Matthew Mercuri, "Nuance and Noise: Lessons Learned from Longitudinal Aggregated Assessment Data," *Journal of Graduate Medical Education* 9, no. 6 (2017): 724–29, https://doi.org/10.4300/jgme-d-17-00086.1.

118. Frank T. Materia et al., "Let's Get Technical: Enhancing Program Evaluation through the Use and Integration of Internet and Mobile Technologies," *Evaluation Program and Planning* 56 (2016): 31–42, https://doi.org/10.1016/j.evalprogplan.2016.03.004.

119. Michelle E. Kiger and Lara Varpio, "Thematic Analysis of Qualitative Data: AMEE Guide No. 131," *Medical Teacher* 42, no. 8 (2020): 846–54, https://doi.org/10.1080/0142159X.2020.1755030.

120. Fink, "Evaluation Reports," in Fink, *Evaluation Fundamentals,* 219–46.

121. Martin V. Pusic et al., "Learning Curves in Health Professions Education," *Academic Medicine* 90, no. 8 (2015): 1034–42, https://doi.org/10.1097/acm.0000000000000681.

122. Ashimiyu B. Durojaiye et al., "Radiology Resident Assessment and Feedback Dashboard," *RadioGraphics* 38, no. 5 (2018): 1443–53, https://doi.org/10.1148/rg.2018170117.

123. Michael T. Brannick, H. Tugba Erol-Korkmaz, and Matthew Prewett, "A Systematic Review of the Reliability of Objective Structured Clinical Examination Scores," *Medical Education* 45, no. 12 (2011): 1181–89, https://doi.org/10.1111/j.1365-2923.2011.04075.x.

124. Madalena Patrício et al., "Is the OSCE a Feasible Tool to Assess Competencies in Undergraduate Medical Education?" *Medical Teacher* 35, no. 6 (2013): 503–14, https://doi.org/10.3109/0142159x.2013.774330.

125. Nasir I. Bhatti, "Assessment of Surgical Skills and Competency," *Otolaryngologic Clinics of North America* 50, no. 5 (2017): 959–65, https://doi.org/10.1016/j.otc.2017.05.007.

126. Anthony S. Thijssen and Marlies P. Schijven, "Contemporary Virtual Reality Laparoscopy Simulators: Quicksand or Solid Grounds for Assessing Surgical Trainees?" *American Journal of Surgery* 199, no. 4 (2010): 529–41, https://doi.org/10.1016/j.amjsurg.2009.04.015.

127. Jillian L. McGrath et al., "Using Virtual Reality Simulation Environments to Assess Competence for Emergency Medicine Learners," *Academic Emergency Medicine* 25, no. 2 (2018): 186–95, https://doi.org/10.1111/acem.13308.

CHAPTER EIGHT

Curriculum Maintenance
and Enhancement

. . . keeping the curriculum vibrant

David E. Kern, MD, MPH, and Patricia A. Thomas, MD

THE DYNAMIC NATURE OF CURRICULA

A successful curriculum is continually developing, undergoing a process of *continuous quality improvement*. A curriculum that is static gradually declines. To thrive, it must undergo ongoing review, as suggested in Figure 1.1, Chapter 1. It must respond to evaluation results and feedback (Step 6), to changes in societal values and needs (Step 1), to changes in the knowledge base and the material requiring mastery (Step 1), to changes in its targeted learners and institutional needs (Step 2), to advances in available educational methodology (Step 4), and to changes in resources (including faculty) (Step 5). Based on the review, goals and objectives may need to be added, revised, or eliminated (Step 3). A successful curriculum requires *understanding*, *management of change*, and *sustenance* to maintain its strengths and to promote further improvement.

Innovations, *networking* with colleagues at other institutions, and *scholarly activity* can also strengthen a curriculum. In addition, accreditation bodies, such as the Liaison Committee on Medical Education[1] in the United States, are likely to require ongoing curriculum review and improvement.

UNDERSTANDING ONE'S CURRICULUM

To appropriately nurture a curriculum and manage change, one must understand the curriculum and appreciate its complexity. This includes not only the written curriculum but also its learners, its faculty, its support staff, the processes by which it is administered and evaluated, and the setting in which it takes place. Table 8.1 provides a list of the various areas related to an ongoing curriculum review. As can be seen, this process involves revisiting several steps of curriculum development. Table 8.2 lists some methods of assessing how a curriculum is functioning. *Formal evaluation* (discussed in Chapter 7) provides objective and representative subjective feedback on some of these areas. Methods that promote *informal information* exchange, such as internal and external reviews, observation of curricular components, and individual or group meetings with learners, faculty, and support staff, can enrich one's understanding of a curriculum. They can also build relationships that help to maintain and further develop a curriculum.

EXAMPLE: *Graduate Medical Education (GME), Preparation for Practice*. Residents in an internal medicine residency program participate in an ambulatory curriculum anchored in their continuity practice at a patient-centered medical home. To ensure that the curriculum leads to desired outcomes, there are many types of formative feedback gathered by the program. Interns are asked to evaluate each module for "usefulness in establishing their primary care practice," articulate specific strengths and weaknesses of each ambulatory block rotation, and self-rate their level of proficiency in key skills. In addition, there are faculty assessments including Mini-CEXs (clinical evaluation exercises) and feedback on patient care notes. Because the faculty teaching in this clinic are the same individuals involved in supporting the residents' ongoing outpatient practice, there is understanding of the practice learning environment and accountability for intern achievement of basic skills. Evaluations are reviewed by the faculty coordinator each year, and potential updates/changes are discussed with designated faculty and clinical preceptors who meet at least quarterly throughout the year. An updated ambulatory curriculum is assembled by the faculty coordinator and course administrator, who then share it with all participating faculty in late spring to ensure that the curriculum remains congruent and cohesive.

EXAMPLE: *Undergraduate Medical Education (UME), Clinical Clerkships*. Case Western Reserve University implemented a major reform of the four-year MD curriculum in 2006, named Western Reserve 2 (WR2). The new curriculum preserved a systems approach to preclerkship study, with an emphasis on small-group case-based learning. In the core clinical year, disciplines, such as surgery and emergency medicine, were "paired" and charged to develop interdisciplinary approaches to teaching and learning the disciplines. Over time, these efforts waned, and clerkships reverted to a block model. Graduation questionnaire results showed less than ideal student satisfaction with the clerkships, and program evaluation indicated problems with comparability of experiences and grading. In 2014, the assistant deans for clerkships convened faculty and staff town halls in each of the major clinical affiliates to identify how the clinical curriculum could more effectively prepare students for modern residencies and health care delivery. Recurrent themes in these discussions were (1) a need for more longitudinal experiences with patients to better understand patient-centered care and chronic disease prevention and management, (2) more longitudinal experiences with faculty preceptors to improve the quality of evaluations, (3) more opportunities to work on interprofessional teams, and (4) more opportunities to explore career options in the third year. In response to these faculty retreats, the deans developed a hybrid longitudinal clerkship model, which included a 12-week ambulatory block at the Cleveland Clinic, and piloted it for two

Table 8.1. Areas for Assessment and Potential Change

The Written or Intended Curriculum

Goals and objectives (Step 3)	Are they understood and accepted by all involved in the curriculum? Are they realistic? Can some be deleted, should some be altered, or do others need to be added, based on review of Steps 1 and 2? Do some address external requirements/accreditation standards, such as milestones or entrustable professional activities (EPAs) (see Chapter 4)? Are the objectives measurable?
Content (Step 4)	Is the amount just right, too little, or too much? Does the content still match the objectives? Can some content be deleted? Should other content be updated or added?
Curricular materials (Step 4)	Are they being accessed and used? How useful are the various components perceived to be? Can some be deleted? Should others be altered? Should new materials be added?
Methods (Step 4)	Are they well executed by faculty and well received by learners? Have they been sufficient to achieve curricular objectives? Are additional methods needed to prevent decay of learning? Do the methods address relevant competencies, milestones, and entrustable professional activities (EPAs) for individual and population care? Are new technologies/educational methodologies available that could enhance the curriculum?
Congruence (Step 5)	Does the curriculum on paper match the curriculum in reality? If not, is that a problem? Does one or the other need to be changed?

The Environment/Setting of the Curriculum

Funding (Step 5)	How is the curriculum funded? Have funding needs changed with addition of new expectations, additional learners, and new technologies or methodologies?
Space (Step 5)	Is there sufficient physical and electronic space to support the various activities of the curriculum? Will added educational methodologies (e.g., simulation, team-based or interprofessional learning, virtual patients) lead to new space demands? For clinical curricula, is there sufficient space for learners to see patients, consult references, and/or meet with preceptors? Do the residents' clinical practices have the space to support the performance of learned skills and procedures?
Equipment and supplies (Step 5)	Are the equipment and supplies sufficient to support the curriculum while in progress, as well as to support and reinforce learning after completion of the curriculum? For example, are there adequate clinical skills space and resources to support learning of interviewing skills? Will new technologies/educational methodologies require additional equipment and supplies (such as virtual reality resources to support the teaching of anatomy or adequate robotic simulators to support learning of surgical skills)? Do learners have access to online resources? Are there sufficient, easily accessible references/electronic resources to support clinical practice experiences? Do the residents' clinical practices have the equipment and support to incorporate learned skills and procedures into routine practice?

Clinical experience (Steps 4 and 5)	Is there sufficient concentrated clinical experience to support learning during the course of the curriculum? Is there sufficient clinical experience to reinforce learning after completion of the main curriculum? If there is insufficient patient volume or case-mix, do alternative clinical experiences need to be found? Do alternative approaches need to be developed, such as simulation or virtual patients? Are curricular objectives and general programmatic goals (e.g., efficiency, cost-effectiveness, customer service, record keeping, communication between referring and consulting practitioners, interprofessional collaboration, and provision of needed services) supported by clinical practice operations? Do support staff members support the curriculum? Is there a competing hidden or informal curriculum?
Learning climate (Step 4)	Is the climate collaborative or competitive? Are learners encouraged to communicate or to hide what they do not know? Is the curriculum sufficiently learner-centered and directed? Is it sufficiently teacher-centered and directed? Are learners encouraged and supported in identifying and pursuing their own learning needs and goals related to the curriculum?
Associated settings (Step 4)	Is learning from the curriculum supported and reinforced in the learners' prior, concomitant, and subsequent settings? If not, is there an opportunity to influence those settings?

Administration of the Curriculum (Step 5)

Scheduling	Are schedules understandable, accurate, realistic, and helpful? Are they put out far enough in advance? Are they adhered to? How are scheduling changes managed? Is there a plan for missed sessions?
Preparation and distribution/electronic posting of curricular materials	Is this being accomplished in a timely and consistent manner?
Collection, collation, and distribution of evaluation information	Is this being accomplished in a timely and consistent manner? If there are several different evaluation forms, can they be consolidated into one form, or administered at one time, to decrease respondent fatigue?
Communication	Are changes in and important information about the curriculum being communicated to the appropriate individuals in a user-friendly, understandable, and timely manner?

Evaluation (Step 6)

Congruence	Is what is being evaluated consistent with the goals, objectives, content, and methods of the curriculum? Does the evaluation reflect the main priorities of the curriculum?
Response rate	Is it sufficient to be representative of learners, faculty, or others involved in or affected by the curriculum?
Accuracy	Is the information reliable and valid?
Usefulness	Does the evaluation provide timely, easily understandable, and useful information to learners, faculty, curriculum coordinators, and relevant others? Is it being used? How?

Table 8.1.   *(continued)*

Faculty (Steps 2, 4, and 5)

Number/type	Are the number and type of faculty appropriate? Do planned revisions (e.g., interprofessional collaboration, simulation) create new needs?
Reliability/accessibility	How reliable are the faculty members in performing their curricular responsibilities? Are they devoting more or less time to the curriculum than expected? How accessible are faculty members in responding to learner questions and individual learner needs? Do faculty members schedule time for discussion?
Teaching/facilitation skills	How skillful are faculty members at assessing learners' needs, imparting information, asking questions, providing feedback, promoting practice-based learning and improvement, stimulating self-directed learning, and creating a learning environment that is open, honest, exciting, and fun? How effective are they at working collaboratively and interprofessionally? Do new educational methodologies (e.g., online teaching, team-based learning, simulation, virtual reality) create a need for new faculty development?
Nature of the learner-faculty relationship	Is the relationship more authoritative or collaborative? Is it more teacher-centered or learner-centered? For clinical precepting, do learners see patients on their own? Do learners observe the faculty member seeing patients or in other roles? Are learners exposed to faculty members' professional life outside the curriculum (e.g., clinical practice, research, community work, ongoing professional development)? Do learners get to know faculty members as people and how they balance professional, family, and personal life? Do faculty members serve as good role models?
Satisfaction	Do faculty members feel adequately recognized and rewarded for their teaching? Do they feel that their role is an important one? Are they enthusiastic? How satisfied are faculty members with clinical practice, teaching, and their professional lives in general?
Involvement	To what extent are faculty members involved in the curriculum? Do faculty members complete evaluation forms in a timely manner? Do faculty members attend scheduled meetings? Do faculty members provide useful suggestions for improving the curriculum?

Learners (Steps 2, 4, and 6)

Needs assessment	Have prior training, preparation, or expectations of learners changed?
Achievement of curriculum objectives	Have cognitive, affective, psychomotor, process, and outcome objectives been achieved? Are learners responsible in meeting their obligations to the curriculum?

Satisfaction	How satisfied are learners with various aspects of the curriculum?
Involvement	To what extent are learners involved in the curriculum? Do they complete evaluation forms in a timely manner? Do they attend scheduled activities and meetings? Do they complete online sessions? Do they provide useful suggestions for improving the curriculum?
Application	Do learners apply their learning in other settings and contexts? Do they teach what they have learned to others?

Table 8.2.   Methods of Assessing How a Curriculum Is Functioning

Formal Evaluation (See Chapter 7, Evaluation and Feedback)
    "Just-in-time" evaluations by learners
    Learner/faculty/staff/patient questionnaires
    Objective measures of skills and performance
    Focus groups of learners, faculty, staff, patients
    Other systematically collected data
    Online tracking of use/completion of activities

Informal Evaluation
    Regular/periodic meetings with learners, faculty, staff
    Special retreats and strategic planning sessions
    Site visits
    Informal observation of curricular components, learners, faculty, staff
    Informal discussions with learners, faculty, staff
    Monitoring of online forums/discussion boards/chat rooms

successive years. Faculty monitored the student and faculty satisfaction, ability of students to fulfill clerkship patient experiences via student logs, and student performance on National Board of Medical Examiners (NBME) shelf examinations. With positive feedback from the stakeholders and evidence of equivalent exam performance to students on traditional block clerkships, the clerkship was implemented for the full cohort of Lerner College of Medicine students in 2017.[2,3]

Electronic curriculum management systems can be used to provide coordinated information for understanding and managing subject-focused curricula, including their integration with other curricula and larger educational programs, such as an entire medical school curriculum.[4,5]

MANAGEMENT OF CHANGE

Overview and Level of Decision-Making

Most curricula require midcourse, end-of-cycle, and/or end-of-year changes. Changes may be prompted by informal feedback, evaluation results, accreditation standards, changes in available technology/methods and resources, or the evolving needs of learners, faculty, institutions, or society (a review of Step 1). Before expending resources to make curricular changes, however, it is often wise to *decide whether the need for change (1) is sufficiently important* (e.g., affects a significant number of people; knowledge-base or clinical approach has significantly changed; external accrediting body mandates change); *(2) is able to be addressed given available resources*; and *(3) will persist if it is not addressed.*

It is also helpful to consider *who should make the changes and at what level they should be addressed.* Minor operational changes that are necessary for the smooth functioning of a curriculum are most efficiently made at the level of the curriculum coordinator or the core group responsible for managing the curriculum. More complicated needs that require in-depth analysis and thoughtful planning for change may best be assigned to a carefully selected task group. Other needs may best be discussed and addressed in meetings of learners, faculty, and/or staff. Before implementing major curricular changes, it is often wise to ensure broad, representative support. It can also be helpful to pilot major or complex changes before implementing them fully.

> **EXAMPLE:** *UME, Coordinated Response to Challenge Arising from Curricular Revision.* The WR2 block core clerkship curriculum[2] (see example above) included a mandatory Friday afternoon curriculum at the medical school, in which students worked through clinical cases according to which clerkship they were currently taking. The cases were developed and taught by clinical faculty from each discipline. This format did not work with the longitudinal clerkship (LC) model, since LC students were not in a block schedule that allowed equivalent exposure to all the case content. In addition, clerkship students were reporting inadequate feedback and direct observation of clinical skills in many of the clerkships. Lastly, the school intended to enhance the teaching of health systems science in the core clerkship year. The associate dean for curriculum identified a clerkship director with a particular interest in clinical reasoning, and together they designed a new 12-month curriculum for Friday afternoon clerkship students. The new course, Sciences and Art of Medicine Integrated, set out to integrate students' knowledge of basic, clinical, and health systems sciences. The course used a series of cases in small groups to allow students to practice clinical skills in the simulation center, explore pathophysiology of symptoms and evidence-based management as a group, and reflect on systems issues, with each small group developing a "mechanism of disease" visual map. Since all students had the same year-long exposure to the case series, the LC students received equivalent exposure to the content as the block clerkship students. The new curriculum was presented to the WR2 Curriculum Committee, and subsequently to the Committee on Medical Education for full approval, and was implemented in 2019–20.[6]

> **EXAMPLE:** *Continuing Medical Education (CME), Response to a Sudden Environmental Change.* A longitudinal faculty development program in teaching skills, with foci on relationship-centered teaching, experiential and collaborative learning, reflective practice, leadership, and career building in health professional education, relied heavily on in-person small-group learning. With the prohibitions against social gathering and the requirements for physical distancing necessitated by the COVID-19 pandemic, it was no longer possible for participants to meet in person. With the assistance of an instructional designer and input from participants, program faculty were able to transition this highly interactive program to an inviting, functional online platform.[7]

Accreditation Standards

Important drivers of change in health professional curricula are the organizations charged with accreditation at each level of the continuum. In the United States, the national medical accrediting bodies are the Liaison Committee on Medical Education (LCME)[8] and the Commission on Osteopathic College Accreditation (COCA)[9] for undergraduate medical education, the Accreditation Council for Graduate Medical Education (ACGME)[10] for graduate (residency and fellowship) education, and the Accreditation Council for Continuing Medical Education (ACCME)[11] for continuing medical education. Many other countries have their own accreditation bodies. FAIMER (the Foundation for Advancement of International Medical Education and Research) maintains the Directory of Organizations that Recognize/Accredit Medical Schools (DORA) internationally.[12] The World Federation for Medical Education (WFME) provides global expert consensus on standards for medical schools and other providers of medical education.[13] It recognizes accrediting agencies that require these standards for the medical schools they accredit. The Accreditation Council for Graduate Medical Education–International (ACGME-I) provides accreditation for residencies and fellowships internationally.[14] Curriculum developers should stay abreast of *changing* accreditation standards that will impact their curricula, since these standards must be explicitly addressed. It is also useful to look at expectations beyond the immediate timeline of the curriculum. For instance, a medical school curriculum that must address the LCME standards should also be aware of the ACGME Common Program Requirements. The adoption of the six ACGME core competencies and more recent emphasis on entrustable professional activities (EPAs) have altered many undergraduate programs' approaches to teaching and assessment[15–18] (see Chapters 4 and 5). Attending to these generic competencies in undergraduate, graduate, and postgraduate/continuing medical education curricula can improve coordination throughout the medical education continuum and permit reinforcement and increasing sophistication of learning at each level. Similar concerns relate to accrediting bodies for other health professions and governmental standards for licensing in many countries (see Chapter 1, "Relationship to Accreditation").

EXAMPLE: *UME Curriculum, Anticipating a New Accreditation Standard.* The ACGME Clinical Learning Environment Review (CLER) expects resident training in patient safety events, including knowing how to report medical errors and near misses, receiving institutional summary information on patient safety reports, and "participating as team members in real and/or simulated interprofessional clinical patient safety activities, such as root cause analyses or other activities that include analysis, as well as formulation and implementation of actions."[19] To better prepare students, a new health systems science curriculum in a medical school was designed to include activities such as performing a root cause analysis and PDSA (plan-do-study-act) quality improvement cycle in the preclerkship curriculum and active learning on reporting patient safety events during the core clerkship year.[20]

Environmental Changes

Changes in the environment in which a curriculum takes place can *create new opportunities* for the curriculum, *reinforce* the learning that has occurred, and *support* its *application* by learners or *create challenges* for curriculum coordinators. Decisions to increase class size or open new campus sites can profoundly affect resources in UME curricula. In both UME and GME, practice development activities often impact clinical curricula. New institutional or extra-institutional resources might be used to benefit a curriculum.

EXAMPLE: *UME, Environmental Changes.* The new undergraduate medical curriculum (see above) at Case Western Reserve University included interprofessional education (IPE) and required every student to be involved in an interprofessional (IP) team.[21] A coordinator was hired to oversee this.

Reinforce Learning. Medical students learned to use an instrument to self-assess their team skills in an online IPE course in year one; the new community-based education activities used the same instrument for faculty to observe and upper-level students to self-assess.

Support and Governance. In the Office of Interprofessional and Interdisciplinary Education and Research (https://case.edu/ipe/), a new vice provost was recruited to oversee IPE in the university; two masters-trained program managers oversaw implementation of the IPE curriculum.

Challenges: New requirements for participation in IPE are challenging for some professions (e.g., nursing and social work), since they cannot add additional credits to the degrees.

EXAMPLE: *CME, Response to a Pandemic Challenge.* See example above under "Overview and Level of Decision-Making."

Early adoption of resources must sometimes be tempered with a need to understand the context of the entire curriculum and strategize for best utilization. Adding on an additional software that seems like a good fit for the new curriculum, for instance, may be perceived by learners as an additional burden, given other software requirements.

EXAMPLE: *UME Curriculum, Electronic Student Portfolios.* The curriculum developers for the new integrated curriculum recommended an electronic student portfolio to track student development of competencies across the four-year curriculum, with inclusion of evaluations, reflective writing, and communications with advisors. The medical school's Educational Policy and Curriculum Committee noted that this was the fourth secured electronic system that would be required in the curriculum and recommended that coordination and programming be further developed to simplify student access and maximize its use.

Faculty Development

One of the most important resources for any curriculum is its faculty. As discussed in Chapter 6, a curriculum may benefit from faculty development efforts specifically targeted toward the needs of the curriculum. Institution-wide, regional, or national faculty development programs (see Appendix B) that train faculty in specific content areas, or in time management, teaching, curriculum development, management, or research skills, may also benefit a curriculum. Introduction of new educational technology invariably requires a plan for faculty development if the technology is to be used effectively.

EXAMPLE: *Rapid Transition to Online Learning.* With prohibitions against social gathering and the requirements for physical distancing necessitated by the COVID-19 pandemic, UME and GME teaching at the Johns Hopkins University had to rapidly transition to online learning. The Office of Faculty Development created several online courses for faculty such as Zoom for Teaching Online. The School of Medicine provided information technology support for faculty in need.

SUSTAINING THE CURRICULUM TEAM

The curriculum team includes not only the faculty but also the support staff and learners, all of whom are critical to a curriculum's success. Therefore, it is important to attend to processes that motivate, develop, and support the team. These processes include orientation, communication, stakeholder involvement, faculty development and team activities, recognition, and celebration (Table 8.3).

EXAMPLE: *GME Curriculum.* Within clinic, internal medicine residents are divided into one of four groups that meet monthly during a noon conference and cover for each other during clinic absences. Each group has a faculty attending who follows the residents longitudinally. The faculty leaders also meet monthly with each other and quarterly with the larger preceptor group responsible for precepting daily clinic sessions. The interprofessional staff are included in preclinic huddles. In addition, an ambulatory chief resident coordinates the outpatient clinical experiences.

EXAMPLE: *Johns Hopkins Faculty Development Program: Programs in Curriculum Development.* These include a 10-month, intense, project-driven course (established in 1987), shorter two-day and half-day

Table 8.3. Methods of Motivating, Developing, and Supporting a Curriculum Team

Method	Mechanisms
Orientation and Communication • Goals and objectives • Guidelines/standards • Evaluation results • Program changes • Rationale for above • Learner, faculty, staff, patient experiences	• Syllabi/handouts • Meetings, in person or online • Email, other forms of electronic communication • Website
Involvement of Faculty, Learners, Staff • Goal and objective setting • Guideline development • Curricular changes • Determining evaluation and feedback needs	• Questionnaires/interviews • Informal one-on-one meetings • Group meetings, in person or online • Online forums/discussion boards • Task group membership • Strategic planning
Faculty Development and Team Activities	• Team teaching/co-teaching • Faculty development activities • Retreats • Task groups to analyze/assess needs • Strategic planning groups
Recognition and Celebration	• Private communication • Public recognition • Rewards • Parties and other social gatherings

workshops (established in the 1990s), an online course (established 2017), and a program on curriculum renewal (implemented in 2020). Debrief meetings after each session and participation in at least annual comprehensive planning sessions keep facilitators involved in program assessment and revision and fine-tuning of their skills on a regular basis. A facilitator-in-training program, in which graduates of the 10-month longitudinal program co-facilitate with seasoned facilitators, prepares future facilitators for the program. Regular electronic communications keep facilitators abreast of all program developments. Sharing of evaluation results and an end-of-year celebration, with oral abstract presentations by longitudinal program participants and recognition of program director, facilitator, and support staff contributions, provide positive feedback for all staff.[22]

THE LIFE OF A CURRICULUM

A curriculum should keep pace with the needs of its learners, its faculty, its institution, patients, and society; adjust to changes in knowledge and practice; and take advantage of developments in educational methodology and technology—i.e., undergo a process of continuous quality improvement. A vibrant curriculum keeps pace with its environment and continually changes and improves.[1,23,24] After a few years, it may differ markedly from its initial form. As health problems and societal needs evolve, even a well-conceived curriculum that has been carefully maintained and developed may appropriately be downscaled or ended.

EXAMPLE: *Evolution of a Curriculum to Meet Societal Needs.* With the increased recognition of the high cost and inefficiencies in US health care,[25] the American Board of Internal Medicine initiated an effort that incorporated more than 60 medical professional societies to identify tests and procedures that incur excess cost and risk to patients without proven benefit. Resources for both physicians and patients were made available online as the Choosing Wisely campaign (http://www.choosingwisely.org). The vice dean for medical education charged the associate dean for curriculum for the medical school and residency program directors to incorporate teaching in high-value care into the clinical epidemiology and clinical decision-making curricula using, when appropriate, Choosing Wisely resources.

EXAMPLE: *Changing Structure of Knowledge and Practice.* In a medical school curriculum revision that adjusted to changing medical knowledge and practice, basic science teaching was reorganized by teaching the science of medicine from societal and genetic perspectives and emphasizing individual variability impacted by genetics, social factors, and environmental factors. The previous dichotomy of normal and abnormal was abandoned. Basic science faculty were pleased by the approach because it modeled translational research. Additional time for basic science teaching was built into the clinical biennium to bring students with appreciation of clinical medicine back to the study of basic science and deepen student understanding of causality.[26]

EXAMPLE: *Need to Integrate Use of New Technology into Internal Medicine Training.* The Department of Medicine at an urban academic medical center recognized that point-of-care ultrasound (POCUS) was becoming part of the standard of care in many medical fields, including internal medicine. Yet most internal medicine faculty, who were an important part of clinical teaching on medical services, had received no (53%) or only informal training (20%) in POCUS. Ninety percent reported minimal to no confidence in their ability to understand and operate ultrasound equipment. After small-group hands-on training by an academic hospitalist who had received certification in POCUS exam techniques, participants in the training showed improvement in the ability to interpret ultrasound images. All participants reported at least moderate comfort in their ability to understand and operate ultrasound equipment.[27]

EXAMPLE: *Replacement of a Curriculum Due to Changing Health Care Environment.* In the 1990s, capitated, or health maintenance organization (HMO), insurance was on the ascendancy in the United States, and most of the community-based practice (CBP) patients in one residency program were covered under HMO insurance. A managed care curriculum was introduced into a residency training program. Subsequently, the prevalence of HMO-insured patients dropped in the United States and in the CBPs. The course was renamed the Medical Practice and Health Systems Curriculum. The curriculum content evolved from one with emphasis on capitated care to one that emphasized systems-based practice, including quality improvement theory and practice; patient safety; health insurance systems; health systems finance, utilization, and costs; medical informatics; practice management; addressing the needs of populations; social determinants of health and health care disparities; and teamwork.

NETWORKING, INNOVATION, AND SCHOLARLY ACTIVITY

A curriculum can be strengthened not only by improvements in the existing curriculum per se, such as environmental changes, new resources, faculty development, and processes that support the curricular team, but also by networking, ongoing innovation, and associated scholarship.

Networking

Faculty responsible for a curriculum at one institution can benefit from and be invigorated by *communication with colleagues at other institutions.*[28,29] Conceptual clarity and understanding of a curriculum are usually enhanced as it is prepared for publication or presentation. New ideas and approaches may come from the manuscript reviewers' comments or from the interchange that occurs after publication or presentation. Multi-institutional efforts can produce scholarly products (see below), such as annotated bibliographies,[30] articles,[31,32] texts,[33,34] and curricula[35,36] that improve upon or transcend the capabilities of faculty at a single institution. The opportunity for such interchange and collaboration can be provided at professional meetings and through professional organizations. Increasingly, social media is being used to rapidly share information, foster collaborations, disseminate work, and develop a professional brand.[37,38]

EXAMPLE: *Online Discussion Group.* DR-ED (https://omerad.msu.edu/about-us/publications/dr-ed-an-electronic-discussion-group-for-medical-educators) is a listserv system maintained by the Office of Medical Education Research and Development at the College of Human Medicine, Michigan State University. Subscription is free for medical educators. It promotes discussion and problem-solving of issues related to medical education, facilitates networking, and provides an electronic forum for disseminating information about resources related to medical education development and research.

EXAMPLE: *Professional Organization.* The Academy of Communication in Healthcare (https://www.achonline.org/) serves as the professional home for researchers, educators, practitioners, and patients committed to improving communication and relationships in health care. Through courses, training programs, conferences, interest groups, and online resources, it provides opportunities for collaboration, support, and personal and professional development.

Innovation and Scholarly Activity

Scholarly inquiry can enrich a curriculum by increasing the breadth and depth of knowledge and understanding of faculty, by creating a sense of excitement among faculty and learners, and by providing the opportunity for learners to engage in scholarly projects. Scholarly activities may include original research or critical reviews in the subject matter of the curriculum or in the methods of teaching and learning that subject matter. Such scholarship can result not only in publications for curriculum developers but other forms of dissemination (see Chapter 9). Scholarship can arise from means other than the original development, implementation, and evaluation of a curriculum. Once developed, curricula provide ongoing opportunities for innovation that can form the basis of scholarship. The need for innovation is often heralded by learner and faculty assessments, as well as opportunities to use new educational methods. Support for innovation can come from networking and the habits of scholarly inquiry.

EXAMPLE: *Systematic Review Related to Interprofessional Education (IPE).* Faculty involved in IPE educational efforts at one medical school collaborated on a systematic review as part of a needs assessment.[39]

EXAMPLE: *Reporting on Integrating Advances in Technology into UME Teaching of Anatomy.* Anatomy faculty reported on and evaluated the introduction of a new augmented reality technology (HoloAnatomy) into anatomy teaching at another medical school.[40,41]

EXAMPLE: *Innovation: Integrating Home Visits and Multidisciplinary Care for High-Risk Patients into Resident Continuity Clinic.* Residents and faculty at one teaching hospital introduced home visits and a multidisciplinary approach to care for high utilizing patients in its internal medicine continuity clinic.[42,43] Subsequently, the opportunity was afforded to develop consistent interdisciplinary teams for high-risk patients as part of a health systems–wide initiative. The latter demonstrated a reduction in hospital readmission rates and costs.[44,45] All were reported upon.

EXAMPLE: *Innovation: Reporting on a Primary Care Track in Internal Medicine Residency to Care for a Vulnerable Population.* Another teaching hospital developed an internal medicine residency track to care for HIV and LGBT (lesbian, gay, bisexual, and transgender) patients. Program developers reported on the program and its results.[46]

CONCLUSION

Attending to processes that maintain and enhance a curriculum helps the curriculum remain relevant and vibrant. These processes help a curriculum to evolve in a direction of continuous improvement.

QUESTIONS

For the curriculum you are coordinating, planning, or would like to be planning, please answer or think about the following questions:

1. As curriculum developer, what methods will you use (see Table 8.2) to *understand* the curriculum in its complexity (see Table 8.1)?

2. How will you implement minor *changes*? Major changes? What changes need to be reviewed by an oversight committee?

3. Will evolving *accreditation standards* affect your curriculum?

4. Could *environment* or *resource changes* provide opportunities for your curriculum? Can you stimulate positive changes or build upon new opportunities? Do environmental or resource changes present new challenges? How should you respond?

5. Is *faculty development* required or desirable?

6. What methods (see Table 8.3) will you use to maintain the *motivation and involvement* of your faculty? Of your support staff?

7. How could you *network* to strengthen the curriculum, as well as your own knowledge, abilities, and productivity?

8. Are there *related scholarly activities* that you could encourage, support, or engage in that would strengthen your curriculum, help others engaged in similar work, and/or improve your faculty's/your own promotion portfolio?

GENERAL REFERENCES

Baker, David P., Eduardo Salas, Heidi King, James Battles, and Paul Barach. "The Role of Teamwork in the Professional Education of Physicians: Current Status and Assessment Recommendations." *Joint Commission Journal on Quality and Patient Safety* 31, no. 4 (2005): 185–202. https://doi.org/10.1016/s1553-7250(05)31025-7.
Review article that describes eight broad competencies of teamwork that may be relevant to sustaining a curricular team: effective leadership, shared mental models, collaborative orientation, mutual performance monitoring, backup behavior, mutual trust, adaptability, and communication.

Duerden, Mat D., and Peter A. Witt. "Assessing Program Implementation: What It Is, Why It's Important, and How to Do It." *Journal of Extension* 50, no. 1 (2012).
Discusses why assessment of program implementation is important (e.g., enhances interpretation of outcome results). Describes five main dimensions of implementation (adherence to operational expectations, dosage, quality of delivery, participant engagement/involvement, and program differentiations—i.e., what components contributed what to the outcomes).

Dyer, W. Gibb, Jeffrey H. Dyer, and William G. Dyer. *Team Building: Proven Strategies for Improving Team Performance*. 5th ed. San Francisco, CA: John Wiley & Sons, 2013.
Practical, easy-to-read book, now in its fifth edition, written by three business professors: a father and his two sons. Useful for leaders and members of committees, task forces, and other task-oriented teams—for anyone engaged in collaboration. 304 pages.

Saunders, Ruth P., Martin H. Evans, and Praphul Joshi. "Developing a Process-Evaluation Plan for Assessing Health Promotion Program Implementation: A How-to Guide." *Health Promotion Practice* 6, no. 2 (2005): 134–47. https://doi.org/10.1177/1524839904273387.
Comprehensive systematic approach to evaluating implementation. Includes a list of useful questions.

Whitman, Neal. "Managing Faculty Development." In *Executive Skills for Medical Faculty*, 3rd ed., edited by Neal Whitman and Elaine Weiss. Pacific Grove, CA: Whitman Associates, 2006.
Managing faculty development to improve teaching skills is discussed as a needed executive function. Five strategies are offered to promote education as a product of the medical school: rewards, assistance, feedback, connoisseurship (developing a taste for good teaching), and creativity. 8 pages.

REFERENCES CITED

1. Liaison Committee on Medical Education, "Standard 1.1. Strategic Planning and Continuous Quality Improvement," in *Functions and Structure of a Medical School: Standards for Accreditation of Medical Education Programs Leading to the MD Degree*, March 2021, accessed October 1, 2021, www.lcme.org/publications/.
2. Terry M. Wolpaw et al., "Case Western Reserve University School of Medicine and Cleveland Clinic," *Academic Medicine* 85, no. 9 Suppl. (2010): S439–45, https://doi.org/10.1097/ACM.0b013e3181ea37d6.
3. Patricia A. Thomas et al., "Case Western Reserve University School of Medicine, Including the Cleveland Clinic Lerner College of Medicine," *Academic Medicine* 95, no. 9S, (2020): S396–401, https://doi.org/10.1097/acm.0000000000003411.
4. Eilean G. Watson et al., "Development of eMed: A Comprehensive, Modular Curriculum-Management System," *Academic Medicine* 82, no. 4 (2007): 351–60, https://doi.org/10.1097/ACM.0b013e3180334d41.
5. Tahereh Changiz et al., "Curriculum Management/Monitoring in Undergraduate Medical Education: A Systematized Review," *BMC Medical Education* 19, no. 1 (2019): 60, https://doi.org/10.1186/s12909-019-1495-0.
6. Kathryn Miller, Kelli Qua, and Amy Wilson-Delfosse, "Sciences and Art of Medicine Integrated: A Successful Integration of Basic and Health Systems Science with Clinical Medicine during Core Clerkships," *Medical Science Educator* (forthcoming).
7. Example from Johns Hopkins Faculty Development Program in Teaching Skills 2020–21, provided by Rachel Levine, MD, MPH, Co-director.
8. Liaison Committee on Medical Education, *Functions and Structure of a Medical School: Standards for Accreditation of Medical Education Programs Leading to the MD Degree*, March 2021, accessed October 6, 2021, https://lcme.org/publications/.

9. "Commission on Osteopathic College Accreditation (COCA)," American Osteopathic Association, accessed October 2, 2021, https://osteopathic.org/accreditation/.

10. "Common Program Requirements (Residency)," Accreditation Council for Graduate Medical Education, 2020, accessed October 6, 2021, https://www.acgme.org/what-we-do/accreditation/common-program-requirements/.

11. "Accreditation Requirements," Accreditation Council for Continuing Medical Education, accessed October 2, 2021, https://www.accme.org/accreditation-rules/accreditation-criteria.

12. "Directory of Organizations That Recognize/Accredit Medical Schools (DORA)," Foundation for the Advancement of International Education and Research (FAIMER), accessed October 2, 2021, https://www.faimer.org/resources/dora/index.html.

13. "Standards," World Federation for Medical Education, accessed October 2, 2021, https://wfme.org/standards/.

14. "What is Accreditation" and "Accreditation Process," Accreditation Council for Graduate Medical Education–International (ACGME-I), accessed October 2, 2021, https://www.acgme-i.org/.

15. Olle ten Cate, "Nuts and Bolts of Entrustable Professional Activities," *Journal of Graduate Medical Education* 5, no. 1 (Mar 2013): 157–58, https://doi.org/10.4300/jgme-d-12-00380.1.

16. Olle ten Cate and Fedde Scheele, "Competency-Based Postgraduate Training: Can We Bridge the Gap between Theory and Clinical Practice?" *Academic Medicine* 82, no. 6 (2007): 542–47, https://doi.org/10.1097/ACM.0b013e31805559c7.

17. Deborah E. Powell and Carol Carraccio, "Toward Competency-Based Medical Education," *New England Journal of Medicine* 378, no. 1 (2018): 3–5, https://doi.org/10.1056/nejmp1712900.

18. "The Core Entrustable Professional Activities (EPAs) for Entering Residency," American Association of Medical Colleges, March 2014, accessed October 2, 2021, https://www.aamc.org/what-we-do/mission-areas/medical-education/cbme/core-epas.

19. "CLER Pathways to Excellence: Expectations for an Optimal Clinical Learning Environment to Achieve Safe and High-Quality Patient Care," Version 2.0, CLER Evaluation Committee (Chicago: Accreditation Council for Graduate Medical Education, 2019), https://doi.org/10.35425/ACGME.0003.

20. Luba Dumenco et al., "Outcomes of a Longitudinal Quality Improvement and Patient Safety Preclerkship Curriculum," *Academic Medicine* 94, no. 12 (2019): 1980–1987, https://doi.org/10.1097/ACM.0000000000002898.

21. Ellen Luebbers et al., "Back to Basics for Curricular Development: A Proposed Framework for Thinking about How Interprofessional Learning Occurs," *Journal of Interprofessional Care* (2021): 1–10, https://doi.org/10.1080/13561820.2021.1897002.

22. David E. Kern and Belinda Y. Chen, "Appendix A: Longitudinal Program in Curriculum Development," in *Curriculum Development for Medical Education: A Six-Step Approach,* 3rd ed., ed. Patricia A. Thomas et al. (Baltimore: Johns Hopkins University Press, 2016), 257–71.

23. Institute of Medicine, *Improving Medical Education: Enhancing the Behavioral and Social Science Content of Medical School Curricula* (Washington: National Academies Press, 2004).

24. Molly Cooke, David M. Irby, and Bridget C. O'Brien, *Educating Physicians: A Call for Reform of Medical School and Residency* (Stanford, CA: Jossey-Bass, 2010).

25. Institute of Medicine, *The Healthcare Imperative: Lowering Costs and Improving Outcomes: Workshop Series Summary* (Washington, DC: National Academies Press, 2010).

26. Charles M. Wiener et al., "'Genes to Society'—the Logic and Process of the New Curriculum for the Johns Hopkins University School of Medicine," *Academic Medicine* 85, no. 3 (2010): 498–506, https://doi.org/10.1097/ACM.0b013e3181ccbebf.

27. Anna Maw et al., "Faculty Development in Point of Care Ultrasound for Internists." *Medical Education Online* 21 (2016): 33287, https://doi.org/10.3402/meo.v21.33287.

28. Scott E. Woods et al., "Collegial Networking and Faculty Vitality," *Family Medicine* 29, no. 1 (Jan 1997): 45–49.

29. Analia Castiglioni et al., "Succeeding as a Clinician Educator: Useful Tips and Resources," *Journal of General Internal Medicine* 28, no. 1 (2013): 136–40, https://doi.org/10.1007/s11606-012-2156-8.

30. Donna M. D'Alessandro et al., "An Annotated Bibliography of Key Studies in Medical Education in 2018: Applying the Current Literature to Pediatric Educational Practice and Scholarship," *Academic Pediatrics* 20, no. 5 (2020): 585–94, https://doi.org/10.1016/j.acap.2020.01.012.

31. William T. Branch et al., "A Multi-institutional Longitudinal Faculty Development Program in Humanism Supports the Professional Development of Faculty Teachers," *Academic Medicine* 92, no. 12 (2017): 1680–86, https://doi.org/10.1097/acm.0000000000001940.

32. Sara B. Fazio et al., "Competency-Based Medical Education in the Internal Medicine Clerkship: A Report from the Alliance for Academic Internal Medicine Undergraduate Medical Education Task Force," *Academic Medicine* 93, no. 3 (2018): 421–27, https://doi.org/10.1097/acm.0000000000001896.

33. Adina Kalet and Calvin L. Chou, *Remediation in Medical Education: A Mid-course Correction* (New York: Springer, 2014).

34. Auguste H. Fortin VI et al., *Smith's Patient-Centered Interviewing: An Evidence-Based Method,* 4th ed. (New York: McGraw-Hill Education, 2018).

35. James L. Perucho et al., "PrEP (Pre-exposure Prophylaxis) Education for Clinicians: Caring for an MSM Patient," *MedEdPORTAL* 16 (2020): 10908, https://doi.org/10.15766/mep_2374-8265.10908.

36. James E. Power, Lorrel E. B. Toft, and Michael Barrett, "The Murmur Online Learning Experience (Mole) Curriculum Improves Medical Students' Ability to Correctly Identify Cardiac Murmurs," *MedEdPORTAL* 16 (2020): 10904, https://doi.org/10.15766/mep_2374-8265.10904.

37. Howard Y. Liu, Eugene V. Beresin, and Margaret S. Chisolm, "Social Media Skills for Professional Development in Psychiatry and Medicine," *Psychiatric Clinics of North America* 42, no. 3 (2019): 483–92, https://doi.org/10.1016/j.psc.2019.05.004.

38. Merry Jennifer Markham, Danielle Gentile, and David L. Graham, "Social Media for Networking, Professional Development, and Patient Engagement," *American Society of Clinical Oncology Educational Book* 37 (2017): 782–87, https://doi.org/10.1200/edbk_180077.

39. Erin M. Spaulding et al., "Interprofessional Education and Collaboration among Healthcare Students and Professionals: A Systematic Review and Call for Action," *Journal of Interprofessional Care* (2019): 1–10, https://doi.org/10.1080/13561820.2019.1697214.

40. Susanne Wish-Baratz et al., "A New Supplement to Gross Anatomy Dissection: HoloAnatomy," *Medical Education* 53, no. 5 (2019): 522–23, https://doi.org/10.1111/medu.13845.

41. Jeremy S. Ruthberg et al., "Mixed Reality as a Time-Efficient Alternative to Cadaveric Dissection," *Medical Teacher* 42, no. 8 (2020): 896–901, https://doi.org/10.1080/0142159x.2020.1762032.

42. Melissa S. Dattalo et al., "Frontline Account: Targeting Hot Spotters in an Internal Medicine Residency Clinic," *Journal of General Internal Medicine* 29, no. 9 (2014): 1305–7, https://doi.org/10.1007/s11606-014-2861-6.

43. Stephanie K. Nothelle, Colleen Christmas, and Laura A. Hanyok, "First-Year Internal Medicine Residents' Reflections on Nonmedical Home Visits to High-Risk Patients," *Teaching and Learning in Medicine* 30, no. 1 (2018): 95–102, https://doi.org/10.1080/10401334.2017.1387552.

44. Scott A. Berkowitz et al., "Association of a Care Coordination Model with Health Care Costs and Utilization: The Johns Hopkins Community Health Partnership (J-Chip)," *JAMA Network Open* 1, no. 7 (2018): e184273, https://doi.org/10.1001/jamanetworkopen.2018.4273.

45. Shannon M. E. Murphy et al., "Going Beyond Clinical Care to Reduce Health Care Spending: Findings from the J-Chip Community-Based Population Health Management Program Evaluation," *Medical Care* 56, no. 7 (2018): 603–9, https://doi.org/10.1097/mlr.0000000000000934.

46. David A. Fessler et al., "Development and Implementation of a Novel HIV Primary Care Track for Internal Medicine Residents," *Journal of General Internal Medicine* 32, no. 3 (2017): 350–54, https://doi.org/10.1007/s11606-016-3878-9.

CHAPTER NINE

Dissemination

. . . making it count twice

David E. Kern, MD, MPH, and Sean A. Tackett, MD, MPH

DEFINITION

Dissemination refers to efforts to promote consideration or use of a curriculum or related products (e.g., needs assessment or evaluation results) by others. It also refers to the delivery of the curriculum or segments of the curriculum to new groups of learners.

WHY BOTHER?

The dissemination of a curriculum or related work can be important for several reasons. Dissemination can do the following:

- *Help address a health problem*: As indicated in Chapter 2, the ultimate purpose of a curriculum in medical education is to address a problem that affects the health of the public or a given population. To maximize the positive impact of a curriculum, it is necessary to share the curriculum or related work with others who are dealing with the same problem.

- *Stimulate change*: Innovative curricular work can create excitement and stimulate change in educational programs and medical institutions.[1] Innovations have particular impact when they are disruptive, essentially changing the nature or venue of educational activities.[2,3] Many opportunities exist for disruptive innovation given emerging concepts in educational theory and science, new educational challenges (see Introduction, Table I.1), evolving learning technologies, and changing practice environments. Examples include the following: using systems to improve patient outcomes, addressing social determinants of health and the needs of targeted populations, improving the value and reducing the cost of health care, using high-fidelity simulators and virtual reality, employing collaborative interprofessional practice models, and including competency-based education. New learning technology should make it easier to extend curricula beyond single institutions or countries, as in the development of online courses.[4] Shared, innovative curricula can contribute to a continuously learning health care system[5] by demonstrating uses for health care data, building decision support, coaching health care professionals and leaders, integrating patient and community perspectives, and improving coordination and communication within and across organizations. Some innovations may also increase the efficiency of learning and reduce the cost of health professions education. The American Medical Association (AMA) initiative Accelerating Change in Medical Education (https://www.ama-assn.org/education/accelerating-change -medical-education) is a nice example that combines funding and networking to stimulate change, and to share and disseminate innovations in medical education.

- *Increase collaboration*: Dissemination efforts may lead to increased exchange of ideas between people within an institution, or in different institutions, who are interested in the same issues. Such interchange may lead to active collaboration. The resulting teamwork is likely to lead to development of an even better curriculum or to other products that would not have been developed by individuals working separately.

- *Prevent redundant work*: By disseminating their work, curriculum developers can minimize the extent to which different people expend time and energy repeating work that has been done elsewhere. Instead, others can devote their time and energy to building on what has already been accomplished.

EXAMPLE: *Prevention of Redundancy.* All internal medicine residency programs must provide training in ambulatory medicine. When a web-based curriculum in ambulatory care medicine was developed for internal medicine residency programs, more than 80 residency programs subscribed to it, and the number has grown over time to approximately 250. By subscribing to the curriculum, residency program directors were able to use an existing resource without each program having to create its own set of learning materials. In addition, the income from subscriptions has permitted the curriculum developers to regularly update the curriculum's topic-based modules, thereby continuing to save time for all users of the curriculum.[6–8]

- *Provide feedback to curriculum developers*: By disseminating curriculum-related work, curriculum developers can obtain valuable feedback from others who may have unique perspectives. This external feedback can promote further development of one's curriculum and curriculum-related work (see Chapter 8).
- *Help curriculum developers achieve recognition and academic advancement*: Faculty may devote a substantial amount of time to the development of curricula but have difficulties achieving academic advancement if this portion of their overall work is not recognized as representing significant scholarship. Properly performed, curriculum development, if disseminated, is a recognized form of scholarship.[9,10] Promotion committees and department chairs report that they value clinician-educators' accomplishments in curriculum development.[11–14] Educational portfolios detailing these accomplishments are used by many institutions to support applications for promotion.[14–16] One important criterion for judging the significance of scholarly work is the degree to which the work has been disseminated, especially in peer-reviewed venues, and has had an impact at a local, regional, national, or international level.

EXAMPLE: *Benefits of Dissemination.* Following attendance at a conference on high-value care, a clerkship director worked with other educators to test a method of introducing discussions of value into all medical notes and oral presentations during clinical clerkships. This was ultimately tested across multiple medical schools and adopted by some. The work was published and presented in multiple venues. This nationally recognized work contributed to a clerkship director's academic promotion.[17]

Are dissemination efforts worth the time and effort required? In many cases, the answer is yes, even for individuals who do not need academic advancement. If the curriculum developer performed an appropriate problem identification and general needs assessment, as discussed in Chapter 2, the curriculum will probably address an important problem that has not been adequately addressed previously. If this is the case, the curriculum is likely to be of value to others. The challenge is to decide how the curriculum should be disseminated and how much time and effort the curriculum developer can realistically devote to dissemination efforts.

PLANNING FOR DISSEMINATION

Curriculum developers should start planning for dissemination when they start planning their curriculum (i.e., *before* implementation).[18] To ensure a product worthy of dissemination, curriculum developers will find it helpful to follow rigorously the principles of curriculum development described in this book, particularly with respect to those steps related to the part of their work they wish to disseminate. For an entire curriculum, each of the following steps relates to one of Glassick's criteria for scholarship:[9] Steps 1 and 2 relate to adequate preparation, Step 3 to clear goals and aims, Step 4 to appropriate methods, and Step 6 to significant results and reflective critique. One can also apply Glassick's criteria to each step.

Curriculum developers may also find it useful to think in advance of the characteristics of an innovation that contribute to its diffusion or dissemination, a final criterion for scholarship.[9] It is important to develop a coherent strategy for dissemination that clarifies the purposes of one's dissemination efforts (see above), addresses ethical and legal issues related to the protection of participants and intellectual property, identifies what is to be disseminated, delineates the target audience, and determines venues for dissemination. A realistic assessment of the time and resources available for dissemination is necessary to ensure that the dissemination strategy is feasible. These topics are discussed in the following sections of this chapter.

DIFFUSION OF INNOVATIONS

If the curriculum developer wants to disseminate all or parts of an actual curriculum, it is worthwhile to review what is known about the diffusion of innovations. Factors identified by Rogers[19] that promote the likelihood and rapidity of adoption of an innovation include the following:

- *Relative advantage*—the degree to which an innovation is perceived as superior to existing practice.
- *Compatibility*—the degree to which an innovation is perceived by the adopter as similar to previous experience, beliefs, and values, and is compatible with the adopter's practice environment.
- *Simplicity*—the degree to which a new idea is perceived as relatively easy to understand and implement.
- *Trialability*—the degree to which an innovation can be divided into steps and tried out by the adopter.
- *Observability*—the degree to which the innovation can be seen and appreciated by others.

Additional factors include impact on existing social relations, modifiability, reversibility, required resources (monetary, time, other), risk/uncertainty, and commitment.[20,21]

> **EXAMPLE:** *Diffusion of Team-Based Learning.* Team-based learning (TBL) is an adaptation of small-group learning and problem-based learning (PBL) that also engages small groups of students in the analysis and solving of problems but permits one or a few faculty facilitators to manage multiple small groups. Developed more than 30 years ago for use in business schools, TBL has been adopted by medical schools in multiple countries. While guidelines related to efficacy of TBL have been established, the problem-based exercises can be adapted by different faculty, for different purposes, and for different subject matter.[22,23] TBL has an advantage over small group and PBL because it requires fewer faculty resources.

According to the conceptual model described by Rogers,[19] individuals pass through *several stages* when deciding whether to adopt an innovative idea. These stages include (1) acquisition of *knowledge* about an innovation, (2) *persuasion* that the innovation is worth considering, (3) a *decision* to adopt the innovation, (4) *implementation* of the innovation, and (5) *confirmation* that the innovation is worth continuing.

One of the main implications of diffusion theory and research is that efforts to disseminate an innovative curriculum should involve more than just making others aware of the curriculum. The dissemination strategy should include efforts to *persuade* individuals of the need to consider the curricular innovation. Efforts at persuasion are best directed at individuals who are most likely to make decisions about implementation of a curriculum or who are most likely to influence other individuals' attitudes or behaviors regarding implementation of a curricular innovation. The dissemination strategy also should include efforts to understand and address barriers and facilitators to curricular transfer at three levels: systems (environmental context, culture, communication processes, external requirements), staff (commitment, understanding, skills/abilities), and ease of intervention (complexity, costs, required resources).[24] Finally, there is the need to support those individuals who decide to implement the curriculum. The fields of implementation practice and science add a perspective in this realm by emphasizing the need to assess readiness, supply coaching, and engage necessary systems support for implementation,[25] as well as address sustainability.[26] Such efforts usually require effective interpersonal communication and ongoing follow-up. Regardless of the mode of communication, it usually is best to identify a specific individual or leadership group who will direct the effort to transfer an innovative curriculum to the targeted institution.

Ideally, a collaborative relationship will develop between the original curriculum developer and the adapting group. A collaborative approach is ideal because most curricula require modifications (adaptation rather than adoption) when transferred to other settings. Moreover, the establishment of an ongoing collaborative relationship generally strengthens the curriculum for all users and stimulates further innovation and products.

PROTECTION OF PARTICIPANTS

If curricular components are shared (e.g., images/photos of patients or trainees, examples of student work), protection of participants is a concern. HIPAA (Health Insurance Portability and Accountability Act) regulations pertain to patients and FERPA (Family Educational Rights and Privacy Act) regulations pertain to students. In general, information about patients and trainees should be de-identified. Sometimes trainees sign blanket consent forms at the beginning of training for the sharing of de-identified information for research or educational purposes. When information cannot be de-identified, formal consent is generally required. Relevant compliance officers and registrars can be consulted at educational and health care institutions related to HIPAA, FERPA, and other regulations.

If curriculum-related work would qualify as educational research, then regulations regarding research on human subjects will need to be considered. In addition, international recommendations for medical journals state that all authors should address ethical issues.[27] Most journals require statements about whether ethical approval from an independent review body was obtained and, if not, why not. Federal regulations governing human subjects research in the United States categorize many educational research projects as exempt from the regulations if the research involves the study of normal educational practices or records information about learners in such a way that they cannot be identified.[28] However, US-based institutional review boards (IRBs) often differ in their interpretation of what is exempt. This can pose a challenge for multi-institutional education research where each institution's IRB may need to make its own determination.[29] Regulations may vary internationally.[30] It is wise for curriculum developers to check in advance with their IRBs or relevant research ethics committee. These boards or committees will be concerned about whether participating learners, faculty, patients, or others could incur harm because of participation and will want to know how the benefit would outweigh the risk for harm. Issues such as informed consent, confidentiality, the use of incentives to encourage participation in a curriculum, and funding sources may need to be considered and reported in an application for formal ethical approval.[31] Failure to consult one's IRB or relevant research ethics committee before implementation of the curriculum-related research can have adverse consequences for the curriculum developer who later tries to publish research about the curriculum.[32] (See Chapter 6, Implementation, "Scholarship," and Chapter 7, Evaluation and Feedback, "Task VII: Address Ethical Concerns," for additional details.)

INTELLECTUAL PROPERTY AND COPYRIGHT ISSUES

When considering dissemination of curriculum-related work, curriculum developers need to address intellectual property issues, with respect to both copyrighted content in the curriculum and protecting their own intellectual property.[33] Online material is covered by the same copyright rules as printed materials. A curriculum that is used locally for one's own learners generally falls under the exceptions contained in the Copyright Act, often referred to as fair use privilege provided by Section 107 of US copyright law (Title 17 of the US Code).[34] "Fair use" provides for use of material without the copyright owner's permission if it is being used for teaching, scholarship, or research, and it generally implies no commercial use of the material.[35] In recent times, with the increasing ease of online dissemination, the law is being interpreted more narrowly by universities. Once work—such as a syllabus, a presentation, or a multimedia site with images—is disseminated, it may no longer fall under fair use guidelines. Careful attention to the proper use of copyrighted materials requires additional citations and/or written permissions from publishers for the use of graphs and images. A curriculum developer who is a member of a university should be familiar with the university's intellectual property policy and seek expertise *before* disseminating the work.

Curriculum developers may wish to protect their disseminated products from unlawful use, alteration, or dissemination beyond their control. One approach is to license the material, and most universities have expertise to assist with this process as well. More recently, there has been growing interest in using the internet to increase the availability of educational and research materials to all. *Open access* refers to free sharing of content on the internet. *Creative Commons* is a nonprofit organization that has designed several copyright licenses to allow creators of content to publish that content with a range of copyright privileges, such as whether sharing and modification is acceptable if attribution is given to the creator. More information about publishing under a Creative Commons license is available at its website (www.creativecommons.org).

Most universities have multiple resources to assist faculty in understanding these issues. A helpful guideline and best practices document is available from the Copyright Clearance Center.[36] Additional resources include the US Copyright Office, the Association of Research Libraries,[37] the American Library Association (www.ala.org), resources developed by universities (such as the "Copyright Crash Course" maintained by the University of Texas[38]), and websites such as Opensource.com.[39]

WHAT SHOULD BE DISSEMINATED?

One of the first decisions to make when developing plans for disseminating curriculum work is to *determine whether the entire curriculum, parts of the curriculum* (e.g., reusable learning objects)[40–42] (see Chapter 5), *or curriculum-related work should be disseminated*. The curriculum developer can refer to the problem identification and general needs assessment to determine the extent of the need for the curriculum and to determine whether the curriculum or related work truly represents a significant contribution to the field. The results of the evaluation of a curriculum may also help identify aspects of the curriculum worth disseminating.

In some cases, dissemination efforts will focus on promoting adoption of a *complete curriculum* or *curriculum guide* by other sites. Usually this requires allowance for modifications to meet the unique needs of the learners at these sites. *Online curricula* lend themselves particularly well to dissemination, either after development and refinement or from the beginning.

> **EXAMPLE:** *Reusable Learning Objects (RLOs).* Four digital RLOs were developed on chronic wound care for nursing students and were used for blended learning (see Chapter 5). They covered introduction to chronic wounds and their etiology, chronic wound care assessment, principles of chronic wound care management, and aftercare management. The RLOs were used and rated highly by over 160 nursing students. Nursing students' self-rated abilities in chronic wound care improved.[43]

> **EXAMPLE:** *Complete Curriculum.* The Healer's Art is a 15-hour, quarter-long elective that has been taught annually at the University of California, San Francisco, since 1992 and has been disseminated to more than 90 medical schools (http://www.rishiprograms.org/healers-art/). The course's educational strategy is based on a discovery model that uses principles of adult education, contemplative studies, humanistic and transpersonal psychology, cognitive psychology, formation education, creative arts, and storytelling. The course addresses professionalism, meaning, and the human dimensions of medical practice. Faculty development workshops, guidebooks, and curricular materials prepare faculty to implement the course at their institutions.[44–46]

> **EXAMPLE:** *Online Curriculum.* A self-paced four-hour introduction to the six steps of curriculum development is available online.[47] It provides a concise overview that can be accessed asynchronously and from diverse geographic locations.

In other cases, it is appropriate to limit dissemination efforts to *specific products of the curriculum development process* that are likely to be of value to others. We provide examples below.

The *problem identification and general needs assessment* (Step 1) may yield new insights about a problem that warrant dissemination. This may occur when a comprehensive review of the literature on a topic has been performed, or when a systematic survey on the extent of a problem has been conducted.

> **EXAMPLE:** *Step 1, Systematic Review.* A team working on a medical student curriculum that used social media to promote humanism and professionalism performed systematic reviews on social media use in medical education and on the teaching of empathy to medical students.[48,49] The reviews helped to identify a wide range of methods used, their efficacies, and associated challenges.

> **EXAMPLE:** *Step 1, Systematic Survey.* A colorectal surgeon and a pediatric urologist surveyed fellowship directors and program graduates in their fields as part of their work in developing a model for surgical subspecialty fellowship curricula. Questions addressed the educational and assessment methods used, how the methods were valued, and the perceived achievement of competencies. The findings were published in three articles and served to inform subspecialty fellowship development.[50–52]

The *targeted needs assessment* (Step 2) may yield unique insights about the need for a curriculum that merits dissemination because the targeted learners are reasonably representative of other potential learners. When this occurs, the methods employed in the needs assessment will need to be carefully described so that other groups can determine whether the results of the needs assessment are supported by validity evidence and applicable to them.

EXAMPLE: *Step 2.* A team of educators surveyed targeted learners in an internal medicine residency program regarding prior training, confidence, and ability to interpret point-of-care ultrasound (POCUS) images. Results helped them build a POCUS curriculum for their residents. Their approach to needs assessment in this rapidly evolving field was thought to be relevant to other programs developing PO-CUS curricula and was published.[53]

In some cases, the formulation of learning objectives for a topic (Step 3) may, by itself, represent an important contribution to a field, thereby calling for some degree of dissemination.

EXAMPLE: *Step 3.* A team of educators, who formed a working group for the Teaching and Training Committee of the American Association for Geriatric Psychiatry, used a systematic iterative process to develop learning objectives in six domains for medical students. Their publication provided justification for the objectives as well as suggested teaching guidelines.[54]

In other cases, it may be worthwhile to focus the dissemination efforts on specific *educational methods* (Step 4) and/or on *implementation* strategies (Step 5).

EXAMPLE: *Steps 4 and 5.* The Harvard Medical School–Cambridge integrated clerkship was piloted in 2004–5 with eight volunteer medical students. The goal of the innovation was to restructure clinical education to address the inadequacies of hospital-based experiences as effective learning opportunities for chronic care, continuity of care, and humanism. A dedicated group of faculty from the medical school collaborated with clinicians to design this unique approach to the clinical year. A variety of obstacles needed to be overcome, including fiscal, cultural, political, and operational ones.[55] This curriculum became a model for longitudinal integrated clerkships nationwide.[56]

Measurement instruments that have been developed for a curriculum and validated in its implementation can be also disseminated. Most often, however, it is the results of the *evaluation* of a curriculum (Step 6) that are the focus of dissemination efforts, because people are more likely to adopt an innovative approach, or abandon a traditional approach, when there is evidence regarding the efficacy of each approach.

EXAMPLE: *Step 6, Evaluation Instrument.* An observational checklist for clinical skills, or the Objective Structured Assessment of Technical Skills, was developed for laparoscopic hysterectomy. Internal structure, content, and relationship to other variable (predictive/discriminant) validity evidence was provided.[57]

EXAMPLE: *Step 6, Evaluation of a Curriculum.* In a randomized controlled trial, participants in a web-based acute pain management curriculum for nurses improved their knowledge and self-rated efficacy compared to the control group, but not their immediate post-intervention attitudes.[58]

WHO IS THE TARGET AUDIENCE?

Dissemination efforts may be targeted at individuals within one's institution, individuals at other institutions, or individuals who are not affiliated with any institution. The ideal target audience for dissemination of a curriculum depends on the nature of the curricular work being disseminated and the reasons for dissemination identified during planning. For example, the ideal audience for disseminating a curriculum for medical students on delivering primary care to a culturally diverse, inner-city, indigent population might be the faculty and deans of medical schools located in major cities. In contrast, a curriculum on public health, health facility, and health professional responses to pandemics would be worth disseminating broadly, both geographically and among different levels and types of health professionals.

HOW SHOULD CURRICULUM-RELATED WORK BE DISSEMINATED?

Once the purpose and content of the dissemination and the target audience have been defined and available resources identified, the curriculum developer must choose the most appropriate modes of dissemination (see Table 9.1 and text below). Ideally, the curriculum developer will use a variety of dissemination modes to maximize impact.

Presentations

Usually, the first mode of dissemination involves *written or oral* presentations to key people *within the setting where the curriculum was developed*. These presentations may be targeted at potential learners or at faculty who will need to be involved in the curriculum. The presentations may also be directed at leaders who can provide important support or resources for the curriculum.

An efficient way to disseminate curriculum-related work to other sites is to present it at regional, national, or international *meetings of professional societies*. A workshop or mini course that engages the participants as learners is an appropriate format for presenting the content or methods of a curriculum. A presentation that follows a research abstract format is appropriate for presenting results of a needs assessment or a curriculum evaluation. General guidelines have been published for oral and poster presentations.[59–63] Specific guidelines are provided by many professional organizations. Sometimes they include additional formats tailored to innovative curricular work.[64] As illustrated in Table 9.2, information from the six-step curriculum development cycle can fit nicely into the format for an abstract presentation.

Interest Groups, Working Groups, and Committees of Professional Organizations

In some cases, presentation of curricular work, collaboration on curricula and publications, sharing of ideas and resources, and back-and-forth communication may oc-

Table 9.1.   Modes of Disseminating Curriculum Work

- Presentations of posters, oral abstracts, workshops, or courses to individuals and groups within specific institutions
- Presentations of posters, oral abstracts, workshops, or courses at regional, national, and international professional meetings
- Involvement in multi-institutional interest groups, working groups, or committees of professional organizations
- Use of digital platforms
    - Submission of curricular materials to a web-based educational clearinghouse
    - Preparation and distribution of instructional audiovisual recordings
    - Preparation and distribution of online educational modules or reusable learning objects (RLOs)
- Publication of an article in a printed or online professional journal
- Publication of a manual, book, or book chapter
- Use of social media
- Preparation of a press release

Table 9.2.   Format for a Curriculum Development Abstract Presentation or Manuscript

I. Introduction
    A. Rationale
        1. Problem identification
        2. General needs assessment
        3. Targeted needs assessment
    B. Purpose
        1. Goals of curriculum
        2. Goals of evaluation: evaluation questions

II. Materials and Methods
    A. Setting
    B. Subjects / power analysis if any
    C. Educational intervention
        1. Relevant specific measurable objectives
        2. Relevant educational strategies
        3. Resources: faculty, other personnel, equipment/facilities, costs*
        4. Implementation strategy*
        5. Display or offer of educational materials*
    D. Evaluation methods
        1. Evaluation design
        2. Evaluation instruments
            a. Reliability measures, if any
            b. Validity measures, if any
            c. Display (or offer) of evaluation instruments
        3. Data collection methods
        4. Data analysis methods

III. Results
    A. Data: including tables, figures, graphs, etc.
    B. Statistical analysis

IV. Conclusions and Discussion
    A. Summary and discussion of findings
    B. Contribution to existing body of knowledge, comparison with work of others*
    C. Strengths and limitations of work
    D. Conclusions/implications
    E. Future directions*

*These items are often omitted from presentations.

cur within multi-institutional interest groups, working groups, and committees of professional organizations. Curriculum developers can create or engage in such groups.

EXAMPLE: *Interest and Working Groups.* The Society of General Internal Medicine has numerous interest groups and other communities that periodically meet, communicate electronically, share resources and work, plan educational events, and collaborate on publications.[65] As mentioned above, a self-created working group of the Teaching and Training Committee of the American Association for Geriatric Psychiatry developed and published learning objectives and corresponding teaching strategies for medical students in geriatric psychiatry.[54] Members of the coaching interest group of the AMA Accelerating

Change in Medical Education consortium medical schools created handbooks for faculty coaches and coachees.[66]

Use of Digital Platforms

Electronic communication systems provide a tremendous opportunity for curriculum developers to share curricular materials with anyone having internet access. Written curricular materials, instructional visual and audio recordings (see RLOs example, above), interactive instructional software, and measurement instruments used for needs assessment and/or curriculum evaluation can be shared widely using digital media. Online modules and courses, including massive open online courses (MOOCs), are broadly available.[4] Interpersonal educational methods used for achieving affective and psychomotor objectives are less amenable to such transfer, although there are increasing exceptions with the advent of interactive software, gaming, and virtual reality. A cautionary note: universities are increasingly liable for ensuring accessibility with online and electronic communications, so curriculum developers should check that the platforms they are using follow current regulations and guidelines.

> **EXAMPLE:** *Online Curricula in Palliative Care.* The Center to Advance Palliative Care (www.capc.org) houses online courses in communication skills, pain and symptom management, and advance care planning. Continuing education and maintenance of certification credits are offered.

Educational clearinghouses, such as MedEdPORTAL (www.mededportal.org), which publishes peer-reviewed curricular materials that are indexed in PubMed and includes curricula from multiple professions, can provide the opportunity to disseminate one's work widely. Information about the existence of an educational clearinghouse for a particular clinical domain generally can be obtained from the professional societies that have a vested interest in educational activities in that domain. (See Appendix B for additional clearinghouse information.)

Publications

One of the most traditional, but still underused, modes of disseminating medical education work is publication in a *medical journal or textbook*, which can be print or digital. When a curriculum developer seeks to disseminate a comprehensive curriculum, it may be wise to consider preparation of a book or manual. On the other hand, the format for original research articles can be used to present results of a needs assessment or a curriculum evaluation (see Table 9.2). The format for review articles or meta-analyses can be used to present results of a problem identification and general needs assessment. An editorial, perspective, or special article format sometimes can be used for other types of work, such as discussion of the most appropriate learning objectives or methods for a needed curriculum.

Many journals will consider articles derived from curriculum-related work. A useful bibliography of journals for educational scholarship has been compiled and updated by the Association of American Medical Colleges (AAMC) Group on Educational Affairs (see General References). Curriculum developers who wish to publish work related to their curriculum should prepare their manuscript using principles of good scientific writing.[18,67] Their manuscript will have an increased chance of being accepted by a journal if the results of the curriculum work are relevant to the journal's intended audience and purpose and if that journal has a track record of publishing medical education articles (Table 9.3). The JANE (Journal/Author Name Estimator) website (https://jane.biosemantics .org/) is a helpful resource where an author can enter the name and/or abstract for a manuscript and be directed to the best matching journals, articles, and authors. The curriculum developer may choose the most appropriate journals for submission of their work by using the JANE website to identify potential journals; Table 9.3 to check each journal's propensity to publish curricular work, its impact factor, and Scimago Journal Rank (SJR); and the AAMC's Annotated Bibliography of Journals for Educational Scholarship to read a description of each journal. Manuscripts should follow the Instructions for Authors provided by the journal to which they will be submitted and, for instructions not specified, by the "Recommendations for the Conduct, Reporting, Editing, and Publication of Scholarly Work in Medical Journals," published by the International Committee of Medical Journal Editors (ICMJE).[68] Curriculum evaluations will most likely be accepted for publication by peer-reviewed journals if they satisfy common standards of methodological rigor.[69–71] Table 9.4 displays criteria that may be considered by reviewers of a manuscript on a curriculum. Several of the criteria listed in Table 9.4 have been combined into a *medical education research study quality instrument*, or *MERSQI*, score,[69] which has been shown in one study to predict the likelihood of acceptance for publication.[70] Seldom do even published curricular articles satisfy all these criteria. Nevertheless, the criteria can serve as a guide to curriculum developers interested in publishing their work. Methodological criteria for reporting controlled trials,[72] systematic review articles and meta-analyses,[73–75] and nonrandomized educational, behavioral, and public health interventions[76] have been published elsewhere. One-stop shopping for reporting guidelines is available at EQUATOR (Enhancing the Quality and Transparency of Health Research) Network (https://www.equator-network.org).

An increasingly prevalent option to publishing in a conventional, subscription-based journal is publishing in an *open access journal*.[77,78] Open access journals remove price barriers to public access, such as subscription fees and pay-per-view charges, and permission barriers, such as most copyright and licensing restrictions. They cover costs in other ways and may charge publication fees after acceptance. In general, reputable open access journals require peer review prior to acceptance. *Open access repositories*, on the other hand, accept both manuscripts that have and have not yet been peer-reviewed. They can be discipline-specific or institutional, and they do not perform peer review themselves. When it seems important to disseminate an innovative model or findings immediately, some open access journals offer the opportunity to publish online after editorial screening and prior to peer review by readers and members of a review panel.[79] Legitimate open access journals and repositories provide additional opportunities to publish and remove access barriers for readers. However, they may not be indexed in search engines such as MEDLINE and have less impact than articles published in established journals. The curriculum developer should be wary of *predatory journals*, who may charge for reviewing as well as publishing articles, who misleadingly use a better-known journal's name or website, or who use deceptive practices to elicit submissions, attract and describe editorial boards, and portray impact. Guidelines and lists have been published for identifying legitimate open access journals.[77] The JANE website mentioned above also tags journals that are currently indexed in MEDLINE and open access journals approved by the Directory of Open Access Journals.

Table 9.3.   Peer-Reviewed Journals and Sites That Are Likely to Publish Curriculum-Related Work

Journal	N*	%†	2-yr IF‡	5-yr IF§	SJR‖	MEDLINE#
Health Professional Education Journals						
Academic Medicine	289	27.7	5.4	6.8	2.0	Yes
Advances in Health Sciences Education	77	22.7	2.5	2.9	1.3	Yes
Advances in Medical Education and Practice	172	35.5	NA	NA	NA	No
Advances in Physiology Education	76	22.0	1.5	2.2	0.5	Yes
American Journal of Pharmaceutical Education	256	34.1	2.4	2.5	0.8	Yes
Anatomical Sciences Education	146	43.3	3.8	3.9	1.1	Yes
Biochemistry and Molecular Biology Education	94	22.5	0.0	0.9	0.3	Yes
BMC Medical Education	574	31.0	1.8	2.2	0.8	Yes
CBE Life Sciences Education	68	16.4	2.2	3.7	1.3	Yes
Clinical Teacher, The	109	24.2	NA	NA	0.4	Yes
Currents in Pharmacy Teaching and Learning	303	36.7	NA	NA	0.6	No
Education for Primary Care	59	19.3	NA	NA	0.4	Yes
European Journal of Dental Education	163	36.7	1.1	1.1	0.6	Yes
International Journal of Medical Education	71	31.6	NA	NA	0.6	Yes
Internet and Higher Education	7	7.4	5.0	6.5	8.8	No
Journal of Cancer Education	105	10.3	1.6	1.7	0.6	Yes
Journal of Continuing Education in the Health Professions	28	12.7	1.4	1.6	0.7	Yes
Journal of Dental Education	235	30.0	1.3	1.4	0.5	Yes
Journal of Graduate Medical Education**	NA	NA	NA	NA	0.5	Yes
Journal of Medical Education and Curricular Development	127	52.0	NA	NA	NA	No
Journal of Nursing Education	140	23.5	1.2	1.5	0.7	Yes
Journal of Nutrition Education and Behavior	31	5.6	2.5	3.3	0.8	Yes
Journal of Surgical Education	259	27.0	2.2	2.5	1.0	Yes
Journal of Veterinary Medical Education	141	41.3	1.2	1.3	0.5	Yes
MedEdPORTAL**	NA	NA	NA	NA	0.3	Yes
Medical Education	115	20.4	4.6	5.5	1.8	Yes
Medical Education Online	113	35.8	2.0	2.3	1.0	Yes
Medical Science Educator	166	44.7	NA	NA	0.3	No
Medical Teacher	340	35.1	2.7	3.1	1.4	Yes
Nurse Education in Practice	141	17.6	1.6	2.0	0.9	Yes
Nurse Education Today	265	19.2	2.5	3.0	1.4	Yes
Pharmacy Education	61	24.0	NA	NA	0.2	No
Science Education	100	17.8	2.9	3.6	4.5	No

Journal	N*	%†	2-yr IF‡	5-yr IF§	SJR‖	MEDLINE#
Simulation in Healthcare/Journal of the Society for Simulation in Healthcare	45	16.2	1.8	2.4	0.7	Yes
Teaching and Learning in Medicine	124	43.1	1.8	2.0	1.6	Yes
Selected General and Specialty Health Professional Journals						
Academic Emergency Medicine	8	1.1	3.1	3.3	1.2	Yes
Academic Pediatrics	41	6.2	2.8	3.2	1.3	Yes
Academic Psychiatry	99	22.3	2.1	2.0	0.8	Yes
Academic Radiology	60	5.6	2.5	2.4	1.0	Yes
American Journal of Clinical Pathology	11	1.2	3.0	3.0	1.4	Yes
American Journal of Hospice and Palliative Care	48	5.3	1.6	1.6	0.8	Yes
American Journal of Medical Quality	27	6.9	1.4	1.6	0.6	Yes
American Journal of Medicine	6	0.6	4.5	5.3	1.1	Yes
American Journal of Obstetrics and Gynecology	11	0.6	6.5	6.1	3.5	Yes
American Journal of Preventive Medicine	12	0.9	4.4	5.4	2.3	Yes
American Journal of Roentgenology	5	0.2	3.0	3.2	1.3	Yes
American Journal of Surgery	83	4.3	2.1	2.4	1.0	Yes
Anesthesia and Analgesia	7	0.4	4.3	4.1	1.4	Yes
Annals of Family Medicine	5	1.5	4.7	6.3	1.9	Yes
Annals of Surgery	15	0.9	10.1	9.3	4.2	Yes
BMJ Quality & Safety	7	1.4	6.1	7.3	2.5	Yes
British Journal of Hospital Medicine	5	0.7	0.4	0.4	0.2	Yes
British Journal of Surgery	8	0.8	5.7	6.1	2.2	Yes
Canadian Family Physician	24	5.2	3.1	2.8	0.6	Yes
Clinical Anatomy	32	4.0	2.0	2.1	0.7	Yes
Evaluation and the Health Professions	5	3.2	1.6	1.9	0.5	Yes
Family Medicine	122	29.5	1.4	1.4	0.5	Yes
Internet Journal of Allied Health Sciences and Practice, The	37	9.0	1.8	NA	0.8	No
Journal of the American College of Surgeons	5	0.5	4.6	4.7	2.3	Yes
Journal of the American Geriatrics Society	26	1.4	4.2	4.9	2.0	Yes
Journal of General Internal Medicine	56	3.9	4.6	5.0	1.7	Yes
Journal of Hospital Medicine	12	1.8	2.2	2.6	1.1	Yes
Journal of Interprofessional Care	116	16.4	1.7	2.1	0.8	Yes
Journal of Medical Ethics	15	2.4	2.0	1.9	0.8	Yes
Journal of the National Medical Association	9	2.8	1.0	0.9	0.3	Yes
Journal of Pain and Symptom Management	35	2.9	3.1	3.5	1.4	Yes
Journal of Palliative Medicine	39	3.6	2.2	2.5	1.0	Yes
Journal of Professional Nursing	86	22.8	2.0	2.1	1.0	Yes
Journal of Surgical Research	49	1.8	1.8	2.1	0.8	Yes
Laryngoscope	14	0.4	2.5	2.5	1.2	Yes
Nursing Ethics	18	3.0	2.9	2.6	0.9	Yes

Table 9.3. *(continued)*

Journal	N*	%†	2-yr IF‡	5-yr IF§	SJR‖	MEDLINE#
Obstetrics and Gynecology	14	0.9	5.5	5.6	2.7	Yes
Patient Education and Counseling	49	3.6	2.6	3.4	1.1	Yes
Postgraduate Medical Journal	30	5.8	1.9	2.4	0.6	Yes
Progress in Community Health Partnerships	19	7.9	0.8	1.0	0.4	Yes
Surgery	29	1.7	3.4	3.7	1.5	Yes
Urology	13	0.6	1.9	2.1	0.9	Yes
Western Journal of Emergency Medicine	68	9.0	1.8	NA	0.8	Yes

Note: Table includes selected journals listed in Web of Science or Scimago, all with ≥5 curriculum-related articles. In addition to considering the journals listed above, curriculum developers are advised to read the instructions for authors of the journals in their subspecialty and to review Web of Science or past issues of those journals to see what types of curriculum-related work, if any, the journals have published. Data in this table are correct as of mid-May 2021. NA = not available.

N = number of curriculum-related ("curricul" searched) publications (articles, reviews) listed in Web of Science for 2016–2020.

†Percentage of total publications (articles, reviews) that were curriculum-related in Web of Science for 2016–2020.

‡2-yr IF = 2-year journal impact factor, as reported by Web of Science Journal Citation Reports for year 2019.

§5-yr IF = 5-year journal impact factor, as reported by Web of Science Journal Citation Reports for year 2019.

‖SJR = Scimago Journal Rank for 2020.

#Currently indexed for MEDLINE, as listed in Journals in NCBI Databases through PubMed.

**Not included in Web of Science.

Social and Print Media

Over the past decade, social media, including blogs, microblogs, networking websites, and podcasts, have become an increasingly important approach to amplify or bring attention to one's scholarly work.[80–83] An individual's posts may be followed by others, and the number of followers counted. Others may note or comment on one's work in their posts. It is generally recommended that one's own posts refer considerably more often to the work of others than to their own, in order not to appear too self-promoting.[80] One should also exercise discretion in that, even with disclaimer, opinions expressed on posts may be interpreted as those of the poster's employing institution.[80] Quality indicators for medical education blogs and podcasts have been published.[82]

Curriculum developers should also consider whether their work would have sufficient interest for the lay public. If there is enough interest to warrant issuing a press release, curriculum developers should contact the public affairs office in their institution to request assistance in preparing the press release. Sometimes a press release will lead to requests for interviews or publication of articles in lay publications, either of which will bring attention to the curricular work.

WHAT RESOURCES ARE REQUIRED?

To ensure a successful dissemination effort, it is important for the curriculum developer to identify the resources that are required. While the dissemination of curricular

Table 9.4.   Criteria That May Be Considered in the Review of a Manuscript on a Curriculum

Rationale
- Is there a well-reasoned and documented need for the curriculum or curriculum-related work? (Problem identification and general needs assessment)
- Is there a theoretical or evidence-based rationale for the educational intervention?

Setting
- Is the setting clearly described?
- Is the setting sufficiently representative to make the article of interest to readers? (External validity)

Subjects
- Are the learners clearly described? (Specific profession and specialty within profession; educational level [e.g., third-year medical students, postgraduate year–2 residents, or practitioners]; needs assessment of targeted learners; sociodemographic information; how recruited and, if different groups, how assigned)
- Are the learners sufficiently representative to make the article of interest to readers? (External validity)

Educational Intervention
- Are the relevant objectives clearly expressed?
- Are the objectives meaningful and congruent with the rationale, intervention, and evaluation?
- Are the educational content and methods described in sufficient detail to be replicated? (If written description is incomplete, are educational materials offered in an appendix or elsewhere?)
- Are the required resources adequately described (e.g., faculty, faculty development, equipment)?
- Is implementation described, including how challenges/barriers were addressed?

Evaluation Methods
- Are the methods described in sufficient detail so that the evaluation is replicable?
- Is the evaluation question clear? Are independent and dependent variables clearly defined?
- Are the dependent variables meaningful and congruent with the rationale and objectives for the curriculum? (For example, is performance/behavior measured instead of skill, or skill instead of knowledge, when those are the desired or most meaningful effects?) Are the measurements objective (preferred) or subjective? Where in the hierarchy of outcomes are the dependent variables (patient/health care outcomes > behaviors > skills > knowledge or attitudes > satisfaction or perceptions)? Is there an assessment of potentially adverse outcomes?
- Is the evaluation design clear and sufficiently strong to answer the evaluation question? Could the evaluation question and design have been more ambitious?
    - Is the design single or multi-institutional? (The latter enhances external validity.)
    - Has randomization and/or a control/comparison group been used?
    - Are long-term as well as short-term effects measured?
- Has a power analysis been conducted to determine the likelihood that the evaluation would detect an effect of the desired magnitude?
- Are raters blinded to the status of learners?
- Are the measurement instruments described or displayed in sufficient detail? (If incompletely described or displayed, are they offered or referenced?)
- Do the measurement instruments possess content validity? (See Chapter 7.) Are they congruent with the evaluation question?

Table 9.4.   *(continued)*

- Have inter- and intra-rater reliability and internal consistency validity been assessed? (See Chapter 7.)
- Are there other forms of validity evidence for the measurement instruments (e.g., relationship to other variables evidence, such as concurrent and predictive validity)? (Desirable, but frequently not achieved in curricular publications; see Chapter 7.)
- Are the reliability and validity measures sufficient to ensure the accuracy of the measurement instruments? Have the measurement instruments been used elsewhere? Have they attained a level of general acceptance? (Rarely are the last two criteria satisfied.)
- Are the statistical methods (parametric vs. nonparametric) appropriate for the type of data collected (nominal, ordinal, numerical; normally distributed vs. skewed; very small vs. larger sample size)? Are the specific statistical tests appropriate to answer the evaluation question? Have potentially confounding independent variables been controlled for by random allocation or the appropriate statistical methods? Is missing data handled appropriately?
- Are the evaluation methods, as a whole, sufficiently rigorous to ensure the internal validity of the evaluation and to promote the external validity of the evaluation?
- For qualitative evaluation, have measures of "trustworthiness" been included? (See Chapter 7.)
- Are data collection methods described?

Results
- Is the response rate adequate?
- Are the results clearly and accurately described/displayed?
- Has educational significance/effect size been assessed? (See Chapter 7.)

Discussion/Conclusions
- Are the results of sufficient interest to be worthy of publication? (The paper's Introduction and Discussion can help address this question.)
- Has the contribution of the work to the literature been accurately described?
- Are the strengths and limitations of the methodology acknowledged?
- Are the conclusions justified based on the methodology/results of the study or report?

Abstract
- Is the abstract clearly written?
- Does it represent well the content of manuscript?
- Are the data congruent with what is reported in the manuscript?

work can result in significant benefits to both curriculum developers and others, it is also necessary for the curriculum developer to ensure that the use of limited resources is appropriately balanced among competing needs.

Time and Effort

Disseminating curriculum-related work almost always requires considerable time and effort of the *individual or individuals responsible*. Unless one is experienced in disseminating curricular work, it is wise to multiply one's initial estimates of time and effort by a factor of two to four, which is likely to be closer to reality than the original estimate. Less time and effort may be required for posting on social media, presentations of abstracts, workshops, and courses. More time is required for the creation of online modules, instructional interactive software, and audiovisual recordings,[4] and maintaining online materials can require additional, ongoing effort. Peer-reviewed publications require considerable time and effort as well.

People

In addition to the curriculum developer, other personnel may be helpful or necessary for the dissemination effort. The creation of instructional audiovisual recordings or computer software for widespread use generally requires the involvement of *individuals with appropriate technical expertise.*[4] Individuals with research and/or statistical expertise are important to making needs assessments and evaluation research publishable. Collaborative approaches with *colleagues* permit the sharing of workload, can help group members maintain interest and momentum, and can provide the type of creative, critical, and supportive interactions that result in a better product than would have been achieved by a single individual. The identification of a *mentor* is helpful to individuals with little experience in disseminating curricular work. Participation in a writing accountability group can also be helpful.[84]

Equipment and Facilities

Equipment needs for dissemination are generally minimal and usually consist of equipment that is already accessible to health professional faculty, such as audiovisual equipment or a personal computer. Occasionally, software programs may need to be purchased. *Facilities or space* for presentations are usually provided by the recipients. Occasionally, a studio or simulation facility may be required for the development of audiovisual recordings.

Funds

Faculty may need to protect time to accomplish a dissemination effort. Technical *consultants* may require support. Funds may also be required for the purchase of necessary new *equipment* or the rental of *facilities*. Sometimes a faculty member's institution is able to provide such funding. Sometimes external sources can provide such funding (see also Chapter 6 and Appendix B). Well-funded curricula are often of higher quality than those that are poorly funded, and they typically fare better when it comes to publishing work related to the curricula.[69,70]

HOW CAN DISSEMINATION AND IMPACT BE MEASURED?

To determine whether dissemination efforts have the desired impact on target audiences, curriculum developers should try to measure the effectiveness of dissemination. Quantitative and qualitative measurements can be helpful in assessing the degree of dissemination and impact of one's work. Such measures can help promotion committees in academic medical centers appreciate the impact of an educator's work.

For *journal articles*, there are several available measures of the influence of the journal in which an article is published:

- *Journal impact factor*—most used measure: average number of citations per article in a given year for articles published during the previous *n* years; two and five years are most frequently used. Available at Web of Science's Journal Citation Reports (JCR).[85] Impact factors vary among fields, depending on the number of people in that field citing publications; for example, impact factors will be lower for medical education journals than for most clinical journals and lower for most subspecialties than for more general clinical fields.

- *Scimago Journal Rank (SJR) indicator*—measure of the scientific influence of a journal that accounts for both the number of citations and the prestige of the journal from which the citations come.[86] It also considers the thematic closeness of the citing and the cited journals and limits journal self-citations. A journal's SJR is a numeric value indicating the average number of weighted citations received during a selected year per document published in that journal during the previous three years. SJRs may have less variation across fields than impact factors.
- *Eigenfactor score*—number of times that articles published in the past five years in a given journal are cited, with citations from highly cited journals influencing the score more than citations from less frequently cited journals. References by one article to another in the same journal are removed. Eigenfactor scores are scaled so that the sum of the Eigenfactor scores of all journals listed in JCR is 100. Available in individual journal profiles in JCR.[85]
- *Article influence score*—journal's Eigenfactor score divided by the number of articles over the same time span, normalized so that the mean score is 1.00. Available in individual journal profiles in JCR.[85]
- *Cited half-life*—median age of articles cited in the JCR year specified. Available in individual journal profiles in JCR.[85]
- *Immediacy index*—average number of citations per article in the year of publication. Frequently issued journals may have an advantage because an article published early in the year has a better chance of being cited than one published later in the year. Available in individual journal profiles in JCR.[85]

Curriculum developers may want to consider such measures of journal influence when choosing a journal for submission of a manuscript. However, measures of journal impact are imperfect and should not be used without taking into consideration how the readership of a targeted journal compares with the audience one wants to reach.

Perhaps a more important measure of dissemination is how often one's work has been accessed or cited by others. A *citation index*, such as Web of Science,[87] Scopus (www .scopus.com), or Google Scholar (https://scholar.google.com), provides information on the number of times journal articles include one's work in its references. Each database has somewhat different characteristics, with Google Scholar retrieving somewhat more citations per article.[88] These databases can also provide a measure, called an *h-index*, for authors who have had many publications. The value of *h* is equal to the number of an author's papers (*n*) that have *n* or more citations. For example, an *h*-index of 20 means there are 20 items that have 20 citations or more. The *h*-index thus reflects both the number of publications an author has had and the number of citations per publication. The index was developed to improve on simpler measures, such as the total number of citations or publications.[89] It is more appropriately used for authors who have been publishing for some time than for relatively junior authors. It is best used in conjunction with a list of publications accompanied by the number of citations for each, since it does not distinguish between authors with the same *h*-index, one of whom has had several publications with many more citations than *h*, and another who has had only publications with a few more citations than *h*. In addition, the *h*-index works properly only for comparing academicians working in the same field, such as education. Desirable *h*-indices vary widely among different fields, such as medical student education, biochemistry, and clinical cardiology research.

For *curricular materials*, one can *keep track of the number of times they have been requested or accessed by others*. This is easiest for online material, where one can build in a tracking mechanism for access and completion. MedEdPORTAL (www.mededportal .org), for example, is a MEDLINE-indexed, peer-reviewed journal of teaching and learning resources in the health professions published by the AAMC, in partnership with the American Dental Education Association. It provides authors with usage reports that give total download counts, educational reasons for downloads, and the downloading user's role, affiliated institution, and country.[90] For other forms of dissemination, impact can be measured in a variety of ways. For *books*, one can keep track of *sales*, *book reviews*, and *communications* regarding the book. Google Scholar includes book as well as journal article citations, as does Scopus to a lesser degree. For *workshops* and *presentations*, one can keep track of the *number* and *locations* of those that are peer-reviewed and requested. For online workshops and webinars, one can ask hosts for audience characteristics, such as kind of learner (e.g., student, trainee, health professional), location, or other collected demographics. Another measure of dissemination is *media coverage* of one's work, which can be assessed by running an internet search for any news coverage of the work.

Fortunately, software metrics have been developed to measure how often one's work (e.g., books, presentations, datasets, videos, and journal articles) are downloaded or mentioned in social media, newspapers, government documents, and reference managers, in addition to being cited in journal articles. One such approach, developed by Altmetric (www.altmetric.com),[91,92] provides quantitative and qualitative information, including a score, about the online attention given to one's work. Online attention can include (but is not limited to) peer reviews on Faculty of 1000, citations on Wikipedia and in public policy documents, discussions on research blogs, mainstream media coverage, bookmarks on reference managers, and mentions on social networks. Altmetric information is now included for articles indexed in some journals.

Most of the above measures provide quantitative information about the dissemination of one's work. Curriculum developers can elect to collect additional information, including qualitative information about how their ideas and curricular materials have been used or reviewed. Friesen et al. describe the value of developing qualitative descriptions of impact using a variety of *gray metrics*, such as widespread application of one's work, translations into different languages, integration of one's contributions into policy, formal recognitions of impact, requests for consultation and presentation, and communications of appreciation.[93] Finally, curriculum developers can use *systematic assessment strategies* to directly evaluate the impact or dissemination of their work.

EXAMPLE: *Systematic Evaluation Strategy to Assess Dissemination.* An online curriculum in ambulatory care medicine was developed for internal medicine residency programs, and approximately 250 residency programs now subscribe to this curriculum. Information on the use of modules and resident performance is routinely collected. Periodic surveys of the program directors or curriculum administrators at each site assess how the curriculum is used.[6–8] The curriculum is also structured to generate reports related to each module.[94–96]

CONCLUSION

The dissemination of a curriculum or the products of a curriculum development process can be valuable to the curriculum developer and curriculum, as well as to others.

It is important to develop a coherent strategy for dissemination that clarifies the purposes of one's dissemination efforts, addresses ethical and legal issues related to the protection of participants and intellectual property, identifies what is to be disseminated, delineates the target audience, and determines venues for dissemination. A realistic assessment of the time and resources available for dissemination is necessary to ensure that the dissemination strategy is feasible.

QUESTIONS

For a curriculum that you are coordinating, planning, or would like to be planning, please answer or think about the following questions and prompts:

1. What are the *reasons* why you might want to disseminate part or all of your work?

2. *Which* steps in your curriculum development process would you expect to lead to a discrete *product* worth disseminating to other individuals and groups?

3. *Describe a dissemination strategy* (target audiences, modes of dissemination) that would fulfill your reasons for wanting to disseminate part or all your work. Usually this requires more than one mode of dissemination (see Table 9.1).

4. *Estimate the resources, in terms of time and effort, personnel, equipment/facilities, and funds*, that would be required to implement your dissemination strategy. Is the strategy feasible? Do you need to identify mentors, consultants, or colleagues to help you develop or execute the dissemination strategy? Do your plans for dissemination need to be altered or abandoned?

5. What would be a *simple strategy for measuring the impact of your dissemination efforts*? Consider your goals for dissemination and the importance of documenting the degree and impact of your dissemination.

6. Imagine the *benefits, pleasures, and rewards* of a successful dissemination effort. Are you willing to invest the time and energy necessary to achieve a dissemination goal?

GENERAL REFERENCES

AAMC-Regional Groups on Educational Affairs (GEA): Medical Education Scholarship, Research, and Evaluation Section. "Annotated Bibliography of Journals for Educational Scholarship." Accessed October 4, 2021. https://www.aamc.org/system/files/2019-11/prodev-affinity-groups -gea-annotated-bibliography-journal-educational-scholarship-110619.pdf.
This bibliography, compiled by medical educators in the AAMC's Group on Educational Affairs, lists over 100 journals and repositories, with structured annotations, including descriptions, topics, types of manuscripts, and audience.

Garson, Arthur, Jr., Howard P. Gutgesell, William W. Pinsky, and Dan G. McNamara. "The 10-Minute Talk: Organization, Slides, Writing, and Delivery." *American Heart Journal* 111, no. 1 (1986): 193–203. https://doi.org/10.1016/0002-8703(86)90579-x.
Classic, and still useful, article that provides practical instruction on giving 10-minute oral presentations before a professional audience.

Gutkin, Stephen W. *Writing High-Quality Medical Publications: A User's Manual*. Boca Raton, FL: CRC Press, 2018.
Discusses the process of writing and reviewing manuscripts and appropriate use of statistical tests. Also has consensus criteria and checklists for quality. 506 pages.

Kern, David E., William T. Branch, Michael L. Green, et al. "Making It Count Twice: How to Get Curricular Work Published." May 14, 2005. Accessed October 5, 2021. www.sgim.org/File%20 Library/SGIM/Communities/Education/Resources/WG06-Making-it-Count-Twice.pdf.
Practical tips from the editors of the first medical education issue of the *Journal of General Internal Medicine* on planning curricular work so that it is likely to be publishable, on preparing curriculum-related manuscripts for publication, and on submitting manuscripts to journals and responding to editors' letters. 33 pages.

Rogers, Everett M. *Diffusion of Innovations*, 5th ed. New York: Free Press, 2003.
Classic text that presents a useful framework for understanding how new ideas are communicated to members of a social system. 551 pages.

Westberg, Jane, and Hilliard Jason. *Fostering Learning in Small Groups: A Practical Guide*. New York: Springer Publishing, 2004.
Practical book, drawing on years of experience, on practical strategies for planning and facilitating small groups. Can be applied to giving workshops. 288 pages.

Westberg, Jane, and Hilliard Jason. *Making Presentations: Guidebook for Health Professions Teachers*. Boulder, CO: Center for Instructional Support, Johnson Printing, 1991.
User-friendly resource for health professionals on all aspects of preparing and giving presentations, stage fright, audiovisuals, and strategies to enhance presentations. 89 pages.

REFERENCES CITED

1. Barbara F. Sharf et al., "Organizational Rascals in Medical Education: Midlevel Innovation through Faculty Development," *Teaching and Learning in Medicine* 1, no. 4 (1989): 215–20, https://doi.org/10.1080/10401338909539414.
2. Neil Mehta et. al., "Just Imagine: New Paradigms for Medical Education*,*" *Academic Medicine* 88, no. 10 (2013): 1418–23, https://doi.org/10.1097/ACM.0b013e3182a36a07.
3. Malathi Srinivasan, "Disruptive and Deliberate Innovations in Healthcare," *Journal of General Internal Medicine* 28, no. 9 (2013): 1117–18, https://doi.org/10.1007/s11606-013-2550-x.
4. Belinda Y. Chen et al., "From Modules to MOOCs: Application of the Six-Step Approach to Online Curriculum Development for Medical Education," *Academic Medicine* 94, no. 5 (2019): 678–85, https://doi.org/10.1097/acm.0000000000002580.
5. Institute of Medicine, *Best Care at Lower Cost: The Path to Continuously Learning Health Care in America* (Washington, DC: The National Academies Press, 2013), https://doi.org/10.17226/13444.
6. Stephen D. Sisson et al., "Multicenter Implementation of a Shared Graduate Medical Education Resource," *Archives of Internal Medicine* 167, no. 22 (2007): 2476–80, https://doi.org/10.1001/archinte.167.22.2476.
7. Stephen D. Sisson and Deepan Dalal, "Internal Medicine Residency Training on Topics in Ambulatory Care: A Status Report," *American Journal of Medicine* 124, no. 1 (2011): 86–90, https://doi.org/10.1016/j.amjmed.2010.09.007.
8. Stephen D. Sisson, Amanda Bertram, and Hsin-Chieh Yeh, "Concurrent Validity between a Shared Curriculum, the Internal Medicine In-Training Examination, and the American Board of Internal Medicine Certifying Examination," *Journal of Graduate Medical Education* 7, no. 1 (2015): 42–47, https://doi.org/10.4300/jgme-d-14-00054.1.

9. Charles E. Glassick, "Boyer's Expanded Definitions of Scholarship, the Standards for Assessing Scholarship, and the Elusiveness of the Scholarship of Teaching," *Academic Medicine* 75, no. 9 (2000): 877–80, https://doi.org/10.1097/00001888-200009000-00007.

10. Deborah Simpson et al., "Advancing Educators and Education by Defining the Components and Evidence Associated with Educational Scholarship," *Medical Education* 41, no. 10 (2007): 1002–9, https://doi.org/10.1111/j.1365-2923.2007.02844.x.

11. Ayese A. Atasoylu et al., "Promotion Criteria for Clinician-Educators," *Journal of General Internal Medicine* 18, no. 9 (2003): 711–16, https://doi.org/10.1046/j.1525-1497.2003.10425.x.

12. Brent W. Beasley et al., "Promotion Criteria for Clinician-Educators in the United States and Canada: A Survey of Promotion Committee Chairpersons," *JAMA* 278, no. 9 (1997): 723–28.

13. Maryellen E. Gusic et al., "Evaluating Educators Using a Novel Toolbox: Applying Rigorous Criteria Flexibly across Institutions," *Academic Medicine* 89, no. 7 (2014): 1006–11, https://doi.org/10.1097/acm.0000000000000233.

14. Michael S. Ryan et al., "How Are Clinician-Educators Evaluated for Educational Excellence? A Survey of Promotion and Tenure Committee Members in the United States," *Medical Teacher* 41, no. 8 (2019): 927–33, https://doi.org/10.1080/0142159x.2019.1596237.

15. Claudia Lucy Dalton, Anthony Wilson, and Steven Agius, "Twelve Tips on How to Compile a Medical Educator's Portfolio," *Medical Teacher* 40, no. 2 (2018): 140–45, https://doi.org/10.1080/0142159x.2017.1369502.

16. Kanade Shinkai et al., "Rethinking the Educator Portfolio: An Innovative Criteria-Based Model," *Academic Medicine* 93, no. 7 (2018): 1024–28, https://doi.org/10.1097/acm.0000000000002005.

17. Eileen M. Moser et al., "SOAP-V: Introducing a Method to Empower Medical Students to Be Change Agents in Bending the Cost Curve," *Journal of Hospital Medicine* 11, no. 3 (2016): 217–20, https://doi.org/10.1002/jhm.2489.

18. David E. Kern et al., "Making It Count Twice: How to Get Curricular Work Published," May 14, 2005, www.sgim.org/File%20Library/SGIM/Communities/Education/Resources/WG06-Making-it-Count-Twice.pdf.

19. Everett M. Rogers, *Diffusion of Innovations*, 5th ed. (New York: Free Press, 2003), 219–66.

20. Ross C. Brownson et al., "Implementation, Dissemination, and Diffusion of Public Health Innovations," in *Health Behavior and Health Education*, 5th ed., ed. Karen Glanz, Barbara K. Rimer, and K. Viswaneth (San Francisco: Jossey-Bass Public Health, 2015), 301–25.

21. James W. Dearing and Jeffrey G. Cox, "Diffusion of Innovations Theory, Principles, and Practice," *Health Affairs* 37, no. 2 (2018): 183–90, https://doi.org/10.1377/hlthaff.2017.1104.

22. Annette W. Burgess, Deborah M. McGregor, and Craig M. Mellis, "Applying Established Guidelines to Team-Based Learning Programs in Medical Schools: A Systematic Review," *Academic Medicine* 89, no. 4 (Apr 2014): 678–88, https://doi.org/10.1097/acm.0000000000000162.

23. Tyler Reimschisel et al., "A Systematic Review of the Published Literature on Team-Based Learning in Health Professions Education," *Medical Teacher* 39, no. 12 (2017): 1227–37, https://doi.org/10.1080/0142159x.2017.1340636.

24. Liesbeth Geerligs et al., "Hospital-Based Interventions: A Systematic Review of Staff-Reported Barriers and Facilitators to Implementation Processes," *Implementation Science* 13, no. 1 (2018): 36, https://doi.org/10.1186/s13012-018-0726-9.

25. Kylie Porritt et al., eds., *JBI Handbook for Evidence Implementation,* JBI, 2020, accessed October 3, 2021, https://jbi-global-wiki.refined.site/space/JHEI.

26. Stephanie Koh et al., "An Orientation for New Researchers to Key Domains, Processes, and Resources in Implementation Science," *Translational Behavioral Medicine* 10, no. 1 (2020): 179–85, https://doi.org/10.1093/tbm/iby095.

27. "Protection of Research Participants," International Committee of Medical Journal Editors (ICMJE), accessed October 3, 2021, http://www.icmje.org/recommendations/browse/roles-and-responsibilities/protection-of-research-participants.html.

28. Electronic Code of Federal Regulations (e-CFR), "Protection of Human Subjects," accessed October 3, 2021, https://ecfr.federalregister.gov/current/title-34/subtitle-A/part-97?toc=1.

29. Ann Schwartz et al., "The Emergence and Spread of Practice-Based Medical Education Research Networks," *Academic Medicine* 95, no. 11S, (2020): S12–13, https://doi.org/10.1097/acm.0000000000003641.

30. "International Compilation of Human Research Standards," Office for Human Research Protections, HHS, accessed October 3, 2021, https://www.hhs.gov/ohrp/international/compilation-human-research-standards/.

31. Laura W. Roberts et al., "An Invitation for Medical Educators to Focus on Ethical and Policy Issues in Research and Scholarly Practice," *Academic Medicine* 76, no. 9 (2001): 876–85, https://doi.org/10.1097/00001888-200109000-00007.

32. John M. Tomkowiak and Anne J. Gunderson, "To IRB or not to IRB?" *Academic Medicine* 79, no. 7 (2004): 628–32.

33. "Copyright Essentials," Copyright Clearance Center, accessed October 3, 2021, http://www.copyright.com/wp-content/uploads/2020/12/Copyright-Essentials.pdf.

34. "Copyright Law of the United States (Title 17)," US Copyright Office, accessed October 3, 2021, https://www.copyright.gov/title17/.

35. "Fair Use Index," US Copyright Office, accessed October 3, 2021, https://www.copyright.gov/fair-use/index.html.

36. "Using Course Management Systems: Guidelines and Best Practices for Copyright Compliance," Copyright Clearance Center, accessed October 3, 2021, https://www.copyright.com/wp-content/uploads/2015/04/Using-Course-Management-Systems.pdf.

37. "Copyright and Fair Use/Fair Dealing," Association of Research Libraries, accessed October 3, 2021, https://www.arl.org/category/our-priorities/advocacy-public-policy/copyright-and-fair-use/.

38. "Copyright Crash Course," University of Texas, accessed October 3, 2021, http://copyright.lib.utexas.edu.

39. "What Is Open Source?" Opensource.com, accessed October 3, 2021, https://opensource.com/resources/what-open-source.

40. Jorge G. Ruiz, Michael J. Mintzer, and S. Barry Issenberg, "Learning Objects in Medical Education," *Medical Teacher* 28, no. 7 (2006): 599–605, https://doi.org/10.1080/01421590601039893.

41. Diane M. Billings, "Using Reusable Learning Objects," *Journal of Continuing Education in Nursing* 41, no. 2 (2010): 54–55, https://doi.org/10.3928/00220124-20100126-08.

42. Ehsan Khan, Maggie Tarling, and Ian Calder, "Reusable Learning Objects for Nurse Education: Development, Evaluation, Challenges and Recommendations," *British Journal of Nursing* 28, no. 17 (2019): 1136–43, https://doi.org/10.12968/bjon.2019.28.17.1136.

43. Catherine Redmond et al., "Using Reusable Learning Objects (RLOs) in Wound Care Education: Undergraduate Student Nurse's Evaluation of Their Learning Gain," *Nurse Education Today* 60 (2018): 3–10, https://doi.org/10.1016/j.nedt.2017.09.014.

44. Michael W. Rabow, Judith Wrubel, and Rachel N. Remen, "Authentic Community as an Educational Strategy for Advancing Professionalism: A National Evaluation of the Healer's Art Course," *Journal of General Internal Medicine* 22, no. 10 (2007): 1422–28, https://doi.org/10.1007/s11606-007-0274-5.

45. Michael W. Rabow, Maya Newman, and Rachel N. Remen, "Teaching in Relationship: The Impact on Faculty of Teaching 'the Healer's Art,'" *Teaching and Learning in Medicine* 26, no. 2 (2014): 121–28, https://doi.org/10.1080/10401334.2014.883982.

46. Michael W. Rabow et al., "Insisting on the Healer's Art: The Implications of Required Participation in a Medical School Course on Values and Humanism," *Teaching and Learning in Medicine* 28, no. 1 (2016): 61–71, https://doi.org/10.1080/10401334.2015.1107485.

47. "Med Ed Curriculum Development," Johns Hopkins School of Medicine, accessed May October 4, 2021, https://learn.hopkinsmedicine.org/learn/course/external/view/elearning/9/curriculum-development-for-medical-education.

48. Christine C. Cheston, Tabor E. Flickinger, and Margaret S. Chisolm, "Social Media Use in Medical Education: A Systematic Review," *Academic Medicine* 88, no. 6 (2013): 893–901, https://doi.org/10.1097/ACM.0b013e31828ffc23.

49. Samantha A. Batt-Rawden et al., "Teaching Empathy to Medical Students: An Updated, Systematic Review," *Academic Medicine* 88, no. 8 (2013): 1171–77, https://doi.org/10.1097/ACM.0b013e318299f3e3.

50. Susan L. Gearhart et al., "Teaching and Assessing Technical Proficiency in Surgical Subspecialty Fellowships," *Journal of Surgical Education* 69, no. 4 (2012): 521–28, https://doi.org/10.1016/j.jsurg.2012.04.004.

51. M. Francesca Monn et al., "ACGME Core Competency Training, Mentorship, and Research in Surgical Subspecialty Fellowship Programs," *Journal of Surgical Education* 70, no. 2 (2013): 180–88, https://doi.org/10.1016/j.jsurg.2012.11.006.

52. Ming-Hsein Wang et al., "Pediatric Urology Fellowship Training: Are We Teaching What They Need to Learn?" *Journal of Pediatric Urology* 9, no. 3 (2013): 318–21, discussion 22, https://doi.org/10.1016/j.jpurol.2012.03.015.

53. Mohammed Elhassan et al., "Internal Medicine Residents' Point-of-Care Ultrasound Skills and Need Assessment and the Role of Medical School Training," *Advances in Medical Education and Practice* 10 (2019): 379–86, https://doi.org/10.2147/amep.S198536.

54. Kirsten M. Wilkins et al., "Six Things All Medical Students Need to Know about Geriatric Psychiatry (and How to Teach Them)," *Academic Psychiatry* 41, no. 5 (2017): 693–700, https://doi.org/10.1007/s40596-017-0691-7.

55. Barbara Ogur et al., "The Harvard Medical School-Cambridge Integrated Clerkship: An Innovative Model of Clinical Education," *Academic Medicine* 82, no. 4 (2007): 397–404, https://doi.org/10.1097/ACM.0b013e31803338f0.

56. Judith N. Hudson et al., "Longitudinal Integrated Clerkships," *Medical Teacher* 39, no. 1 (2017): 7–13, https://doi.org/10.1080/0142159x.2017.1245855.

57. Mona M. Savran et al., "Objective Assessment of Total Laparoscopic Hysterectomy: Development and Validation of a Feasible Rating Scale for Formative and Summative Feedback," *European Journal of Obstetrics & Gynecology and Reproductive Biology* 237 (2019): 74–78, https://doi.org/10.1016/j.ejogrb.2019.04.011.

58. Jebog Yoo et al., "Development and Evaluation of a Web-Based Acute Pain Management Education Program for Korean Registered Nurses: A Randomized Controlled Trial," *Nurse Education in Practice* 38 (2019): 7–13, https://doi.org/10.1016/j.nepr.2019.05.013.

59. Arthur Garson Jr. et al., "The 10-Minute Talk: Organization, Slides, Writing, and Delivery," *American Heart Journal* 111, no. 1 (1986): 193–203, https://doi.org/10.1016/0002-8703(86)90579-x.

60. Kurt Kroenke, "The 10-Minute Talk," *American Journal of Medicine* 83, no. 2 (1987): 329–30, https://doi.org/10.1016/0002-9343(87)90704-2.

61. Philip E. Bourne, "Ten Simple Rules for Making Good Oral Presentations," *PLoS Computational Biology* 3, no. 4 (2007): e77, https://doi.org/10.1371/journal.pcbi.0030077.

62. Thomas C. Erren, "Ten Simple Rules for a Good Poster Presentation," *PLoS Computational Biology* 3, no. 5 (2007): e102, https://doi.org/10.1371/journal.pcbi.0030102.

63. Wendy H. Vogel and Pamela H. Viale, "Presenting with Confidence," *Journal of the Advanced Practitioner in Oncology* 9, no. 5 (2018): 545–48.

64. "AMEE Fringe" and "PechaKucha 20×20™," AMEE Conferences, accessed October 4, 2021, https://amee.org/conferences/amee-2018/abstracts.

65. "Communities," Society of General Internal Medicine, accessed October 4, 2021, https://www.sgim.org/communities.

66. "Coaching/Coachee Handbooks for Educators and Students," Accelerating Change in Medical Education, American Medical Association, accessed October 4, 2021, https://www.ama-assn.org/education/accelerating-change-medical-education/academic-coaching-medical-education.

67. Stephen W. Gutkin, *Writing High-Quality Medical Publications: A User's Manual* (CRC Press, 2018).

68. "Recommendations for the Conduct, Reporting, Editing, and Publication of Scholarly Work in Medical Journals," International Committee of Medical Journal Editors (ICMJE), December 2019, accessed October 4, 2021, www.icmje.org.

69. Darcy A. Reed et al., "Association between Funding and Quality of Published Medical Education Research," *JAMA* 298, no. 9 (2007): 1002–9, https://doi.org/10.1001/jama.298.9.1002.

70. Darcy A. Reed et al., "Predictive Validity Evidence for Medical Education Research Study Quality Instrument Scores: Quality of Submissions to JGIM's Medical Education Special Issue," *Journal of General Internal Medicine* 23, no. 7 (2008): 903–7, https://doi.org/10.1007/s11606-008-0664-3.

71. Darcy Reed et al., "Challenges in Systematic Reviews of Educational Intervention Studies," *Annals of Internal Medicine* 142, no. 12 Pt. 2 (June 21, 2005): 1080–9, https://doi.org/10.7326/0003-4819-142-12_part_2-200506211-00008.

72. Consolidated Standards of Reporting Trials (CONSORT), accessed October 4, 2021, www.consort-statement.org.

73. David Moher et al., "Preferred Reporting Items for Systematic Reviews and Meta-analyses: The PRISMA Statement," *PLoS Medicine* 6, no. 7 (2009): e1000097, https://doi.org/10.1371/journal.pmed.1000097.

74. Morris Gordon and Trevor Gibbs, "STORIES Statement: Publication Standards for Healthcare Education Evidence Synthesis," *BMC Medicine* 12 (2014): 143, https://doi.org/10.1186/s12916-014-0143-0.

75. Risha Sharma et al., "Systematic Reviews in Medical Education: A Practical Approach: AMEE Guide 94," *Medical Teacher* 37, no. 2 (2015): 108–24, https://doi.org/10.3109/0142159x.2014.970996.

76. Don C Des Jarlais et al., "Improving the Reporting Quality of Nonrandomized Evaluations of Behavioral and Public Health Interventions: The TREND Statement," *American Journal of Public Health* 94, no. 3 (2004): 361–66, https://doi.org/10.2105/ajph.94.3.361.

77. Eileen F. Baker et al., "Open Access Medical Journals: Promise, Perils, and Pitfalls," *Academic Medicine* 94, no. 5 (2019): 634–39, https://doi.org/10.1097/acm.0000000000002563.

78. Peter Suber, "Open Access Overview," accessed October 4, 2021, http://legacy.earlham.edu/~peters/fos/overview.htm.

79. MedEdPublish, an Official AMEE Journal, accessed October 4, 2021, https://www.mededpublish.org/home.

80. Howard Y. Liu, Eugene V. Beresin, and Margaret S. Chisolm, "Social Media Skills for Professional Development in Psychiatry and Medicine," *Psychiatry Clinics of North America* 42, no. 3 (2019): 483–92, https://doi.org/10.1016/j.psc.2019.05.004.

81. Heather J. Logghe et al., "The Academic Tweet: Twitter as a Tool to Advance Academic Surgery," *Journal of Surgical Research* 226 (2018): viii–xii, https://doi.org/10.1016/j.jss.2018.03.049.

82. Michelle Lin et al., "Quality Indicators for Blogs and Podcasts Used in Medical Education: Modified Delphi Consensus Recommendations by an International Cohort of Health Professions Educators," *Postgraduate Medical Journal* 91, no. 1080 (2015): 546–50, https://doi.org/10.1136/postgradmedj-2014-133230.

83. Nathan Evaniew et al., "The Scholarly Influence of Orthopaedic Research According to Conventional and Alternative Metrics: A Systematic Review," *Journal of Bone and Joint Surgery Reviews* 5, no. 5 (2017): e5, https://doi.org/10.2106/jbjs.Rvw.16.00059.

84. Alisha H. Redelfs, Juan Aguilera, and Sarah L. Ruiz, "Practical Strategies to Improve Your Writing: Lessons Learned from Public Health Practitioners Participating in a Writing Group," *Health Promotion Practice* 20, no. 3 (2019): 333–37, https://doi.org/10.1177/1524839919838398.

85. "Journal Citation Reports," Web of Science, accessed February 12, 2022, https://www.webofscience.com/wos/woscc/basic-search.

86. "Scimago Journal and Country Rank," Scimago, accessed February 12, 2022, https://www
    .webofscience.com/wos/woscc/basic-search.
87. "Author Search," Web of Science, accessed October 5, 2021, https://apps.webofknowledge
    .com.
88. Abhaya V. Kulkarni et al., "Comparisons of Citations in Web of Science, Scopus, and Google
    Scholar for Articles Published in General Medical Journals," *JAMA* 302, no. 10 (2009): 1092–
    96, https://doi.org/10.1001/jama.2009.1307.
89. J. E. Hirsch, "An Index to Quantify an Individual's Scientific Research Output," *Proceedings
    of the National Academies of Science of the United States of America* 102, no. 46 (2005):
    16569–72, https://doi.org/10.1073/pnas.0507655102.
90. "MedEdPORTAL Author Handbook," MedEdPORTAL, accessed October 5, 2021, https://www
    .adea.org/uploadedFiles/ADEA/Content_Conversion_Final/mededportal/Documents
    /authorhandbook2012.pdf.
91. "What Are Altmetrics?," accessed October 25, 2021, https://www.altmetric.com/about
    -altmetrics/what-are-altmetrics.
92. Margaret S. Chisolm, "Altmetrics for Medical Educators," *Academic Psychiatry* 41, no. 4 (2017):
    460–66, https://doi.org/10.1007/s40596-016-0639-3.
93. Farah Friesen et al., "Approaching Impact Meaningfully in Medical Education Research," *Academic Medicine* 94, no. 7 (2019): 955–61, https://doi.org/10.1097/acm.0000000000002718.
94. Stephen D. Sisson and Amanda Bertram, "Changes in Knowledge of Diabetes Guidelines during Internal Medicine Residency Training," *Primary Care Diabetes* 4, no. 3 (2010): 193–95,
    https://doi.org/10.1016/j.pcd.2010.06.002.
95. Jessie K. Marshall et al., "Residents' Attitude, Knowledge, and Perceived Preparedness toward
    Caring for Patients from Diverse Sociocultural Backgrounds," *Health Equity* 1, no. 1 (2017):
    43–49, https://doi.org/10.1089/heq.2016.0010.
96. Carl G. Streed Jr. et al., "Assessment of Internal Medicine Resident Preparedness to Care for
    Lesbian, Gay, Bisexual, Transgender, and Queer/Questioning Patients," *Journal of General
    Internal Medicine* 34, no. 6 (2019): 893–98, https://doi.org/10.1007/s11606-019-04855-5.

CHAPTER TEN

Curriculum Development
for Larger Programs

Patricia A. Thomas, MD, and David E. Kern, MD, MPH

INTRODUCTION

Thus far, this book has focused on the application of concepts to smaller curricular projects, often contained within larger educational programs. The natural history of educators, however, is that with increasing experience and broadening of interest, they become responsible for larger educational programs—often extending, for individual learners, over many years. Examples include degree-bearing programs, residency or fellowship training programs, certificate programs, and maintenance of certification programs.

In addition to the inherent complexity of these programs, many are in need of systematic curriculum development. The move to competency-based education (see Chapter 4) across the health professions has required a reassessment of educational objectives, educational methods, and evaluation approaches. Interest in shortening and reducing the cost of medical training has prompted alternative program structures, such as the combined baccalaureate and medical degree programs in the United States[1,2] and the 0+5 surgical subspecialty training programs.[3,4] Introducing new content has also driven structural changes. Examples include the use of an integrated internship in ophthalmology, which has allowed the introduction of health systems science[5] and a community-based family residency program, which emphasizes care of underserved populations and health equity.[6] In the early twenty-first century, several landmark white papers, accreditation statements, and consensus reports articulated a vision for how health professions education can better address societal health care needs.[7-16] These guidelines and reports are driving curriculum renewal across the breadth of health professions education and often require major redesign to meet new program objectives.

As an example of new design, *integrated* curricula have become the norm for many health professions curricula.[17-19] Integration can refer to the integration of a topic, such as ethics or geriatrics, across multiple courses, or the integration of major disciplines, such as anatomy, physiology, and pathophysiology, into single units of the curriculum. These are examples of *horizontal integration*. *Vertical integration* refers to the integration of clinical sciences, including patient care and management previously taught in later years, into the basic, social, and health systems sciences of the early years of a curriculum and a return to the basic sciences in the later years of the curriculum.[19,20] Harden has described the continuum of integration from siloed, discipline-based courses to a transdisciplinary (or real-world experience) curriculum as an 11-step ladder.[21] As curricular designs progress up the ladder, there is increasing need for a central curriculum organizational structure, broad participation of faculty, content experts in curriculum planning, and strong communication lines.[17,21]

This chapter discusses curriculum development, maintenance, and enhancement for large educational programs, using the six-step model as a framework for the discussion. The chapter builds on Chapters 2 through 7, which provide detailed explanation of individual steps and will be referenced throughout.

In addition to the bedrock of good curriculum design that has evolved from the six-step model, there are unique aspects to the successful design and implementation of larger programs, such as external accreditation systems, curriculum integration and mapping, resource utilization, and succession planning. Management requires the assembly and maintenance of a collaborative team of educators and stakeholders and the use of modern practices of organizational management. One of these practices is active monitoring of the various elements of the program. As discussed below, *curricu-*

lum mapping, which tracks the congruence of objectives, methods, content, and assessments, is key to effective curriculum development and management in large and long programs. *Table 10.1 highlights these elements within the six-step framework.*

STEP 1: PROBLEM IDENTIFICATION AND GENERAL NEEDS ASSESSMENT: UNDERSTANDING SOCIETAL NEEDS, HEALTH WORKFORCE COMPETENCIES NEEDED, AND ACCREDITATION REQUIREMENTS

The numerous calls for health professions education reform frequently cite the gaps in delivery of a properly skilled health care workforce. As with smaller curricular projects, the leadership of health professions education degree or certification programs needs to be aware of how well societal health needs are being met or not being met by the existing programs. For larger programs, these needs are often framed in terms of producing a workforce that matches the current and future health care needs of the population.[14,22] Are programs producing enough graduates who are appropriately trained and committed to serving the target populations? Or is there a mismatch between the competencies of graduates and societal health care needs?

If there is a mismatch between the competencies of current graduates and the current and anticipated workforce needs, program directors need to understand the root causes of that mismatch.[22] Examples that have been named include the length and cost of school attendance;[15,23,24] the primacy of graduate medical education training in hospital-based settings, even though the most critical need is chronic disease in outpatient-based settings;[14,25] learning environments that result in graduates with less empathy and compassion than matriculants; [26,27] training in silos that leaves graduates with a poor understanding of other health professionals' contributions to quality care;[28,29] a paucity of training in behavioral and population health that results in graduates untrained in managing population health, chronic care, or vulnerable populations;[30] and a lack of clinical role models in systems thinking, population management, high-value care, and cultural humility.[31] Understanding these root causes enables the curriculum developer to be strategic about which of these areas might be addressed in the curriculum.

Many of the gaps between curricula and the delivery of a properly skilled health care workforce relate less to discipline-specific knowledge, attitude, and psychomotor skills and more to generalizable skills and behaviors that are relevant across many curricula in an educational program, such as adaptive problem-solving, cultural humility, commitment to quality improvement, and shared interprofessional (defined as the presence of members of more than one health care and/or social care profession)[13] values. For an educational program to address these skills, the leadership team needs to articulate the problem and the gaps (i.e., general needs assessment), create a vision for addressing them, and begin the work of designing a consistent and developmental approach across a time-limited educational program.

Chapter 2 refers to the accrediting bodies and standards as *resources* for Step 1. For large programs, attention to accreditation and regulatory boards is not an option but rather a *requirement*. Program leaders need to have a thorough awareness of the language and intent of accreditation standards that apply to their program.

A truly visionary medical education leadership is attuned not only to today's problems but also to anticipated future problems in improving the health of the public.

Table 10.1.   Special Considerations in the Development and Maintenance of Larger Educational Programs

Step 1: Problem Identification and General Needs Assessment: Understanding Societal Needs, Health Workforce Competencies Needed, and Accreditation Requirements
- Understanding the numbers, distribution, and competencies of graduates required to meet the health care needs of the population
- Understanding regulatory and accrediting body requirements and standards
- Anticipating new competencies that graduates will need

Step 2: Targeted Needs Assessment: Aligning with Institutional Mission, Selecting Learners, Assessing Targeted Learners, and Assessing the Targeted Learning Environment
- Articulating a vision that communicates need for the program and provides narrative for its identity
- Understanding the mission of the institution(s) in which the program resides
- Recruiting and selecting learners likely to meet program requirements, enhance the professional learning community, and meet the needs of served populations
- Assessing the knowledge, skills, preparation for self-directed learning, familiarity with learning methods, and other needs of diverse learners
- Assessing capacity for flexibility and individualization of learning
- Assessing system-level factors that impact learner well-being
- Assessing the degree of alignment of the following with educational program mission and goals:
  - Institutional (university, school, and health system) policies and procedures
  - Clinical, research, and business mission goals
  - Institutional culture (e.g., hidden and informal curricula)
- Assessing a wide variety of stakeholders: administrators, faculty, staff, and others who need to provide resources or other support to, need to participate in, or will otherwise affect the educational program
- Assessing adequacy of physical and electronic facilities and resources for learning

Step 3: Goals and Objectives: Prioritizing Objectives, Defining Level of Mastery, and Ensuring Congruence
- Aligning program mission and goals with societal needs and external standards/requirements
- Communicating program goals effectively to all stakeholders
- Ensuring different levels of goals and objectives (e.g., program, individual curricular, individual session) are congruent with one another
- Reaching consensus on level of mastery expected for learners
- Emphasizing core ideas
- Working in competency-based frameworks (competencies, milestones, EPAs*)
- Monitoring congruence of goals and objectives with educational strategies and assessments
- Using curriculum mapping and management systems to help accomplish the above

Step 4: Educational Strategies: Aligning and Integrating Educational Content and Choosing Educational Methods
- Aligning educational content and methods with institutional and program values, mission, and goals
- Using curriculum mapping and management systems to support alignment and integration of content
- Providing educational strategies to support diverse learner needs and developmental levels, ensuring the achievement of desired milestones, competencies, and EPAs*
- Aligning educational strategies with institutional resources and feasibility
- Incorporating online learning

Step 5: Implementation: Establishing Governance, Ensuring Quality, and Allocating Resources
- Establishing an effective leadership team and governance structure that is participatory, transparent, and equitable
- Addressing unique governance needs: for integrated, interdisciplinary, and interprofessional programs; for geographically distributed campuses
- Using curriculum mapping and management systems to make data-driven decisions
- Incorporating quality assurance into governance
- Rewarding faculty and staff effort
- Planning for leadership succession
- Monitoring curricular time and facility needs
- Understanding and managing funding resources

Step 6: Evaluation and Feedback: Supporting Competency Development and an Adaptive Health Education Program
- Tracking competency development of individual and groups of learners over time
- Managing multiple types of evaluation data from multiple sources
- Using evaluation data to modify and further improve the educational program

---

*Entrustable professional activities.

A changing demographic of one's population, the increase in global interconnected-ness, the increased access to information, and the power of social media, demand mastery of new content and skills in the next generation of health providers. Leaders can remain abreast of these societal needs through journals, professional networking, and attention to accreditation and regulatory standards.

STEP 2: TARGETED NEEDS ASSESSMENT

The final product of Step 2, coupled with Step 1, will be a concise vision for the curriculum or program that inspires stakeholders in its creation and promotion, and forms the ongoing narrative identity for the program.

Aligning with Institutional Mission

As noted in Chapter 2, program leaders need to confirm that the program is sup-porting the mission and vision of the institution within which it resides. A state-funded school or residency program may have a more defined population (e.g., a rural or un-derserved urban population) that is a primary mission focus. Another school or program may choose to focus on its contribution to the next generation of physician-scientists. These different missions will necessitate different approaches. Making the connection to institutional mission will build institutional support and facilitate the allocation of suf-ficient resources in Step 5 (described below).

Selecting Learners

For curriculum developers of smaller curricula, the learners for a given program have already been selected. For larger programs, the selection of learners is a significant step in the design of the program. Decisions about who is an appropriate learner for a given program can have an impact far beyond the time course of the program itself. Selection of the appropriate students into medical schools has been described as a critical step in the transformation of US health care into a system that achieves greater patient access, lower cost, and higher quality.[32,33] Similarly, selection of graduates into residency training programs impacts the disciplines for decades beyond the training program. The Accreditation Council for Graduate Medical Education (ACGME) now requires that residency training programs systematically cultivate a more diverse workforce.[34]

Medical school admission committees must consider not only the academic skills but also the interpersonal and intrapersonal competencies of applicants. While assessing individual applicants' qualifications and characteristics, the admissions committee must also have an eye toward building an optimal learning community that addresses the institutional mission. Many programs are striving to achieve gender, racial, and ethnic diversity that better reflects the populations or the geographic areas served by the medical school. Evidence suggests that diversity in the student body generates a workforce that can better meet the needs of the population.[34–38] Achieving diversity in medical school matriculants has been a challenge, however.[37] To ensure a diverse and qualified group of learners, a process must be created that minimizes biases in the selection procedure. Efforts to reduce bias may include active recruitment of groups not currently represented in the student body, education of the selection committee on unconscious bias and the error inherent in overvaluing standardized testing, and monitoring the diversity of the selection committee itself.[39]

Beyond recruitment, both undergraduate medical education (UME) and graduate medical education (GME) programs have capacity for and are charged with *building a pipeline* into their programs, ensuring an inclusive learning environment, and investing in the success of recruited learners.[34,40]

Persons with disabilities are increasingly recognized as underrepresented in the health professions, with multiple calls for their inclusion in the health care workforce.[41,42] As of 2019, only 4.9% of US medical students self-reported disability, with the majority reporting nonapparent disability such as attention-deficit/hyperactivity disorder (ADHD), learning disability, and psychological disability; mobility, visual, and hearing disabilities and other functional impairments were a minority of self-reported disabilities.[43] Reasons to facilitate entry of persons with disabilities into the professions include the following: they improve the care of persons with disabilities, they educate their near peers through daily interactions, and their entry fulfills a legal obligation under the Americans with Disabilities Act for schools not to discriminate. For medical schools, one of the barriers has been the required technical standards, which have not kept pace with the technology advances that support persons with mobility or sensory impairments.[44,45] Once the school or program commits to entry of learners with disabilities, it is required by law to support those students with reasonable accommodations that allow equivalent learning experiences.[46] Preparing for inclusion of learners with disabilities requires not only openness to disability in the admissions process but also clear policies for reporting disability and determining accommodations, peer and mentor supports, and attention to educational and assessment methods[42] (see also Meeks and Neal-Boylan in General References).

Assessing Targeted Learners

The complexity of Step 2 for large programs is increased by the number and diversity of learners, since the program must ensure that each learner has the maximum opportunity for success. A typical US medical school entering class can have an age range from 22 to 40 years, suggesting that students arrive with a range of premedical school educational and life experiences. Each student in this class, however, is expected to attain competence in several domains within a narrow timeline. At the UME level, addressing learners' needs may mean offering enrichment programs to students with nonscience backgrounds, coaching in new educational methods unfamiliar to some students, or acknowledging previously learned content with more flexible coursework. GME programs recruit from a breadth of medical schools with differing curricula, educational methods, and assessment systems. (The educational disruption in 2020 resulting from the COVID-19 pandemic further exacerbated the variation in learners' preparation for residency, prompting a toolkit for UME and GME educators to assess and address preparation for residency.)[47] The learners in nursing programs range from baccalaureate to midcareer professionals in graduate degree programs. All health profession education programs are accepting students with very different skills than even a decade ago, including individuals with undergraduate experiences in team learning and "flipped classrooms," international experiences, familiarity with technology, and social media expertise. Understanding that the learners are changing requires a reassessment of a program's overall philosophy and educational methods in concert with its incoming students.[48,49] Is there enough engagement with learning and tapping into students' resources, cultural identities, and life experiences? Have expectations about the locus of responsibility for learning shifted, and, if so, have administrators clearly articulated them? Does the assessment system reflect these changes?

Step 2 is also a challenge for board certification and maintenance of certification programs, whose participants span decades of educational backgrounds and a variety of practice patterns.[50]

> **EXAMPLE:** *Participation in Maintenance of Certification.* Maintenance of Certification (MOC) was adopted by the American Board of Medical Specialties in 2000 to move board certification from a model of self-directed lifelong learning and recertification to a model of continuous quality improvement and accountability. The American Board of Family Medicine (ABFM) began its transition of diplomates into MOC in 2003. An analysis of participants seven years after this transition found that 91% of active, board-certified family physicians were participating in MOC. Physicians who practiced in underserved areas, worked as solo practitioners, or were international medical graduates, however, were less likely to participate in MOC.[51] This data prompted the ABFM to further research the root causes of lack of participation in MOC and identify changes in MOC that can improve participation.[52]

A review of challenges in MOC implementation has found the best educational practices for MOC participants are to ensure the activities are based on *needs of individual learners*, are learner-driven and learner-centered, and incorporate deliberate practice and reflective practice[53] (see Chapter 5).

Assessing the Targeted Learning Environment

The targeted learning environment of large programs may include a variety of venues: classrooms, small-group learning spaces, laboratories, virtual learning platforms, and lecture halls (environments generally under program control), as well as office and clinical practices, clinical sites, and affiliated health systems (less controlled by the program). The educational leadership needs to understand and to strengthen lines of communication with the disparate stakeholders of the program in these various venues, engage representatives in curriculum design and quality control, be explicit about educational objectives, and provide resources and feedback on performance. For large programs especially, the failure to engage actively or sufficiently with these educational partners can facilitate a hidden or "collateral" curriculum that undermines the objectives of the formal curriculum. Ongoing analysis of the learning environment may identify factors that need greater attention.

Studies have shown that up to 50% of medical students and 60% of residents have symptoms of burnout, 30% have depressive symptoms, and 1 in 10 medical students is suicidal.[54] Dyrbye, Lipscomb, and Thibault have described multiple *system-level factors* that impact learner well-being, including work intensity, finding meaning in work, flexibility and control, an organizational culture with adequate diversity, mentoring and support of teaching, a learning environment and grading schema that rewards collaboration rather than competition, faculty teaching behaviors, social supports, family and personal leave policies, and educational debt.[54] Promoting learner well-being requires redesign, as suggested by the authors, and monitoring of all domains in this complex system.[54]

Health systems are essential to medical education at the UME and GME levels, but they can be unequal partners to the educational programs. The educational program leadership needs to be aware of an affiliated health system's mission, policies, procedures, and culture. Accreditation standards require that clinical affiliation agreements stipulate a "shared responsibility for creating and maintaining an appropriate learning environment."[55] Affiliation agreements may not be sufficiently nimble, however, to respond to conflicts between educational and clinical missions, and mechanisms should be in place for the leadership to address these issues as they arise. A case in point was the introduction of the electronic medical record (EMR) into academic medical centers and GME training just as duty-hour restrictions were increased. Residents often experienced a professional conflict in time management when they were told not to use the "cut and paste" function but to remain within duty-hour limits, and they experienced conflict in communication when they were urged to use "billable" terms rather than more descriptive language. Medical student education was also affected. In a rapidly changing health system environment, the alignment of mission and goals for education often needs assessment and renewal.

> **EXAMPLE:** *Conflict between Health System Policy and Educational Program Goals.* Medical schools have a responsibility to teach students skills in electronic documentation. Health systems' issues of provenance, integrity of information, patient privacy, and compliance with billing have frequently limited medical students' access to EMRs during clinical rotations. As recently as 2014, medical schools in North America reported that while 108 schools allowed medical students information entry and modification in the EMR during their inpatient hospital rotations, 47 schools allowed "read only" access.[56] In addition to limiting students' training and competence in use of the EMR, these policies introduced issues of professionalism into the learning environment, as students found other ways to access the records.

In 2018, the Centers for Medicare and Medicaid Services issued new guidelines, which allow teaching physicians to verify (and not redocument) student documentation for billable activities in the EMR, facilitating student EMR documentation in many health systems. As the student role in the EMR expanded, medical school programs increased teaching of EMR skills with workshops and simulated environments to better prepare medical students for use of the EMR during clinical rotations.[57,58]

Another aspect of assessing the learning environment relates to the adequacy of *facilities* for learning. Accreditation standards stipulate that a medical education program must have adequate buildings and facilities to support the program. Expanding class sizes, technology-enhanced learning methods (such as virtual reality), and increasing use of active and online learning approaches can make existing facilities obsolete. Residency programs need space for in-person and online teaching conferences, call rooms, and safe storage of personal belongings in clinical spaces. The ability to deliver online learning may require the provision of personal devices and is also driven by institutional resources such as information technology (IT) support, access to bandwidth, privacy and security standards, instructional design support, and faculty development (see Chapter 5).

STEP 3: GOALS AND OBJECTIVES

Prioritizing Objectives

By virtue of their size and duration, large and/or integrated programs often have expansive, multidimensional goals. This can be problematic in writing objectives at the program level, particularly as content experts and other stakeholders petition for the inclusion of additional content. Long, unwieldy lists of learning objectives that are useful neither to learners nor to faculty can result from attempts to reflect all the content in a large program. In addition, inclusion of all the potential *measurables* may result in a loss of generalizable goals that are the core values or goals of the program (such as problem-solving, critical thinking, and self-directed learning) and may unintentionally prioritize content that can be assessed.[59,60] If the program developers write specific measurable objectives intended to describe terminal objectives for the entire program, these objectives may be too advanced to inform program matriculants about what is expected.

In a long program, building a bridge between the broad expansive goals of the program—such as "to graduate physicians who are altruistic, dutiful, skillful, and knowledgeable and who will best meet the needs of our state and local communities"[61]—and the specific, measurable course or event objectives requires, in effect, several *levels of objectives*. Different levels of objectives should be written for individual educational events (such as a lecture or simulation activity); for a course, block, or rotation; for a year or milestone; and, finally, for summative objectives or competencies of the program. These different levels communicate increasing specificity as one drills down to the individual events and increasing inclusiveness and integration of content as one builds toward the overall program goal, and together they create a roadmap that guides faculty and learners toward achievement of the overall program goals.

Defining Level of Mastery

The *knowledge* domain has been especially problematic in this process of defining a level of specificity for level of learner. The nature of medical knowledge in the twenty-first century is undergoing exponential change. Discipline-based faculty are often distressed that there is not sufficient time to teach their discipline, but this has probably always been an issue in higher education, which historically has experienced tension between subject matter specialists and those who argue for relevance.[60,62] Rather than gauge one discipline's time against another's, it is more useful to step back and reflect on the *overall goal of the educational program*. For example, Tanner and Tanner define curriculum not as the presentation of a body of knowledge but rather as the "reconstruction of knowledge and experience that enables the learner to grow in exercising intelligent control over subsequent knowledge and experience."[59] With this overall goal, comprehensive coverage of content is not appropriate. Tyler challenges content experts in larger educational programs with the question "What can your subject contribute to the field of young people who are *not* going to be specialists in your field?"[60]

Before objectives can be defined, then, faculty need to reach a consensus regarding *level of mastery* (i.e., the amount of content that the program can reasonably expect learners to master), which entails a balance of specificity and generalizability. This involves a process of prioritization at the program level, in view of overall program mission and goals.

> **EXAMPLE:** *Level of Mastery in a Master's Degree.* A medical school planned to offer a new Master of Science in Physician Assistant (PA) Studies. The state Board of Regents required that all courses in the degree program be at the graduate level. The existing graduate-level Pharmacology course designed for PhD students focused on topics such as drug development and was not a good match for the needs of the PA program students, who needed more practical knowledge for prescribing. The Pharmacology faculty worked with the PA program leadership to design a Pharmacology for Physician Assistants course that contained appropriate content and level of mastery.

The good news is that true expertise seems to be grounded in a deep understanding of big ideas and concepts.[63] Educational programs, then, should clearly articulate these big ideas in the program goals and learning objectives and provide opportunities to *repeatedly apply* these concepts in new contexts. This changing understanding of the nature of knowledge and learning has directed many long educational programs to emphasize *core ideas* and release students from rote memorization of minutiae. Integrating the core concepts across disciplines and making explicit their relationships supports complex clinical decision-making and the building of expertise[64,65] (see Chapter 5).

> **EXAMPLE:** *Preparation for Future Learning as a UME Curricular Goal.* During a curriculum renewal process, the faculty of a medical school challenged previous assumptions of the "2+2" model of UME learning and assessment and designed a new approach specifically to build students' adaptive expertise. Preparation for future learning is defined as a capacity to learn from practice, use resources effectively, and invent new strategies for problem-solving in clinical practice. The preclerkship curriculum is structured with 72 weekly cases, with increasing complexity over time. With each clinical scenario, students work in small groups through guided discovery of cases using embedded questions, followed by guidance from expert instructors. Basic science is taught not as an independent discipline but rather as a causal mechanism for clinical signs and symptoms presented in the clinical scenarios. Explicit presentations of the relationships between the disciplines are made. Challenging cases allow opportunities to experience "productive failure," as students attempt multiple solutions.[66] The cases are organized sequentially into blocks with progressive complexity, thus presenting a spiral curriculum.[21,67]

Ensuring Congruence

Because of the complexity and numbers of stakeholders, the curricula of large programs are constantly under threat of *drifting* from their intended goals and objectives. Once program objectives have been adopted, it is important to ensure that implementation of the program is congruent with its intended goals and objectives. Sometimes advances in learning theory, educational methods, and content in various elements of the curriculum precede and necessitate changes in overall program goals. In the example above, faculty purposefully set out to prepare learners for future learning in changing and complex clinical situations. The new curriculum aligned educational methods, student assessments, and student experience to this preparation-for-future-learning goal[66,67] (see Chapter 5).

The move to *competency-based* frameworks in medical education has facilitated articulation of an appropriate level of educational program objectives (see Chapter 4).

The *competency domains*, *milestones*, and *the entrustable professional activities (EPAs)* serve to communicate the desired outcomes in these programs (see Chapter 4). Implementing a competency-based approach for a larger program is not a small undertaking, however. Competency-based education requires major investments in understanding the developmental nature of the competency, in designing the opportunities to achieve competence across multiple educational venues (Step 4), and in assessing the achievement of milestones for each learner (Step 6).

Regardless of whether a program's educational objectives are framed in competencies or in other core ideas, curriculum developers will need to demonstrate that the educational strategies and assessments of each component of the curriculum are congruent with these objectives. This activity is now frequently achieved with curriculum mapping software, as described below.

STEP 4: EDUCATIONAL STRATEGIES

Chapter 5 defines educational strategies as *content* and *methods*. Nothing conveys a stronger message regarding the core values of an educational program than the educational strategies that the program employs.

> **EXAMPLE:** *Internal Medicine Residency and Patient-Centered Care.* An internal medicine program introduced a unique general inpatient service rotation in which teams cared for a smaller number of patients but were asked to incorporate several patient-centered activities into the care of every patient. These activities included medication reconciliation, communications with the outpatient physician, post-discharge phone follow-up, and participation in multidisciplinary care teams. The exposure of every resident to this model of care communicated the value of patient-centered care in the mission and goals of the program.[68]

Telemedicine is increasingly recognized as a tool to improve access to health care. The commitment of time in the curriculum for students to be competent in telemedicine communicates the program's commitment to improved access to health care.[69]

> **EXAMPLE:** *An Interprofessional Rotation in Telehealth for Vulnerable Patients.* Faculty in medicine and pharmacy collaborated on the development of a telehealth rotation for medical and pharmacy students to address patients vulnerable to the effects of COVID-19 and delaying medical care. Goals for the rotation were to (1) engage in interprofessional collaboration and practice specific communication skills; (2) perform medication reconciliation and provide medication counseling; (3) review social determinants of health and their impact on chronic disease in the context of a global pandemic; (4) administer health screenings for depression, intimate partner violence, and tobacco use; and (5) provide telephone outreach to vulnerable patients. Patients were identified by participating faculty from their panels. Students participated in interprofessional huddles, collaborated on patient interviews, and screened for mental health issues.[70]

Aligning and Integrating Educational Content

The decisions about educational *content* in large programs follow from the discussions above regarding goals and objectives. The usual approach is to decide on the "big concepts" that the program will strive to have learners master, and then to develop a sequential delivery with time-limited courses, blocks, or rotations that have more specific learning goals and objectives. Within each course or block, smaller events, such as lectures, small-group sessions, or simulation exercises, will have more specific learning objectives and, therefore, more specific content. These more specific learning objectives should support the development of the course, block, or rotation learning objectives, which in turn support the development of the overall program objectives and competencies. This relationship is referred to as *curricular mapping*.

Curricular mapping is the system that allows content to be mapped across the curriculum and adjusted to minimize gaps and unnecessary redundancies. Software is increasingly used for these curricular mapping functions in large, integrated medical education programs. Typically, curricular events are entered into a calendar. *Key concepts* or *keywords* are identified within each event, as well as the *instructional method*. The event and its objectives are linked to the next higher level of objective, such as the course objectives, which in turn is linked to the next higher level of objective, such as the year or milestone objectives, and so on. When the overall curriculum is placed into curriculum management software, the location of content can be identified and quantified across multiple courses, rotations, and years.[71,72]

Both the World Federation for Medical Education (WFME)[73] and the Liaison Committee on Medical Education (LCME)[74] have accreditation standards mandating a system of curriculum management. There are proprietary curriculum management systems, and the Association of American Medical Colleges (AAMC) maintains its Curriculum Inventory,[75] but most UME programs have tailored their curriculum management systems to the individual programs and objectives. Knowing where content is taught is critical not only to the curriculum leadership but also to individual teaching faculty and students. One of the major challenges in an *integrated curriculum* that is taught by interdisciplinary (i.e., integrating knowledge from different disciplines) faculty is presenting content with appropriate sequencing and scaffolding that facilitates learning[17,76] (see Chapter 5). Effective systems allow learners and faculty to make data-driven decisions regarding the effectiveness of the curriculum in the progression of learning.[76]

> **EXAMPLE:** *Use of Curriculum Mapping to Improve Quality of UME.* A new medical school using an integrated clinical presentation curriculum adopted curriculum mapping software and fully incorporated it into the course review process. The visualization features of the software facilitated identification of unnecessary redundancies and important gaps in the curriculum. As examples, the renal course was found to have a gap in presenting pharmacologic management of urinary incontinence, and the hematology course was found to have redundant presentations of major histocompatibility complex. Both issues were subsequently addressed by the Office of Medical Education.[77]

Choosing Educational Methods

Choosing educational methods for large programs requires attention to the core values of the program, the needs of learners, the developmental nature of longer programs, the effectiveness of learning methods, the congruence of educational methods with objectives, the available experiences and faculty expertise, and the availability of resources. Decisions about *educational methods* are important in large programs. The choice made for each of these methods conveys a strong message to learners about the core values of the curriculum. Large integrated programs are known more for their educational methods than for the specific content delivered. As examples, the McMaster University Michael G. DeGroote School of Medicine is known for the use of problem-based learning to foster critical thinking skills; the University of Virginia's Next Generation ("NxGen") curriculum and Johns Hopkins University's "Genes to Society" curriculum emphasize systems thinking; and the Geisinger Commonwealth School of Medicine uses an experiential community-based curriculum to promote community-based care.

As discussed above and in Chapter 5, the *diversity of students* also drives a need for *multiple educational methods*, so that each student has the greatest likelihood of successful learning. *Flexibility* in educational methods communicates a respect for individual student preferences and needs and provides *redundant support in changing situations*. The immediate loss of face-to-face education and access to clinical sites during the COVID-19 pandemic is an example of a rapidly changing situation that required temporary conversion of most UME to online learning. Since the learners are constantly changing, the curriculum leadership must understand the needs of the new matriculants with each cohort.

Attention to the *developmental* nature of the curriculum is an additional issue in long-term curricula. Grow describes staged levels of self-directed learning, from the dependent learner to the interested, the involved, and, finally, the self-directed learner.[78] The nature of the educational method and the work of the teacher at each of these stages similarly evolves. It is rare in short educational programs to see this development, but it is critical in longer programs to anticipate and encourage self-directedness to facilitate the necessary lifelong learning required of health professionals. In medical education programs, this means that reliance on one method throughout the program is inappropriate. For example, curriculum developers may be excited to introduce a new form of active learning, such as practice in a virtual reality simulated experience. Incoming learners, however, may never have learned with simulation and may need appropriate preparation for this methodology to develop a sense of comfort and motivation to learn with it. With time, these same learners may tire of simulation and be eager for real-life clinical experiences. In GME, attention to increasing levels of responsibility needs to be built across the curriculum, even though rotations are occurring in the same sites throughout the calendar year.

The *feasibility* of an educational method often determines its adoption in a larger program (see Step 5, below). What may have worked in a pilot program with smaller numbers of self-selected learners and committed faculty may not work when scaled up to an entire class or cohort. Facilities such as standardized patients or simulation center time may be constrained. There may be too few rooms for interprofessional small groups to meet. Additional faculty may need to be identified, released from other duties, and trained in the new method. The introduction of a new method may be disruptive to other components of the curriculum, and there may be a transient drop in performance during a transition. For all these reasons, changes in methodology should incorporate robust evaluation plans to assist the leadership in understanding both positive and negative impacts on all stakeholders (see Step 6, below).

If a program anticipates extensive use of *online learning*, several issues must be managed at the program or school level and are usually met with explicit policies. What personal devices are required for student learning? Who determines the specifications? How is internet access assured, especially if students are expected to learn at home? Are there limitations in what software students can load onto their school devices? Will the devices be used for testing? Who will provide support for hardware, software, and IT issues? Does the school have a policy on professional behavior (online, on campus, in the classroom), security, and communications related to online learning? What do the clinical affiliates require with respect to remote access to the EMR and other clinical systems? Responding to these concerns requires input from many stakeholders to develop a coordinated and effective adaptation to online learning.

STEP 5: IMPLEMENTATION

Large, integrated, and longitudinal programs are often described as complex machines with many moving parts. Implementing these curricula requires attention to the many details of these moving parts, as well as appreciation of the coherent whole and its impact on and relation to even larger institutions, such as the overall university or health system or the population served by the graduates of the program. Skilled leadership of these programs requires the ability to *delegate* the implementation details to appropriate individuals and groups, while attending to the perspectives of a range of stakeholders. For example, stakeholders for a medical school curriculum may include government funders with concerns about the career selection of graduates and population health outcomes, university leadership and alumni with concerns about national rankings and reputation, faculty with concerns about academic freedom, staff with concerns about changing workflow and skill sets, and residency training program directors with concerns about preparedness for residency roles and responsibilities. Educational program leaders should also feel accountable to current learners and their patients, often seen as the most vulnerable participants of these complex systems.

Establishing Governance

No single person or leadership role can provide adequate oversight of implementation in these complex systems. These programs require effective governance structures.[79] Governance, which is often invisible to the learners, has powerful implications for curricular quality and outcomes. It needs to be carefully constructed for large, integrated programs to reflect the core values of the school or program. Traditional hierarchical, bureaucratic governance centralizes authority and decision-making and emphasizes standardization. A flat or networked governance structure gives faculty and students access to authority and decision-making; it facilitates innovation and adaptation to change. The governance structure powerfully communicates institutional values about the relationship among students, faculty, and administration.

In discipline-based curricula, courses are governed within individual departments. Course names often reflect the names of the department, such as "Pharmacology" and "Pediatrics." The department chair assigns the course leadership and allocates faculty teaching effort. Departmental faculty determine course content and methods; budgets for teaching are contained within departmental budgets.

Moving to organ system–based curricula in UME was the first step toward integrating disciplines across an extended period, such as a year of the curriculum. Integration is now seen across four years of the curriculum in areas such as ethics, patient safety, and clinical reasoning. With highly integrated curricula, governance and decision-making no longer rest within individual departments. Blocks of curricula in integrated frameworks are designed by interdisciplinary faculty who determine appropriate levels of objectives, plan content and methods, and review evaluations. The work can be tedious and contentious but is critical to the success of the curriculum. Without true integration, students experience a disjointed and fragmented presentation of content, rather than a developmental or "scaffolded" presentation.[17] Correcting this can be problematic because an unintended consequence of the integrated design can be a disengagement of departmental discipline-based leadership from a curriculum that no longer reflects specific departmental effort.

The lesson for integrated curricula is that governance needs to be structured as *transparent*, *participatory*, and *equitable*. Effective governance includes robust program evaluation and quality assurance processes that provide feedback on performance to individual faculty, their academic supervisors, the course and content leaders, and the budgetary process for teaching and evaluation (see Step 6). This flow of information supports transparency and equity. In North America, the LCME mandates a centralized curriculum governance structure that has the authority and resources to implement and maintain a high-quality curriculum.[74] Schools often structure the curriculum governance to reflect the "structure" of the curriculum. For instance, there may be a centralized committee with subcommittees that reflect the major content areas or competencies within the curriculum, such as basic science, clinical sciences, health systems sciences, and the thesis requirement. These subcommittees are made up of interdisciplinary design teams, which monitor objectives, methods, and assessments for the relevant content areas. Other schools use structures with a combination of elected and appointed faculty to oversee the curriculum.

Charged with expansion of the health care workforce and increasing the number of learners, many schools and universities are developing geographically distributed campuses. Governance again is critical to the development, maintenance, and quality of these campuses.[80]

Moving health professions education to *interprofessional health education* requires extensive work at higher levels of organization. The Institute of Medicine categorized enabling or interfering factors for successful interprofessional education as professional culture, institutional culture, workforce policy, and financing policy.[81] Each of these areas must be addressed not only at a school level but also at the university, community, and national levels, which requires broad participation of stakeholders and committed and effective leadership. A 2019 Health Professions Accreditors Collaborative report noted the importance of *leadership* to drive the work required in a collaborative environment and detailed several examples of institutional commitment to interprofessional education (IPE) for collaborative practice.[82]

Ensuring Quality

A common issue in large programs is who has access to program outcome data, including learner performance, faculty and course or rotation performance, and graduate outcomes, and who has authority to act on this data. *Continuous quality improvement* (CQI) is vital to a large curriculum, and that role often rests in another peer committee of faculty who oversee student assessments, achievement, and program evaluation. (See discussion of curriculum mapping and management above). For learner assessment, promotion, and remediation, the program needs clear policies and guidelines that are broadly publicized, as well as additional resources of faculty coaching, testing options, and accommodations (see Kalet and Chou in General References). Inclusion or broad representation of stakeholders in the governance structure is the first step toward *participatory leadership*, a key feature of successful curricular innovation and renewal[83] (see Chapter 8).

As an example of this broader view of governance, there is increasing recognition that mentoring, advising, and the informal curriculum are an integral part of the overall curriculum, especially as it relates to the competency domain of personal and professional development (see Chapter 5). Several medical schools have instituted longitudinal faculty-student structures, termed *learning communities*, to address student professional identity formation, wellness, academic and career advising, and, at times, clinical skills and humanities courses.[84] Similarly, longitudinal *coaching* programs have been used at the GME level to foster professional development.[85,86] At a minimum, those charged with professional development and professional identity formation need to be aware of the curriculum's flow, work demands, and milestones and should be included as active members of curriculum and program planning and governance.

In GME, the role of quality oversight often falls to an associate program director, charged with ongoing monitoring of performance outcomes. Residency programs are also broadening the representation of stakeholders in their governance structures by including nursing and hospital administration staff, and board certification programs are including patients and patient advocates as members of their governance.

Allocating Resources

The issues of *personnel, time, facilities*, and *funding* are shared by new curricula, ongoing curricula, and curricula during change. *Personnel* issues include identifying appropriate faculty to lead and implement a curriculum, having an overall program of acknowledging and rewarding faculty effort in teaching,[87–89] and developing a staff workflow that maximizes available resources. Educational leaders may have to enlist and support individuals not under their supervisory control; this requires political skill.

Forward-thinking leaders will also recognize that there should be a *succession plan* for important educational roles in a complex curriculum.[90,91] Planning for succession means using an open, fair process to identify faculty or staff who could eventually assume leadership roles, providing these individuals the opportunities to develop leadership or advanced educator skills, and aligning roles with institutional needs and plans. Medical teaching faculty may not have had access to leadership development or may not have thought to use it, and it may fall to the program director to encourage it. Many universities and health systems have local leadership development skills training. If not available locally, faculty can explore their own professional societies for this training. (See also Appendix B for faculty development opportunities.)

Decisions about the allotment of *curricular time* include monitoring the informal as well as formal hours in a curriculum, to ensure that there is adequate time for students' self-directed learning, reflection, and other enrichment activities, and explicitly addressing the perception of many that time equals importance in a curriculum. Once again, a curricular management system can be very helpful in tracking program-level information (such as the number of formal curricular hours per week or the amount of time spent in didactic vs. active learning) and identifying conflicts when faculty or students organize "optional" events.

Facilities are critical to curriculum effectiveness and have an impact on the learning environment, as discussed above. Educational methods, such as immersive simulation or team-based learning, can fail if the facilities are not appropriate to the task or to the number of learners. Large programs need policies and mechanisms to efficiently use and distribute facility resources. At a time when virtual space has become as important as actual space for learning, facilities must now include optimal *informational technology* access and design of virtual learning environments.

Perhaps the most important task at the program level is the *allocation of funds* in the educational program. Despite calls for increased investment in health professions education, both in the United States and abroad, the financial model has not changed for decades.[14,92,93] Less grant money is available for research and development in health professions education than in biomedical research; almost no external funding is available for ongoing core curriculum functions (see Appendix B, "Funding Resources"). State funding is increasingly at risk in a climate of conservative fiscal policy. The curriculum, then, must often be funded by tuition, philanthropy, or clinical revenue sources. Given the average indebtedness of US medical school graduates, there is tremendous pressure to limit any further increases in tuition.[24] Decisions to incur new costs in a program must be carefully balanced with the goal of delivering high-value education at the lowest cost possible.

Residency education in the United States is funded primarily through Medicare and Medicaid payments to hospital systems through a complex formula dependent on number of inpatient bed-days. The Veterans Health Administration and Health Resources and Services Administration also contribute significant financial support to GME. Lastly, some positions are supported by state governments, industry, and private sources.[14] This financial model results in unintended consequences, such as a lack of support for non-hospital-based training, prompting calls for a restructure of the system.[14,93]

STEP 6: EVALUATION AND FEEDBACK

As with smaller curricula, large educational programs must have an overall plan for evaluation and must monitor that evaluation in real time.

Supporting Competency Development

With respect to learners, a program that has moved to a competency-based framework needs to track competency development by multiple learners over long time periods, often using a variety of assessments. *Programmatic assessment* of learners is a system design that continually collects low-stakes assessments with periodic higher-stakes assessments. High-stakes decisions are supported by the richness of multiple and varied assessments over time. The dual goal is to drive learning with the assessment process and facilitate robust decision-making.[94] A review of programmatic assessment found that it has been implemented most often in workplace or clinical programs, and while it supports the dual goals, problems of overload of information, workload, and lack of supportive personal relationships may impair its effectiveness.[95]

Other approaches to competency assessment include the adoption of *learning portfolios* to track documentation of learner achievement[96–98] (see Chapter 7). Electronic portfolios allow individual learners to upload "exhibits" (i.e., documentation of achievement of competence), share with faculty evaluators, and receive feedback.[96,99]

> **EXAMPLE:** *Aligning Assessment System with Program Goals in Preparation for Future Learning Curriculum.* A curriculum restructured its assessment system to improve frequency and usefulness of feedback to students. Low-stakes weekly exams as well as narrative feedback are used for ongoing assessment. Students access an "e-portfolio," review their academic progress periodically with an academic coach, and then submit reflective personal learning plans at key points in the curriculum. Students receive early and frequent feedback and coaching on improving learning behaviors. A student progress committee reviews a compilation of data to make high-stakes decisions about students' progress in the program.[67]

When collected data from evaluation and assessment systems are organized, often through a variety of data analysis techniques (including natural language processing and visualization of data), electronic systems can also track the achievement of learner milestones at the aggregate or program level (*learning analytics*).[100]

An Adaptive Health Education Program

With respect to program evaluation, evaluation data should be engineered to support an adaptive or learning system. Larger health profession education programs generate not only learners' performance data but also data such as learner and faculty satisfaction, environmental surveys, faculty time, budgets, utilization of rooms, simulation space, benchmarks with peer institutions and programs, candidate interest in programs, and surveys of nonattenders to a program. The challenge with this data is to transform it into "actionable intelligence" that serves to make timely corrections, supports CQI, and identifies the program's readiness for change in a rapidly changing health care environment.[101] While *dashboards* can be used to monitor key performance indicators of a program in real time, it is critical that the program engages a broad group of stakeholders to synthesize, analyze, and interpret data, with the goal of CQI and innovation[101–104] (see also Chapter 7, "General Considerations").

LEADING CURRICULUM ENHANCEMENT AND RENEWAL IN LARGER EDUCATIONAL PROGRAMS

Major reform efforts, which have been widespread in health professions education over the past two decades, can be disruptive and resource-intensive, and require creative engagement of stakeholders. The role of the leader in curriculum reform is critical to managing the climate and expectations during the reform and in seeing a reform effort through to its successful implementation.

Understanding the factors that promote successful organizational change efforts is therefore an important attribute for the curriculum leader.[105,106] These factors include the following:

- Development and communication of a shared vision and rationale
- Collaboration with and engagement of key stakeholders
- Openness to data and diverse perspectives
- Flexibility
- Formation of an effective leadership team
- Provision of necessary support/protection for others to act on the vision
- Beginning with successes, even if small, and building on them with multiple activities
- Alignment with institutional culture, policies, and procedures to the degree possible; institutionalization of changes
- Effective communication throughout the process with all stakeholders

Familiarity with the community of stakeholders and their needs is important and is aided by the ability to appreciate one's organization through *multiple perspectives*. Bolman and Deal have termed these perspectives "frames" and describe organizational frames as (1) structural: the formal roles and relationships; (2) human resource: the needs of the organization's people, such as development, training, and rewards; (3) political, such as the need to allocate resources; and (4) symbolic/value-based.[107] When conflicts and barriers affect organizational functioning, the ability to view the situation from more than one perspective allows a deeper understanding of the root cause and creative solutions.

Numerous leadership skills are relevant to directors of larger educational programs, some of which are mentioned in previous sections of this chapter. They include being an effective change agent (see Chapter 6),[108,109] communication,[110,111] motivation,[112,113] collaboration,[114–116] working in teams,[111,117,118] delegation,[119,120] feedback,[121,122] coaching,[123–125] conflict management,[126,127] and succession planning.[91,128]

Effective leaders are also cognizant of different leadership styles and approaches, as well as the complexity of health care and educational organizations (see General References, "Leadership").[129] They are able to match their approach to situational needs and engage the staff and stakeholders for creative, innovative responses to change. Leadership style can have an impact on the organizational climate, which can result in either an effective, adaptive, and learning organization or an organization riddled with problems and paralyzed in the face of change. Leaders who are visionary, inclusive, socially intelligent, and supportive develop more positive learning climates than those who are more authoritative.[130,131]

> **EXAMPLE:** *Using Organizational Understanding and Leadership Skills to Address Conflict in Curriculum Reform.* A medical school planned a new curriculum with a vision to enhance the systems thinking of its graduates, necessitating inclusion of more social and behavioral science. Basic science faculty who had less allotted time expressed concern that the curriculum was less rigorous and would diminish the reputation of the school—that is, would not uphold the core value of research and discovery. Recognizing that the discussions about allocation of time (a political frame) were value-based, the dean responded to faculty concerns by articulating a vision for the new curriculum in symbolic and value-based terms, noting a new research requirement and plans to enhance the development of physician-scientists.[132]

Because of the broad skill set required to effectively oversee large educational programs and organizational change efforts, it behooves those responsible to develop themselves in the areas noted above. As previously mentioned, leadership development programs are available locally at many universities and through professional societies (see Appendix B).

CONCLUSION

The size and complexity of large, longitudinal programs present challenges, so it is perhaps most useful to think of them as complex systems or organizations. Effective systems and structures are critical to ensure that a program is meeting its goals. The field of organizational development has much to offer educators in understanding the nature and functions of their curricular systems. Special considerations applied to the six-step approach can provide a foundation for developing, implementing, sustaining, and enhancing large or longitudinal programs.

QUESTIONS

For the program you are coordinating, planning, or would like to be planning, please answer or think about the following questions and prompts:

1. Cite the evidence that the program promotes societal health care needs and the institutional mission. What do you see as future changes in health care delivery, and how can the curriculum address these?

2. Describe the trends you see in the demographics, preparedness, or motivations of learners in your program. How can you structure your selection process to recruit the best learning community for your program? What characteristics of learners do you need to monitor to address their learning needs?

3. Describe the learning environment in which this program resides. Who are the stakeholders in this environment? How is the learner experience, learner well-being, and the hidden curriculum being monitored?

4. Describe how the educational program objectives were developed for the program and how they relate to national competency frameworks. Have several levels of objectives been developed for the program?

5. What is the predominant educational method used in the program, and what does that convey about the core values of the program? Does the diversity of educational methods used promote the achievement of desired competencies by all learners? Do they allow for flexibility in the face of changing situations?

6. What system is in place for monitoring the curriculum for congruence of objectives, methods, and assessments; sequencing and coordination of content; and vertical and horizontal integration?

7. Describe the governance for the curriculum, and how transparency, participation, and equity are ensured in the governance.

8. Describe how faculty are developed, supported, and rewarded for teaching in your program. How are faculty needs and actual faculty effort monitored to ensure there is an appropriate match?

9. How is information on learner and program outcomes used to improve the quality of the program? Is the system of program evaluation sufficiently robust to make data-based decisions?

10. If a curriculum renewal process is in progress, note any conflicts or barriers to its success. How can these be addressed by leadership, faculty, and students?

GENERAL REFERENCES

Bland, Carole J., Sandra Starnaman, Lisa Wersal, Lenn Moorhead-Rosenberg, Susan Zonia, and Rebecca Henry. "Curricular Change in Medical Schools." *Academic Medicine* 75, no. 6 (2000): 575–94. https://doi.org/10.1097/00001888-200006000-00006.
   This systematic study of the published literature on medical curricular change, although looking at twentieth-century reforms, has not been replicated, and its lessons are still timely. The authors synthesized their review into characteristics that contribute to success. These include the organization's mission and goals, history of change, politics, organizational structure, need for change, scope and complexity of the innovation, cooperative climate, participation, communication, human resource development, evaluation, performance dip, and leadership.

Bolman, Lee G., and Terrence E. Deal. *Reframing Organizations: Artistry, Choice, and Leadership*. 6th ed. San Francisco: Jossey-Bass, 2017.
   An updated synthesis of the authors' framework for organization theory, with examples. The four frames discussed are (1) the Structural Frame, the social architecture of the organization; (2) the

Human Resource Frame, the properties of people and organizations; (3) the Political Frame, the allocation of resources and struggles for power; and (4) Organizational Symbols and Culture. The book concludes with Leadership in Practice. 526 pages.

Hafferty, Frederick W., and Joseph F. O'Donnell, eds. *The Hidden Curriculum in Health Professional Education*. Lebanon, NH: Dartmouth College Press, 2014.
This book examines the history, theory, methodology, and application of hidden curriculum theory in health professional education. Includes chapters devoted to professional identity formation, social media, and longitudinal integrated clerkships. 322 pages.

Institute of Medicine. *Graduate Medical Education That Meets the Nation's Health Needs*. Washington, DC: National Academies Press, 2014.
The Institute of Medicine committee's report proposes significant revisions to rectify current shortcomings and to create a GME system with greater transparency, accountability, strategic direction, and capacity to innovate.

Interprofessional Education Collaborative Expert Panel. *Core Competencies for Interprofessional Collaborative Practice: Report of an Expert Panel: 2016 Update*. Washington, DC: Interprofessional Education Collaborative, 2016. Accessed October 8, 2021. https://www.ipecollaborative.org/ipec-core-competencies.
The Interprofessional Education Collaborative consists of multiple health professions educational organizations. In 2011, the IPEC consensus report described the need for development of collaborative practice and proposed four competency domains—roles and responsibilities, shared values and ethics, interprofessional communication, and teamwork—and learning objectives within each domain. The 2016 update recognized the overarching domain of interprofessional collaboration and modified the competencies to more directly address the Triple Aim.

Kalet, Adina, and Calvin C. Chou, eds. *Remediation in Medical Education: A Mid-course Correction*. New York: Springer Publishing, 2014.
This multiauthor text collates the literature and experience to date in the context of defined competencies for physicians, the limitations of assessment, and approaches to remediation. One section, authored by a student affairs dean, looks at program-level issues such as privacy, technical standards, fitness for duty, and the official academic record.

Meeks, Lisa M., and Leslie Neal-Boylan, eds. *Disability as Diversity: A Guidebook for Inclusion in Medicine, Nursing and the Health Professions*. New York: Springer International Publishing, 2020.
Intended for deans, student affairs faculty, disability officers, and program leaders, this text provides practical examples and best practices for planning and implementing an inclusive learning environment for students with disability, including writing policy, addressing the learning climate, maintaining accreditation standards, and remaining compliant with the Americans with Disabilities Act.

Leadership

Goleman, Daniel. "Leadership That Gets Results." *Harvard Business Review*, March–April 2000. Accessed April 16, 2021. https://hbr.org/2000/03/leadership-that-gets-results.
Describes different management styles (coercive, authoritative, affiliative, democratic, pacesetting, coaching—Hay Group) and the importance of being able to flex one's management style. Also discusses emotional intelligence.

Merton, Robert K. "The Social Nature of Leadership." *American Journal of Nursing* 69, no. 12 (1969): 2614. https://doi.org/10.2307/3421106.
A good article on the relational aspects of leadership. Distinguishes authority from leadership. Authority involves the legitimated rights of a position that require others to obey; leadership is an interpersonal relation in which others comply because they want to, not because they have to.

Northouse, Peter G. *Leadership: Theory and Practice*. 8th ed. SAGE Publications, 2018.
Comprehensive text on classic and contemporary approaches to leadership, described in a reader-friendly, evidence-based manner. Includes chapters on trait, skills, behavioral, and situational

approaches; transformational, authentic, servant, and adaptive leadership; path-goal theory; and leader-member exchange theory, as well as chapters on team leadership, gender, and culture.

Palmer, Parker. "Leading from Within." In *Let Your Life Speak: Listening for the Voice of Vocation*. San Francisco: John Wiley & Sons, 2000. Accessed April 16, 2021. http://www.couragerenewal .org/PDFs/Parker-Palmer_leading-from-within.pdf.
Describes inner work and knowledge that is an underpinning of enlightened, enabling leadership. Discusses undesirable shadows that leaders can cast: personal insecurity (can lead to behaviors that deprive others of their identities to buttress one's own); belief that the universe is a battle-ground (can lead to unnecessary competition when what is needed is collaboration); functional atheism (belief that ultimate responsibility for everything rests on oneself, which leads to burnout, depression, despair, imposition of one's will on others, lack of empowerment of others); fear of chaos (leads to excessive control); and denial of death/fear of failure (leads to maintaining/resus-citating things that are no longer alive or needed). Palmer advocates for doing the inner work that promotes a work environment embodying collaboration, respect, empowerment, flexibility, enjoyment.

Organizational/Culture Change

Kotter, John P. *Leading Change*. Boston: Harvard Business School Press, 2012.
An excellent book on leading change in today's fast-paced, global market. Although oriented toward business, it is applicable to most organizations. Based on his years of experience and study, Dr. Kotter, professor emeritus at Harvard Business School, discusses eight steps critical to creat-ing enduring *major change in organizations*.

Westley, Frances, Brenda Zimmerman, and Michael Q. Patton. *Getting to Maybe: How the World Is Changed*. Toronto: Random House Canada, 2006.
This book is complementary to Kotter's work. It focuses on complex organizations and social change, and it addresses change that occurs from the bottom up as well as from the top down. Richly illustrated with real-world examples, it explains an approach to complex, as distinct from simple or complicated, problems.

Examples of Institutional/Culture Change Efforts

Cottingham, Ann H., Anthony L. Suchman, Debra K. Litzelman, Richard M. Frankel, David L. Moss-barger, Penelope R. Williamson, DeWitt C. Baldwin, and Thomas S. Inui. "Enhancing the In-formal Curriculum of a Medical School: A Case Study in Organizational Culture Change." *Journal of General Internal Medicine* 23, no. 6 (2008): 715–22. https://doi.org/10.1007 /s11606-008-0543-y.
The Indiana University School of Medicine (IUSM) culture change initiative to improve the informal or hidden curriculum.

Krupat, Edward, Linda Pololi, Eugene R. Schnell, and David E. Kern. "Changing the Culture of Academic Medicine: The C-Change Learning Action Network and Its Impact at Participating Medical Schools." *Academic Medicine* 88, no. 9 (2013): 1252–58. https://doi.org/10.1097 /ACM.0b013e31829e84e0.

Pololi, Linda H., Edward Krupat, Eugene R. Schnell, and David E. Kern. "Preparing Culture Change Agents for Academic Medicine in a Multi-institutional Consortium: The C-Change Learning Ac-tion Network." *Journal of Continuing Education in Health Professions* 33, no. 4 (2013): 244–57. https://doi.org/10.1002/chp.21189.
These two papers present a culture change project shared by five medical schools. Institutional leadership and faculty met regularly as a consortium to create a learning community that would foster a collaborative, inclusive, and relational culture in their constituent institutions.

REFERENCES CITED

1. Marlene P. Ballejos et al., "Combined Baccalaureate/Medical Degree Students Match into Family Medicine Residencies More than Similar Peers: A Matched Case-Control Study," *Family Medicine* 51, no. 10 (2019): 854–57, https://doi.org/10.22454/FamMed.2019.110812.
2. Ellen M. Cosgrove et al., "Addressing Physician Shortages in New Mexico through a Combined BA/MD Program," *Academic Medicine* 82, no. 12 (2007): 1152–57, https://doi.org/10.1097/acm.0b013e318159cf06.
3. Mohamed A. Zayed, Ronald L. Dalman, and Jason T. Lee, "A Comparison of 0 + 5 Versus 5 + 2 Applicants to Vascular Surgery Training Programs," *Journal of Vascular Surgery* 56, no. 5 (2012): 1448–52, https://doi.org/10.1016/j.jvs.2012.05.083.
4. Adam Tanious, "Traditional (5 + 2) Versus Integrated (0–5) Vascular Surgery Training: The Effect on Case Volume and the Trainees Produced," *Seminars in Vascular Surgery* 32, no. 1–2 (2019): 27–29, https://doi.org/10.1053/j.semvascsurg.2019.05.004.
5. Thomas A. Oetting et al., "Integrating the Internship into Ophthalmology Residency Programs," *Ophthalmology* 123, no. 9 (2016): 2037–41, https://doi.org/10.1016/j.ophtha.2016.06.021.
6. Lawrence Family Medicine Residency, "Developing Physician Leaders for Underserved Communities," accessed October 7, 2021, https://glfhc.org/residency/curriculum/.
7. Kenneth M. Ludmerer, "The History of Calls for Reform in Graduate Medical Education and Why We Are Still Waiting for the Right Kind of Change," *Academic Medicine* 87, no. 1 (2012): 34–40, https://doi.org/10.1097/acm.0b013e318238f229.
8. Susan E. Skochelak, "A Decade of Reports Calling for Change in Medical Education: What Do They Say?" *Academic Medicine* 85 (2010): S26–33, https://doi.org/10.1097/acm.0b013e3181f1323f.
9. Molly Cooke, David M. Irby, and Bridget C. O'Brien, *Educating Physicians: A Call for Reform of Medical School and Residency* (San Francisco: Jossey-Bass, 2010).
10. Thomas J. Nasca et al., "The Next GME Accreditation System—Rationale and Benefits," *New England Journal of Medicine* 366, no. 11 (2012): 1051–56, https://doi.org/10.1056/nejmsr1200117.
11. Jason Russell Frank, Linda Snell, and Jonathan Sherbino, *CanMEDS 2015 Physician Competency Framework*, (Ottawa: Royal College of Physicians and Surgeons of Canada, 2015).
12. Julio Frenk et al., "Health Professionals for a New Century: Transforming Education to Strengthen Health Systems in an Interdependent World," *The Lancet* 376, no. 9756 (2010): 1923–58, https://doi.org/10.1016/s0140-6736(10)61854-5.
13. Interprofessional Education Collaborative, *Core Competencies for Interprofessional Collaborative Practice: 2016 Update* (Washington, DC: Interprofessional Education Collaborative, 2016), accessed October 7, 2021, https://www.ipecollaborative.org/ipec-core-competencies.
14. Committee on the Governance and Financing of Graduate Medical Education; Board on Health Care Services; Institute of Medicine; Jill Eden, Donald Berwick, and Gail Wilensky, eds., *Graduate Medical Education That Meets the Nation's Health Needs* (Washington, DC: National Academies Press, 2014), https://doi.org/10.17226/18754.
15. Institute of Medicine (US) Committee on the Robert Wood Johnson Foundation Initiative on the Future of Nursing, at the Institute of Medicine, *The Future of Nursing: Leading Change, Advancing Health* (Washington, DC: National Academies Press, 2011), accessed October 7, 2021, https://www.ncbi.nlm.nih.gov/books/NBK209885/.
16. Ryan L. Crass and Frank Romanelli, "Curricular Reform in Pharmacy Education through the Lens of the Flexner Report of 1910," *American Journal of Pharmaceutical Education* 82, no. 7 (2018): 6804, https://doi.org/10.5688/ajpe6804.
17. Jessica H. Muller et al., "Lessons Learned about Integrating a Medical School Curriculum: Perceptions of Students, Faculty and Curriculum Leaders," *Medical Education* 42, no. 8 (2008): 778–85, https://doi.org/10.1111/j.1365-2923.2008.03110.x.

18. Theo J. Ryan et al., "Design and Implementation of an Integrated Competency-Focused Pharmacy Programme: A Case Report," *Pharmacy* 7, no. 3 (2019): 121, https://doi.org/10.3390/pharmacy7030121.

19. David G. Brauer and Kristi J. Ferguson, "The Integrated Curriculum in Medical Education: AMEE Guide No. 96," *Medical Teacher* 37, no. 4 (2014): 312–22, https://doi.org/10.3109/0142159x.2014.970998.

20. Richard Hays, "Integration in Medical Education: What Do We Mean?" *Education For Primary Care* 24, no. 3 (2013): 151–52, https://doi.org/10.1080/14739879.2013.11494358.

21. R. M. Harden, "The Integration Ladder: A Tool for Curriculum Planning and Evaluation," *Medical Education* 34, no. 7 (2000): 551–57, https://doi.org/10.1046/j.1365-2923.2000.00697.x.

22. Melanie Raffoul, Gillian Bartlett-Esquilant, and Robert L. Phillips, "Recruiting and Training a Health Professions Workforce to Meet the Needs of Tomorrow's Health Care System," *Academic Medicine* 94, no. 5 (2019): 651–55, https://doi.org/10.1097/acm.0000000000002606.

23. James J. Youngclaus, Sarah A. Bunton, and Julie Fresne, *An Updated Look at Attendance Cost and Medical Student Debt at U.S. Medical Schools* (Washington, DC: Association of American Medical Colleges, 2017), accessed October 7, 2021, https://www.aamc.org/data-reports/analysis-brief/report/updated-look-attendance-cost-and-medical-student-debt-us-medical-schools.

24. Monique Simone Pisaniello et al., "Effect of Medical Student Debt on Mental Health, Academic Performance and Specialty Choice: A Systematic Review," *BMJ Open* 9, no. 7 (2019): e029980, https://doi.org/10.1136/bmjopen-2019-029980.

25. American College of Osteopathic Internists, *White Paper: The Phoenix Physician* (American College of Osteopathic Internists, 2011), accessed October 7, 2021, https://www.acoi.org/public/acoi-position-statements/the-phoenix-physician-white-paper.

26. Adam J. McTighe et al., "Effect of Medical Education on Empathy in Osteopathic Medical Students," *Journal of Osteopathic Medicine* 116, no. 10 (2016): 668–74, https://doi.org/10.7556/jaoa.2016.131.

27. Melanie Neumann et al., "Empathy Decline and Its Reasons: A Systematic Review of Studies with Medical Students and Residents," *Academic Medicine* 86, no. 8 (2011): 996–1009, https://doi.org/10.1097/acm.0b013e318221e615.

28. George E. Thibault, "Reforming Health Professions Education Will Require Culture Change and Closer Ties Between Classroom and Practice," *Health Affairs* 32, no. 11 (2013): 1928–32, https://doi.org/10.1377/hlthaff.2013.0827.

29. Tanya Rechael Lawlis, Judith Anson, and David Greenfield, "Barriers and Enablers that Influence Sustainable Interprofessional Education: A Literature Review," *Journal of Interprofessional Care* 28, no. 4 (2014): 305–10, https://doi.org/10.3109/13561820.2014.895977.

30. Patricia A. Cuff and Neal A. Vanselow, eds., *Improving Medical Education: Enhancing the Behavioral and Social Science Content of Medical School Curricula* (Washington, DC: National Academies Press, 2004).

31. Jed D. Gonzalo, Anna Chang, and Daniel R. Wolpaw, "New Educator Roles for Health Systems Science," *Academic Medicine* 94, no. 4 (2019): 501–6, https://doi.org/10.1097/acm.0000000000002552.

32. Kelly E. Mahon, Mackenzie K. Henderson, and Darrell G. Kirch, "Selecting Tomorrow's Physicians," *Academic Medicine* 88, no. 12 (2013): 1806–11, https://doi.org/10.1097/acm.0000000000000023.

33. Rachel H. Ellaway et al., "A Critical Scoping Review of the Connections between Social Mission and Medical School Admissions: BEME Guide No. 47," *Medical Teacher* 40, no. 3 (2017): 219–26, https://doi.org/10.1080/0142159x.2017.1406662.

34. Alda Maria R. Gonzaga et al., "A Framework for Inclusive Graduate Medical Education Recruitment Strategies," *Academic Medicine* 95, no. 5 (2020): 710–16, https://doi.org/10.1097/acm.0000000000003073.

35. Cynthia X. Yuen and Donovan Lessard, "Filling the Gaps: Predicting Physician Assistant Students' Interest in Practicing in Medically Underserved Areas," *Journal of Physician Assistant Education* 29, no. 4 (2018): 220–25, https://doi.org/10.1097/jpa.0000000000000219.

36. Somnath Saha, "Student Body Racial and Ethnic Composition and Diversity-Related Outcomes in US Medical Schools," *JAMA* 300, no. 10 (2008): 1135, https://doi.org/10.1001/jama.300.10.1135.

37. John K. Iglehart, "Diversity Dynamics—Challenges to a Representative U.S. Medical Workforce," *New England Journal of Medicine* 371, no. 16 (2014): 1471–74, https://doi.org/10.1056/nejmp1408647.

38. Ben Kumwenda et al., "Relationship between Sociodemographic Factors and Specialty Destination of UK Trainee Doctors: A National Cohort Study," *BMJ Open* 9, no. 3 (2019): e026961, https://doi.org/10.1136/bmjopen-2018-026961.

39. Association of American Medical Colleges, *Roadmap to Diversity and Educational Excellence: Key Legal and Educational Policy Foundations for Medical Schools*, 2nd ed. (Washington, DC: Association of American Medical Colleges, 2014).

40. "LCME Consensus Statement Related to Satisfaction with Element 3.3, Diversity/Pipeline Programs and Partnerships," Liaison Committee on Medical Education, March 2015, accessed October 7, 2021, https://lcme.org/publications/.

41. Lisa M. Meeks, Kurt Herzer, and Neera R. Jain, "Removing Barriers and Facilitating Access," *Academic Medicine* 93, no. 4 (2018): 540–43, https://doi.org/10.1097/acm.0000000000002112.

42. Lisa M. Meeks et al., "Realizing a Diverse and Inclusive Workforce: Equal Access for Residents with Disabilities," *Journal of Graduate Medical Education* 11, no. 5 (2019): 498–503, https://doi.org/10.4300/jgme-d-19-00286.1.

43. Lisa M. Meeks et al., "Change in Prevalence of Disabilities and Accommodation Practices among US Medical Schools, 2016 vs. 2019," *JAMA* 322, no. 20 (2019): 2022, https://doi.org/10.1001/jama.2019.15372.

44. Laura B. Kezar et al., "Leading Practices and Future Directions for Technical Standards in Medical Education," *Academic Medicine* 94, no. 4 (2019): 520–27, https://doi.org/10.1097/acm.0000000000002517.

45. Raymond H. Curry, Lisa M. Meeks, and Lisa I. Iezzoni, "Beyond Technical Standards: A Competency-Based Framework for Access and Inclusion in Medical Education," *Academic Medicine* 95, no. 12S (2020): S109–12, https://doi.org/10.1097/acm.0000000000003686.

46. Philip Zazove et al., "U.S. Medical Schools' Compliance with the Americans with Disabilities Act," *Academic Medicine* 91, no. 7 (2016): 979–86, https://doi.org/10.1097/acm.0000000000001087.

47. "Transition in a Time of Disruption: Practical Guidance to Support the Move from Undergraduate Medical Education to Graduate Medical Education," AACOM, AAMC, ACGME, ECFMG/FAIMER, March 2021, accessed October 7, 2021, https://www.acgme.org/covid-19/transition-to-residency/.

48. Laura Hopkins et al., "To the Point: Medical Education, Technology, and the Millennial Learner," *American Journal of Obstetrics and Gynecology* 218, no. 2 (2018): 188–92, https://doi.org/10.1016/j.ajog.2017.06.001.

49. Valerie N. Williams et al., "Bridging the Millennial Generation Expectation Gap: Perspectives and Strategies for Physician and Interprofessional Faculty," *The American Journal of the Medical Sciences* 353, no. 2 (2017): 109–15, https://doi.org/10.1016/j.amjms.2016.12.004.

50. David G. Nichols, "Maintenance of Certification and the Challenge of Professionalism," *Pediatrics* 139, no. 5 (2017): e20164371, https://doi.org/10.1542/peds.2016-4371.

51. Imam M. Xierali et al., "Family Physician Participation in Maintenance of Certification," *Annals of Family Medicine* 9, no. 3 (2011): 203–10, https://doi.org/10.1370/afm.1251.

52. Paul V. Miles, "Maintenance of Certification: The Profession's Response to Physician Quality," *Annals of Family Medicine* 9, no. 3 (2011):196–97, https://doi.org/10.1370/afm.1254.

53. Ligia Cordovani, Anne Wong, and Sandra Monteiro, "Maintenance of Certification for Practicing Physicians: A Review of Current Challenges and Considerations," *Canadian Medical Journal* 11, no. 1 (2020): e70–80, https://doi.org/10.36834/cmej.53065.

54. Liselotte N. Dyrbye, Wanda Lipscomb, and George Thibault, "Redesigning the Learning Environment to Promote Learner Well-Being and Professional Development," *Academic Medicine* 95, no. 5 (2020): 674–78, https://doi.org/10.1097/acm.0000000000003094.

55. Liaison Committee on Medical Education, "Standard 1.4," in *Functions and Structure of a Medical School: Standards for Accreditation of Medical Education Programs Leading to the MD Degree*, March 2021, accessed October 7, 2021, http://www.lcme.org/publications/.

56. AAMC Curriculum Inventory Report, *EHR System Use by Medical Students: Number of Medical Schools with Level of Medical Student Access to Electronic Health Record System by Academic Year*, Association of American Medical Colleges, (2014), accessed October 7, 2021, https://www.aamc.org/data-reports/curriculum-reports/interactive-data/ehr-system-use-medical-students.

57. Jillian Zavodnick and Tasha Kouvatsos, "Electronic Health Record Skills Workshop for Medical Students." *MedEdPORTAL* 15, no. 1 (2019), https://doi.org/10.15766/mep_2374-8265.10849.

58. Akshay Rajaram et al., "Training Medical Students and Residents in the Use of Electronic Health Records: A Systematic Review of the Literature" *Journal of the American Medical Informatics Association* 27, no. 1 (2020): 175–80, https://doi.org/10.1093/jamia/ocz178.

59. Daniel Tanner and Laurel Tanner, *Curriculum Development* (Upper Saddle River, NJ: Pearson Merrill/Prentice Hall, 2007).

60. Ralph W. Tyler, *Basic Principles of Curriculum and Instruction* (Chicago, IL: University of Chicago Press, 2013).

61. Association of American Medical Colleges, *Learning Objectives for Medical School Education: Guidelines for Medical Schools,* 1998, accessed October 7, 2021, https://www.aamc.org/what-we-do/mission-areas/medical-education/msop.

62. Greer Williams, *Western Reserve's Experiment in Medical Education and Its Outcome* (New York: Oxford University Press, 1980).

63. John D. Bransford, Ann L. Brown, and Rodney R. Cocking, eds., *How People Learn: Brain, Mind, Experience and School: Expanded Edition* (Washington, DC: National Academies Press, 2000).

64. Nicole N. Woods, Lee R. Brooks, and Geoffrey R. Norman, "The Role of Biomedical Knowledge in Diagnosis of Difficult Clinical Cases," *Advances in Health Sciences Education* 12, no. 4 (2007): 417–26, https://doi.org/10.1007/s10459-006-9054-y.57.

65. Nicole N. Woods and Maria Mylopoulos, "On Clinical Reasoning Research and Applications: Redefining Expertise," *Medical Education* 49, no. 5 (2015): 543, https://doi.org/10.1111/medu.12643.

66. Maria Mylopoulos et al., "Preparation for Future Learning: A Missing Competency in Health Professions Education?" *Medical Education* 50, no. 1 (2015): 115–23, https://doi.org/10.1111/medu.12893.

67. Kulamakan Kulasegaram et al., "The Alignment Imperative in Curriculum Renewal," *Medical Teacher* 40, no. 5 (2018): 443–48, https://doi.org/10.1080/0142159x.2018.1435858.

68. Laura Hanyok et al., "The Johns Hopkins Aliki Initiative: A Patient-Centered Curriculum for Internal Medicine Residents," *MedEdPORTAL* 8, no. 1 (2012), https://doi.org/10.15766/mep_2374-8265.9098.

69. Shayan Waseh and Adam P. Dicker, "Telemedicine Training in Undergraduate Medical Education: Mixed-Methods Review," *Journal of Medical Internet Research Medical Education* 5, no. 1 (2019): e12515, https://doi.org/10.2196/12515.

70. Christopher A. Bautista et al., "Development of an Interprofessional Rotation for Pharmacy and Medical Students to Perform Telehealth Outreach to Vulnerable Patients in the COVID-19 Pandemic," *Journal of Interprofessional Care* 34, no. 5 (2020): 694–97, https://doi.org/10.1080/13561820.2020.1807920.

71. R. M. Harden, "AMEE Guide No. 21: Curriculum Mapping: A Tool for Transparent and Authentic Teaching and Learning," *Medical Teacher* 23, no. 2 (2001): 123–37, https://doi.org/10.1080/01421590120036547.

72. Tahereh Changiz et al., "Curriculum Management/Monitoring in Undergraduate Medical Education: A Systematized Review," *BMC Medical Education* 19, no. 1 (2019), https://doi.org/10.1186/s12909-019-1495-0.

73. World Federation for Medical Education, *Basic Medical Education WFME Global Standards for Quality Improvement* (Copenhagen, Denmark: WFME, 2015).

74. Liaison Committee on Medical Education, "Standard 8.1," in *Functions and Structure of a Medical School: Standards for Accreditation of Medical Education Programs Leading to the MD Degree*, March 2021, accessed October 7, 2021, http://www.lcme.org/publications/.

75. "Association of American Medical Colleges (AAMC) Curriculum Inventory," accessed October 7, 2021, https://www.aamc.org/what-we-do/mission-areas/medical-education/curriculum-inventory.

76. Eilean G. S. Watson et al., "Development of eMed: A Comprehensive, Modular Curriculum-Management System," *Academic Medicine* 82, no. 4 (2007): 351–60, https://doi.org/10.1097/acm.0b013e3180334d41.

77. Ghaith Al-Eyd et al., "Curriculum Mapping as a Tool to Facilitate Curriculum Development: A New School of Medicine Experience," *BMC Medical Education* 18, no. 1 (2018), https://doi.org/10.1186/s12909-018-1289-9.

78. Gerald O. Grow, "Teaching Learners to Be Self-Directed," *Adult Education Quarterly* 41, no. 3 (1991): 125–49, https://doi.org/10.1177/0001848191041003001.

79. Oscar Casiro and Glenn Regehr, "Enacting Pedagogy in Curricula: On the Vital Role of Governance in Medical Education," *Academic Medicine* 93, no. 2 (2018): 179–84, https://doi.org/10.1097/acm.0000000000001774.

80. David Snadden et al., "Developing a Medical School: Expansion of Medical Student Capacity in New Locations: AMEE Guide No. 55," *Medical Teacher* 33, no. 7 (2011): 518–29, https://doi.org/10.3109/0142159x.2011.564681.

81. IOM (Institute of Medicine), *Measuring the Impact of Interprofessional Education on Collaborative Practice and Patient Outcomes* (Washington, DC: National Academies Press, 2015).

82. Health Professions Accreditors Collaborative, *Guidance on Developing Quality Interprofessional Education for the Health Professions* (Chicago, IL: Health Professions Accreditors Collaborative, 2019), accessed October 7, 2021, https://healthprofessionsaccreditors.org/wp-content/uploads/2019/02/HPACGuidance02-01-19.pdf

83. Karen E. Pinder and Jennifer A. Shabbits, "Educational Leadership During a Decade of Medical Curricular Innovation and Renewal," *Medical Teacher* 40, no. 6 (2018): 578–81, https://doi.org/10.1080/0142159x.2018.1440079.

84. Robert Shochet et al., "Defining Learning Communities in Undergraduate Medical Education: A National Study," *Journal of Medical Education and Curricular Development* 6 (2019), https://doi.org/10.1177/2382120519827911.

85. Kerri Palamara et al., "Professional Development Coaching for Residents: Results of a 3-Year Positive Psychology Coaching Intervention," *Journal of General Internal Medicine* 33, no. 11 (2018): 1842–44, https://doi.org/10.1007/s11606-018-4589-1.

86. Kevin Parks, Jennifer Miller, and Amy Westcott, "Coaching in Graduate Medical Education," in *Coaching in Medical Education: A Faculty Handbook*, ed. Nicole Deiorio and Maya Hammoud (American Medical Association, 2017), 50–54.

87. Daniel Weber et al., "Current State of Educational Compensation in Academic Neurology," *Neurology* 93, no. 1 (2019): 30–34, https://doi.org/10.1212/wnl.0000000000007664.

88. Linda Regan, Julianna Jung, and Gabor D. Kelen, "Educational Value Units: A Mission-Based Approach to Assigning and Monitoring Faculty Teaching Activities in an Academic Medical Department," *Academic Medicine* 91, no. 12 (2016): 1642–46, https://doi.org/10.1097/acm.0000000000001110.

89. Steven Stites et al., "Aligning Compensation with Education: Design and Implementation of the Educational Value Unit (EVU) System in an Academic Internal Medicine Department," *Academic Medicine* 80, no. 12 (2005): 1100–106, https://doi.org/10.1097/00001888-200512000-00006.

90. Sandra K. Collins and Kevin S. Collins, "Changing Workforce Demographics Necessitates Succession Planning in Health Care," *Health Care Manager* 26, no. 4 (2007): 318–25, https://doi.org/10.1097/01.hcm.0000299249.61065.cf.

91. Michael Timms, *Succession Planning That Works: The Critical Path of Leadership Development* (Victoria, BC: FriesenPress, 2016).

92. Kieran Walsh, "Medical Education: The Case for Investment," *African Health Sciences* 14, no. 2 (2014): 472, https://doi.org/10.4314/ahs.v14i2.26.

93. Institute of Medicine (US) Division of Health Sciences Policy, "Financing Medical Education," in *Medical Education and Societal Needs: A Planning Report for the Health Professions* (Washington, DC: National Academies Press, 1983), accessed April 16, 2021, https://www.ncbi.nlm.nih.gov/books/NBK217691/.

94. L. Schuwirth, C. van der Vleuten, and S. J. Durning, "What Programmatic Assessment in Medical Education Can Learn from Healthcare," *Perspectives on Medical Education* 6, no. 4 (2017): 211–15, https://doi.org/10.1007/s40037-017-0345-1.

95. Suzanne Schut et al., "Where the Rubber Meets the Road—an Integrative Review of Programmatic Assessment in Health Care Professions Education," *Perspectives on Medical Education* 10, no. 1 (2020): 6–13, https://doi.org/10.1007/s40037-020-00625-w.

96. Jan Van Tartwijk and Erik W. Driessen, "Portfolios for Assessment and Learning: AMEE Guide No. 45," *Medical Teacher* 31, no. 9 (2009): 790–801, https://doi.org/10.1080/01421590903139201.

97. Tracey McCready, "Portfolios and the Assessment of Competence in Nursing: A Literature Review," *International Journal of Nursing Studies* 44, no. 1 (2007): 143–51, https://doi.org/10.1016/j.ijnurstu.2006.01.013.

98. Hayley Croft et al., "Current Trends and Opportunities for Competency Assessment in Pharmacy Education—a Literature Review," *Pharmacy* 7, no. 2 (2019): 67, https://doi.org/10.3390/pharmacy7020067.

99. Elaine F. Dannefer, "Beyond Assessment of Learning toward Assessment for Learning: Educating Tomorrow's Physicians," *Medical Teacher* 35, no. 7 (2013): 560–63, https://doi.org/10.3109/0142159x.2013.787141.

100. Teresa Chan et al., "Learning Analytics in Medical Education Assessment: The Past, the Present, and the Future," *AEM Education and Training* 2, no. 2 (2018): 178–87, https://doi.org/10.1002/aet2.10087.

101. Constance M. Bowe and Elizabeth Armstrong, "Assessment for Systems Learning: A Holistic Assessment Framework to Support Decision Making across the Medical Education Continuum," *Academic Medicine* 92, no. 5 (2017): 585–92, https://doi.org/10.1097/ACM.0000000000001321.

102. Jeremy A. Epstein, Craig Noronha, and Gail Berkenblit, "Smarter Screen Time: Integrating Clinical Dashboards into Graduate Medical Education," *Journal of Graduate Medical Education* 12, no. 1 (2020): 19–24, https://doi.org/10.4300/jgme-d-19-00584.1.

103. Brent Thoma et al., "Developing a Dashboard to Meet Competence Committee Needs: A Design-Based Research Project," *Canadian Medical Education Journal* 11, no. 1 (2020): e16–34, https://doi.org/10.36834/cmej.68903.

104. Christy Boscardin et al., "Twelve Tips to Promote Successful Development of a Learner Performance Dashboard within a Medical Education Program," *Medical Teacher* 40, no. 8 (2017): 855–61, https://doi.org/10.1080/0142159x.2017.1396306.

105. Frances Westley, Brenda Zimmerman, and Michael Q. Patton, *Getting to Maybe: How the World is Changed* (Toronto: Random House Canada, 2006).

106. John P. Kotter, *Leading Change* (Boston, MA: Harvard Business Review Press, 2012).

107. Lee G. Bolman and Terrence E. Deal, *Reframing Organizations: Artistry, Choice and Leadership* (Hoboken, NJ: Jossey-Bass, 2017).

108. Debra E. Meyerson and Maureen A. Scully, "Tempered Radicalism and the Politics of Ambivalence and Change," *Organization Science* 6, no. 5 (1995): 585–600, https://doi.org/10.1287/orsc.6.5.585.

109. Herb A. Shepard, "Rules of Thumb for Change Agents," in *Organization Development and Transformation*, 6th ed., ed. Wendell L. French, Cecil Bell, and Robert A. Zawacki (New York: McGraw-Hill/Irwin, 2005), 336–41.

110. John P. Kotter, "Leading Change: Why Transformation Efforts Fail," *Harvard Business Review*, May-June 1995, https://hbr.org/1995/05/leading-change-why-transformation-efforts-fail-2.

111. Ken Blanchard, Donald Carew, and Eunice P. Carew, *The One Minute Manager Builds High Performing Teams* (New York: Harper Collins, 2009).

112. Kara A. Arnold, "Transformational Leadership and Employee Psychological Well-Being: A Review and Directions for Future Research," *Journal of Occupational Health Psychology* 22, no. 3 (2017): 381–93, https://doi.org/10.1037/ocp0000062.

113. Matthew R. Fairholm, "Themes and Theory of Leadership: James MacGregor Burns and the Philosophy of Leadership (Working Paper CR01-01)," January 2001, https://www.researchgate.net/publication/283049025_Themes_and_Theories_of_Leadership.

114. Gilbert Steil and Nancy Aronson, *The Collaboration Response: Eight Axioms That Elicit Collaborative Action for a Whole Organization, a Whole Community, a Whole Society* (Scotts Valley, CA: CreateSpace Independent Publishing Platform, 2017).

115. Joe Raelin, "Does Action Learning Promote Collaborative Leadership?" *Academy of Management Learning & Education* 5, no. 2 (2006): 152–68, https://doi.org/10.5465/amle.2006.21253780.

116. Morten Hansen, *Collaboration: How Leaders Avoid the Traps, Build Common Ground, and Reap Big Results* (Boston: Harvard Business Review Press, 2009).

117. David P. Baker, Rachel Day, and Eduardo Salas, "Teamwork as an Essential Component of High-Reliability Organizations," *Health Services Research* 41, no. 4p2 (2006): 1576–98, https://doi.org/10.1111/j.1475-6773.2006.00566.x.

118. Patrick Lencioni, *Overcoming the Five Dysfunctions of a Team: A Field Guide for Leaders, Managers, and Facilitators* (San Francisco: Jossey-Bass, 2005).

119. Ken Blanchard and Spencer Johnson, *The New One Minute Manager* (New York: William Morrow, 2015).

120. Richard A. Luecke and Perry McIntosh, *The Busy Manager's Guide to Delegation*, WorkSmart Series (New York: Amacom, 2009).

121. Rachel Jug, Xiaoyin "Sara" Jiang, and Sarah M. Bean, "Giving and Receiving Effective Feedback: A Review Article and How-To Guide," *Archives of Pathology & Laboratory Medicine* 143, no. 2 (2019): 244–50, https://doi.org/10.5858/arpa.2018-0058-ra.

122. Christopher J. Watling and Shiphra Ginsburg, "Assessment, Feedback and the Alchemy of Learning," *Medical Education* 53, no. 1 (2018): 76–85, https://doi.org/10.1111/medu.13645.

123. John Sargeant et al., "Facilitated Reflective Performance Feedback," *Academic Medicine* 90, no. 12 (2015): 1698–706, https://doi.org/10.1097/acm.0000000000000809.

124. J. Preston Yarborough, "The Role of Coaching in Leadership Development," *New Directions for Student Leadership* 158 (2018): 49–61, https://doi.org/10.1002/yd.20287.

125. Deepa Rangachari et al., "Clinical Coaching: Evolving the Apprenticeship Model for Modern Housestaff," *Medical Teacher* 39, no. 7 (2016): 780–82, https://doi.org/10.1080/0142159x.2016.1270425.

126. Kenneth W. Thomas, *Introduction to Conflict Management: Improving Performance Using the TKI* (Mountain View, CA: CPP, 2002).

127. Roger Fisher, William L. Ury, and Bruce Patton, *Getting to Yes: Negotiating Agreement Without Giving In* (New York: Penguin Books, 2011).

128. Sandra K. Collins and Kevin S. Collins, "Succession Planning and Leadership Development: Critical Business Strategies for Healthcare Organizations," *Radiology Management* 29, no. 1 (2007): 16–21.
129. Zakaria Belrhiti, Ariadna Nebot Giralt, and Bruno Marchal, "Complex Leadership in Healthcare: A Scoping Review," *International Journal of Health Policy and Management* 7, no. 12 (2018): 1073–84, https://doi.org/10.15171/ijhpm.2018.75.
130. Daniel Goleman, Richard E. Boyatzis, and Anne McKee, *Primal Leadership: Realizing the Power of Emotional Intelligence* (Boston: Harvard Business Review Press, 2002).
131. Daniel Goleman and Richard E. Boyatzis, "Social Intelligence and the Biology of Leadership," *Harvard Business Review*, September 2008, https://hbr.org/2008/09/social-intelligence-and-the-biology-of-leadership.
132. Charles M. Wiener et al., "'Genes to Society'—the Logic and Process of the New Curriculum for the Johns Hopkins University School of Medicine," *Academic Medicine* 85, no. 3 (2010): 498–506, https://doi.org/10.1097/ACM.0b013e3181ccbebf.

CHAPTER ELEVEN

Curricula That Address Community Needs and Health Equity

Heidi L. Gullett, MD, MPH, Mamta K. Singh, MD, MS,
and Patricia A. Thomas, MD

> Of all the forms of inequality, injustice in health is the most shocking
> and the most inhuman.
> —Martin Luther King Jr.

> Education either functions as an instrument that is used to facilitate
> integration of the younger generation into the logic of the present
> system and bring about conformity to it, *or* it becomes "the practice of
> freedom," the means by which men and women deal critically and
> creatively with reality and discover how to participate in the
> transformation of their world.
> —Richard Shaull

INTRODUCTION: HEALTH SYSTEMS SCIENCE, DEFINITIONS AND SHARED LANGUAGE, AND THE IMPERATIVE FOR HEALTH EQUITY CURRICULA

In a classic parable, a witness observes a man being swept downstream in a river and jumps in to rescue him but then realizes there are multiple people in the river in need of rescue. Having struggled with multiple rescues, the witness eventually walks upstream to learn what is causing so many to fall into the river.[1] As in the parable, health professions education traditionally aims to provide the skills to care for individual patients within a narrow context of disease or illness episode (i.e., rescuing those who have fallen in the river, one at a time). Attention to the upstream events has been relegated to the fields of public health and preventive medicine. This fragmented approach to health care, however, has contributed to suboptimal and stark differences in health outcomes for individuals, communities, and populations.

Health equity is the just and fair opportunity for everyone to achieve their optimal health.[2] In this chapter, we define *community* as any configuration of individuals, families, and groups whose values, characteristics, interests, geography, and/or social relations unite them in some way.[3] Health professionals, to advance health equity for individuals and communities, must effectively address all determinants of health. Typically, these determinants are clustered into three groups: (1) the *downstream*, immediate health needs for individuals, such as access to quality care for acute and chronic conditions; (2) the *midstream*, intermediary determinants for individuals, such as the environments in which people live and work, education, employment, housing, nutrition, public safety, and transportation (termed the *social determinants of health, or SDOH*); and (3) the *upstream*, *structural determinants* or *community conditions*, such as public policies, economic class, and biases based on race, gender, country of origin, sexual orientation, religion, immigration status, disability, or language.[3-6] These various determinants are interdependent components of *complex, dynamic systems*.[7-8] Increasing evidence highlights the pivotal impact these determinants have on the health of individuals and communities,[9-11] prompting multiple calls for transformative health systems and health professions education.[12-14]

The study of population health, public health, and SDOH furthers the understanding of health equity, and together these elements form one domain of the evolving research and educational field of *health systems science (HSS)*.[15] HSS has emerged as a conceptual approach to understanding health determinants, how care is delivered, and how health care professionals work together for care delivery and improvement.[15] Other domains of HSS include health system improvement, value in health care, health care structure and processes, health policy, clinical informatics, and health technology.[15] Regardless of the domain, HSS curricula require learners to develop the habits of *systems thinking* in analyzing clinical problems and to develop *professional identities* as leaders, advocates, and change agents for improving the health of patients, communities, and populations. HSS builds upon and augments the basic and clinical sciences, expanding the clinician's view beyond the individual patient and into the community and population. Unlike teaching traditional medical curricula, teaching HSS requires overcoming an array of barriers, harnessing unique resources, and developing a complex curriculum, including an experiential learning environment and attention to reflection and mentoring of learners.[16]

Curricula addressing the complexity of HSS, especially health equity, require learners to develop systems thinking habits. *Systems thinking* (ST), the interlinking domain of HSS, is defined as a comprehensive approach to understanding systems' component parts, the interrelatedness of these parts, and how systems work and evolve over time.[15,17] Curricula that address this competency require educators and learners to take a holistic approach to patients and populations and to appreciate the larger system and context of care. Health professionals who demonstrate this competency by appreciating the big picture and the interconnectedness of system components have a greater impact on their patients and exhibit more empathy.[18] While ST is a foundational construct, it is not meant to be taught in isolation.[19] Learning ST occurs informally and experientially.[19] ST can be conceived of as a learning strategy for a given setting, a method for analysis or a shared language for problem-solving that involves pattern and habits (Table 11.1), but it is not a curriculum or a specific teaching program.[20] As with other elements of health equity curricula, supporting the development of ST requires broad engagement across the curriculum and institutional culture.

This chapter will use the six-step model as a systematic approach to the development, implementation, and evaluation of health equity curricula, highlighting their unique challenges (Table 11.2). Since shared language is critical for this work, the authors present a glossary of terms in Table 11.3. Readers should refer to Chapters 2 through 7 for background and in-depth discussions and resources for each of the steps.

STEP 1: PROBLEM IDENTIFICATION AND GENERAL NEEDS ASSESSMENT: ARTICULATING THE HEALTH PROBLEM AND EDUCATIONAL GAPS

Step 1 is the identification and analysis of a health need (see Chapter 2). In the context of health equity, this requires a clear description of health outcomes for various populations, highlighting health disparities, current data, and trends and what is known about the determinants of health for individuals and populations. The general needs assessment involves an assessment of what is currently being done and what should ideally be implemented to address the problem of health inequities. Stakeholders unique to health equity considerations include policymakers, health system leaders,

Table 11.1.   Habits of a Systems Thinker

- Seeks to understand the big picture
- Observes how elements within systems change over time, generating patterns and trends
- Changes perspectives to increase understanding
- Recognizes the impact of time delays when exploring cause and effect relationships
- Considers how mental models affect current reality and the future
- Considers an issue fully and resists the urge to come to a quick conclusion
- Uses understanding of the system structure to identify possible leverage actions
- Identifies the circular nature of complex cause and effect relationships
- Recognizes that a system's structure generates its behavior
- Considers short-term, long-term, and unintended consequences of actions
- Checks results and changes actions if needed: "successive approximation"
- Surfaces and tests assumptions
- Pays attention to accumulations and their rates of change
- Makes meaningful connections within and between systems

Source: Adapted with permission, Habits of a Systems Thinker®, Waters Center for Systems Thinking, WatersCenterST.org.

Table 11.2.   Considerations in the Development of Health Equity Curricula

Step 1: Problem Identification and General Needs Assessment: Articulating the Health Problem and Educational Gaps
Problem Identification
- Identify population health outcomes and their differences among various groups.
- Describe historical context of population health outcomes, including medicine's role in addressing health outcomes.
- Describe the history of social accountability in medicine and its impact on society, patients, health care professionals, and educators.
- Identify the systemic issues and multiple determinants of health that impact health outcomes at individual, institutional,* population, local, regional, state, national, international levels.

Current Approach
- Identify the intersection of individual and structural/systemic bias and its impact on health outcomes at the individual and population levels.
- Investigate alignment of local institutional and school curricular missions to the needs of society/community, as identified through a structured community health/population-level assessment.
- Describe how relevant stakeholders—policymakers, health systems leaders, community structures, and leaders and influencers—address or fail to address health disparities.
- Describe what health professions educators and educational institutions are doing to address—or how they are failing to address—equity, diversity, and inclusion.

Ideal Approach
- Identify national examples of institutions that foster equity as an organizational value by addressing institutional composition, inclusive organizational values, and attention to equity, diversity, and inclusion.
- Include nontraditional health professions partners and stakeholders, such as public health departments, community-based organizations, policy organizations, and philanthropists.
- Assemble and use a common vocabulary for equity, diversity, and inclusion, including professional development for institutional leadership and faculty.

- Address relevant accreditation standards regarding equity, diversity, and inclusion, as well as social accountability.
- Review national examples of equity curricula that have effectively integrated this content.
- Identify published competencies, educational strategies, assessments, and evaluations across the health professions continuum that address health equity.

Step 2: Targeted Needs Assessment: Selecting Learners and Assessing the Learners and Learning Environment
- Assess institutional culture and readiness or existing commitment to equity, diversity, and inclusion.
- Confirm institutional effort to diversify health care workforce through admissions and selection of learners and by building a diverse institutional community.
- Assess targeted learners for cultural attitudes, prior knowledge and lived experience, explicit and implicit bias, empathy, and attitudes toward poverty.
- Systematically examine the current curriculum for structural racism.
- Identify the intersection of individual and structural/systemic bias and its impact on local learners, faculty, staff, and the learning environment, as well as the current local curriculum, learner experience, and the learning environment with regard to equity, diversity, and inclusion.
- Assess internal change management processes to continually ensure an equitable learning environment.

Step 3: Goals, Objectives, and Competencies
- Ensure alignment of health equity goals and specific, measurable objectives with societal needs and institutional values and mission identified in Step 1.
- Write equity-grounded goals and objectives that illustrate concepts and foster change agency while minimizing bias.
- Assess and align goals and objectives with learner lived experience identified in Step 2.
- Identify competencies for systems thinking, change agency, and equity-grounded health professions practice.
- Engage nontraditional health professions partners and stakeholders, including learners, in review of curricular goals, objectives, and course activities.
- Align goals and objectives with external requirements.

Step 4: Educational Strategies: Aligning and Integrating Content and Choosing Methods
- Implement curricular activities that emphasize the overarching concepts of systems thinking, advocacy, and change agency while minimizing bias.
- Present the historical context of structural and social determinants of health.
- Provide frameworks and tools that prompt learners to challenge assumptions and understand alternative perspectives.
- Develop cross-cultural communication skills, cultural humility, and cultural safety.
- Develop learners' awareness of implicit bias and its impact on clinical care; teach the psychologic basis of bias.
- Facilitate systems thinking approaches to problem-solving.
- Provide learners longitudinal authentic experiences that foster empathy, trust, and partnership with vulnerable populations.
- Consider use of a longitudinal portfolio model to build reflective capacity and commitment to health equity in professional identity formation.
- Assess and align content with learner lived experience identified in Step 2 and goals and objectives identified in Step 3.
- Link content and competency development to societal/community, school/program, and learner needs.

Table 11.2.   *(continued)*

Step 5: Implementation
- Anticipate barriers to implementation from faculty and students, as well as due to resource limitations.
- Recruit and recognize nontraditional faculty members as part of the education team.
- Assess the opportunity cost of addressing health equity in the formal curriculum.
- Share resources for equity, diversity, and inclusion within health professions schools across admissions, learning environment, faculty and staff development, curriculum, and student affairs.
- Establish effective governance structure and coordination with a diverse, interdisciplinary, and nontraditional curricular team.
- Adopt principles of community engagement when working with community partners; support community engagement by sharing curricular and program outcomes.
- Develop all faculty in skills for enhancing an equitable learning environment.
- Pilot or phase in innovative content with robust program evaluation design.
- Plan formal acknowledgment/celebration of faculty and stakeholder curricular leaders.

Step 6: Evaluation and Feedback
- Adopt a framework that includes learner assessment and program outcomes and links curricular evaluation elements to societal/community, school/program, and learner needs.
- Plan just-in-time as well as summative learner evaluations of the curriculum.
- Identify mechanisms by which bias is continually assessed throughout course content, methods, and assessments.
- Assess changes in learners' knowledge, biases, reflective capacity, self-awareness, systems thinking, and structural competency.
- Assess practice behaviors that demonstrate cultural humility, structural competency, reflexivity, advocacy, and systems thinking.
- Align competency assessment across the medical education continuum with consistent focus on equity, diversity, and inclusion.
- Measure and report the "added value" of the health equity curriculum to the community.
- Assess and monitor the social accountability of the home institution and educational program.
- Include comprehensive evaluation data sources, including nontraditional data, to foster continual improvement in curriculum.

*Institution refers to a university, health system, community organization, or governmental agency.

the community-as-the-patient, and public health professionals. The general needs assessment evolves from the key differences between the current and ideal approaches, which builds the argument for curricular development in this area.

The Health Problem: Historical Context and Causes

The problem of interest in health equity curricula is the systemic health differences between groups of patients that are the consequence of bias and unjust allocation of resources.[6] In the United States, which has the world's highest per capita costs for health care, racial and ethnic minorities suffer higher rates of chronic disease, premature death, and infant mortality than white people.[3] Over many decades, life expectancy remains substantially lower and infant mortality higher for Black people as compared with white counterparts. For Indigenous Peoples, mortality rates are 50% higher than white counterparts, and they experience 1.5 times the infant mortality rate of white people.[3,36] The

Table 11.3.   Glossary of Terms Used in Health Systems Science and Health Equity

advocacy. Action to promote social, economic, educational, and political changes that ameliorate the suffering and threats to human health and well-being identified through professional expertise (adapted definition).[21]

community. "Any configuration of individuals, families, and groups whose values, characteristics, interests, geography, and/or social relations unite them in some way."[3]

community-engaged medical education (CEME). Alignment of community needs with the learning objectives of the curriculum through active community engagement.[23]

community engagement. "The process of working collaboratively with and through groups of people affiliated by geographic proximity, special interest, or similar situations to address issues affecting the well-being of those people."[22]

cultural competence. Set of communication skills and practice behaviors that facilitate patient-centered care in multicultural encounters.[24]

cultural humility. Framework that includes a "life-long commitment to self-evaluation and self-critique," analysis and correction of the power dynamics in a patient-provider relationship, and the development of "mutually beneficial partnerships with communities."[25]

cultural safety. Example of systems thinking that extends beyond cultural competence training to focus on the structural, social, and power inequities in patient-provider relationships, and encourages providers to challenge those power relationships.[26]

diversity. "Various backgrounds and races that comprise a community, nation, or grouping."[27]

downstream determinants of health. Immediate health needs for individuals, such as access to quality care for acute and chronic conditions.[3]

equity. Providing all people with fair opportunities to achieve their full potential. Justice in the way people are treated.[11,28]

health care disparities. "Racial or ethnic differences in the quality of healthcare that are not due to access-related factors or clinical needs, preferences and appropriateness of intervention."[29]

health disparities. Systemic health differences between socially disadvantaged groups;[11] "a particular type of health difference that is closely linked with social, economic, and/or environmental disadvantage."[30]

health equity. Just and fair opportunity for everyone to achieve their optimal health;[2] "attainment of the highest level of health for all people," which requires "valuing everyone equally with focused and ongoing societal efforts to address avoidable inequalities, historical and contemporary injustices, and the elimination of health and health care disparities."[30]

health inequities. Differences in health outcomes due to the impact of bias within systems and structures leading to health outcomes that are preventable and unjust based on their systemic etiologies.[11]

health systems science (HSS). "The study of how health care is delivered, how health care professionals work together to deliver care and how the health system can improve patient care and health delivery."[15]

implicit association test (IAT). A tool that "measures attitudes and beliefs that people may be unwilling or unable to report."[31]

inclusion. "Refers to how diversity is leveraged to create a fair, equitable, healthy, and high-performing organization or community where all individuals are respected, feel engaged and motivated, and their contributions toward meeting organization and society goals are valued."[32]

individual racism. "Face-to-face or covert actions toward a person that intentionally express prejudice, hate or bias based on race."[27]

institutional racism. "Policies and practices within and across institutions that, intentionally or not, produce outcomes that chronically favor" or disadvantage a racial group.[27]

Table 11.3.   *(continued)*

---

midstream determinants of health. Intermediary determinants for individuals, such as the environments in which people live and work, education, employment, housing, nutrition, public safety, and transportation (termed the social determinants of health).[3]

social determinants of health (SDOH). "Conditions in the places where people live, learn, work and play that affect a wide range of health risks and outcomes."[3,30]

structural competency. Skills that enable health providers to recognize that clinical presentations can represent the downstream effects of societal factors such as stress, food insecurity, environmental exposures, inadequate education, housing, and racism.[33]

structural determinants of health. Community conditions such as public policy, economic class, and biases.[4]

structural racism. "A system in which public policies, institutional practices, cultural representations, and other norms work in various, often reinforcing ways to perpetuate racial group inequity";[27] "system of structuring opportunity and assigning value based on the social interpretation of how one looks (. . . 'race'), that unfairly disadvantages some individuals and communities, unfairly advantages other individuals and communities, and saps the strength of the whole society through the waste of human resources."[34]

systems thinking (ST). "A transformational approach to learning, problem-solving and understanding the world" (see Table 11.1, "Habits of a Systems Thinker").[20]

underrepresented in medicine (URM). "Those racial and ethnic populations that are underrepresented in the medical profession relative to their numbers in the general population."[35]

upstream determinants of health. Structural determinants or community conditions, such as public policies, economic class, and biases based on race, gender, country of origin, sexual orientation, religion, immigration status, disability, and language.[3-6]

COVID-19 pandemic brought stark reality to the complexity of health disparities and their attendant vulnerabilities, with communities of color experiencing exceptional burdens of morbidity and mortality.[37] After one year of the pandemic, in the United States, people who are white lost 0.8 years of life expectancy; Latino, 1.9 years; and Black, 2.7 years.[38]

Historically, societal interest in health equity dates to the mid-nineteenth century writings in social medicine by Rudolph Virchow and others, followed by a series of initiatives.[39] The World Health Organization (WHO) first addressed the "social condition" in 1946 and then launched "Health for All" in 1978, which resulted in several regional activities to address patterns of illness in populations. In 1992, the WHO Regional Office for Europe published "The Concepts and Principles of Equity and Health," describing seven main determinants of health.[9] In 2002, the Institute of Medicine published "Unequal Treatment," summarizing differences in health and health outcomes between patients in minority and majority US populations.[29] The US Department of Health and Human Services launched the Healthy People Initiative in 2000 with the goal of reducing health disparities; in 2010, the goal was adjusted to eliminating health disparities.[40]

Despite this attention, progress in reducing health disparities has been meager.[41] This is in part because the societal response to health inequities is aimed at policy levels, such as assuring secure housing and nutrition, education, access to care, and equal opportunities in the workforce. The 2010 Patient Protection and Affordable Care Act, for example, improved health insurance coverage and access to care for 20 million Americans, a positive but insufficient correction to the system.

Additionally, the response to health inequity has also been hampered by a historical break between public health and health professions education, which has resulted in a focus in medical school curricula on the individual, while public health education focused on the population.[42–44] This dichotomy in approach between disciplines resulted in polarized thinking around the scope of professional identity despite the reality that both individuals and populations live in complex, dynamic systems with multiple determinants of health.

The twenty-first century has seen numerous calls for health professions education to be *socially accountable*.[29,45,46] The WHO defined social accountability of medical schools as "the obligation to direct their education, research and service activities toward addressing priority health concerns of the community, the region or the nation they have a mandate to serve."[47] One set of criteria for social accountability of medical schools, published in 2012, includes documentation of organizational social accountability plans and documentation of positive impacts resulting from their education, research, service, graduates, and partnerships in the health care of the community.[48]

Building the current argument for an enhanced health equity curriculum begins with presenting data from multiple levels of context, such as data from the individual, institutional (university, health system, community organization, or governmental agency), population, local, regional, state, national, and/or international levels. Three key indicators of the health of a population—infant mortality rate, age-adjusted death rate, and life expectancy—are frequently used as health outcomes of interest. Periodic community health needs assessments conducted by health care systems and territorial, state, and local health departments provide excellent sources of data on community population health outcomes.[16,49,50] In many cases, such assessments employ a health equity lens, providing a unique platform to ground curricular development in local community context.[51,52]

> **EXAMPLE:** *Data Used to Support a Health Equity Curricular Need and Link to Broader Community Health Improvement Planning.* To emphasize the importance of addressing health equity in a medical school curriculum reform, a faculty educator used several data sources to highlight the problem of health disparities in local communities: results from a combined public health and health care system community health assessment, national and regional data, and trends in health care outcomes from the Agency for Healthcare Research and Quality (AHRQ) National Healthcare Quality and Disparities Report.[51,52] As an example of local context, the data supported that a marked difference in life expectancy existed in two zip codes proximate to the medical school and the academic medical center.[51]

Current Approach: Structural Issues and Stakeholder Responses

Targeted approaches have addressed some of the root causes of health disparities, but few have captured the historical context, complexity, interdependencies, and dynamic nature of the problem. Not surprisingly, these approaches have shown no impact on health disparities. One approach to explain the upstream causes of health disparities is to examine intersection of individual and systemic biases and their impact on the health of both individuals and populations.

> **EXAMPLE:** *Describing the Impact of Individual and Systemic Bias on the Health of Neighborhoods.* A health equity course for medical students introduced the impact of "redlining" on the built environment in a local community. Using maps, researchers showed that neighborhoods with poor health outcomes can be traced to those that were "redlined" by the banking industry in the 1930s. Redlining was the Federal Housing Authority (FHA) practice of rejecting mortgages from specific neighborhoods on the

basis of racial discrimination.[53] Although the practice became illegal in the civil rights era, the legacy of redlining has resulted in racial segregation, less investment, increased poverty, and loss of employment. With respect to health issues, redlining has resulted in shorter life expectancy, increased infant mortality and incidence of cancer, lead poisoning in children, asthma, and lack of health care access.[54]

The current approach considers how a particular issue is addressed by various stakeholders, including patients or the community-as-patient in the context of health equity, health care professionals, medical educators, and society. Mission statements may signal a current alignment of an institution (e.g., regional health system, professional group, or educational organization) with the needs of society and the identified community. Some health systems have recently acknowledged their role in addressing the needs of communities they serve by forming public-private partnerships to address both upstream and midstream determinants of health, such as housing, education, transportation, and built environment.[55,56] Other health systems have also committed to tracking patient SDOH, using data to monitor and address emerging needs at a community level.[57]

EXAMPLE: *Academic Medical Center Commitment to End Racism.* Froedtert Health and the Medical College of Wisconsin have partnered in a comprehensive plan to end racism through the following actions identified in their mission statement:

"1. Treating people with dignity and respect
2. Examining our own biases
3. Measuring, tracking and reviewing our policies and practices to meet the needs of everyone we serve
4. Leading change in our communities."[58]

They are also part of the national #123forEquity campaign, a joint effort of the American Hospital Association, Association of American Medical Colleges, and others, that commits to increasing the collection and use of race, ethnicity, language preference, and other sociodemographic data. These efforts are aimed at increasing cultural competency training, increasing diversity in leadership and governance, and strengthening community partnerships.[59]

The health professions' response to health disparities has focused primarily on ensuring that care is equitable and evidence-based for all patients at the individual level. As research has emerged that unequal care occurs at the individual patient and provider level,[60] as well as the health system level, health professions have begun to address the importance of providing culturally appropriate care, such as in licensure and credentialing requirements. In 2005, New Jersey was the first of five states to mandate that all physicians receive cultural competency training for licensure. Most large health care systems followed with required cultural competence training for all health care providers. Continuing medical education providers also sought effective cultural competence training but noted many barriers to behavior change.[61] Evidence for effectiveness of this training shows increased knowledge and skills on the part of providers but a paucity of evidence for improvement in patient outcomes.[62,63]

Health professions educational programs have several problematic areas related to their curricula, learning environments, and selection of learners and trainees. Although evidence is clear that social conditions and the structures within systems impact individual and population health in profound ways, the impact of upstream determinants of health has not been traditionally taught in health professions education. Few health professions educational programs have emphasized ST approaches to problem-solving.

Most health educators introduce health disparities through SDOH curricula.[64] The Association of American Medical Colleges (AAMC) Curriculum Inventory Report notes that 87% of reporting schools require SDOH curriculum in year 1 and 24% have required SDOH content in year 3, likely due to accreditation requirements for inclusion.[64] SDOH content is most frequently limited by its priority in the curriculum and lack of vertical and longitudinal integration, and it remains an area of need in curricular development.[65,66]

One example of the lack of integration of SDOH into the curriculum is manifest as presentation of *race as biology*, often used as an example of *structural racism* embedded in health professions education.[67] For instance, a pathophysiology course that presents racial disparities in the prevalence, onset, or survival of specific diseases implies that there are biologic bases for these differences. These courses rarely provide the alternative explanation that the lived experience of people who are Black, Indigenous, or people of color in a racist society has its own consequences of lifelong stress, access to health care, and other impacts that influence outcomes. Over time, these presentations add to students' preconceived beliefs about racial differences resulting in worsening stereotyping and bias.[68]

Another example of *structural racism* in medical education occurs in teaching and assessment of *clinical skills*. Students have traditionally been taught that the medical history should include documentation of race, which is known from a subjective, often inaccurate, observation. The inclusion of provider-described race in a case presentation opens the opportunity for "racial profiling" and bias in the delivery of care and may further perpetuate individual clinician biases.[68–71] An alternative approach is to discourage the documentation of race, unless there is a clear and compelling reason to do so and, rather, encourage an exploration of patient-described identity, ancestry, cultural beliefs, and health-related practices.[69]

An additional critique of current health professions' education is that it is not producing a workforce that meets the societal health care needs. This begins with the selection of learners who are committed and prepared to care for an increasingly diverse population. Educational institutions have sought increased student diversity for several reasons.[72–76] There is a well-documented maldistribution of health professionals and a mismatch of specialty needs.[77] Underrepresented in medicine (URM) students, however, are more likely to report an interest in working with vulnerable populations and in primary care.[78] Furthermore, there is growing evidence about the importance of patient-provider race concordance in addressing health disparities.[79] URM learners enhance their educational programs, including attitudinal educational outcomes for their peers.[80,81] The increased presence of URM learners in health professions programs has been an intentional goal to foster health equity.[82]

Advancing diversity in the health professions has been difficult and variably successful. In the United States, while the number of female matriculants to medical schools has reached parity with male matriculants, the number of "Black or African American" and "American Indian or Alaska Native" matriculants has remained the same.[83] The number of male Black applicants has decreased since 1978. In academic year 2019, Black or African American applicants constituted 8.4% of the applicant pool and applicants who were Hispanic, Latino, or of Spanish origin, 6.2%.[83] Black or African American males' entry into the health professions seems to be especially burdened by *structural racism* and stereotyping barriers.[84] There are less data for other forms of diversity, such as sexual and gender minorities, disability, first-generation college, and educationally disadvantaged.

Ideal Approach

Health equity curricula thrive when embedded in an institutional culture committed to *equity, diversity, and inclusion* (EDI). The underlying premise of health equity training is that *every* health care professional recognizes inequities and can serve as an advocate and change agent. Shared language and a common vocabulary for EDI, as well as shared understanding of the concepts, requires engagement at the institutional and school levels, as well as with student affairs, faculty affairs, and partner organizations. Broad engagement can promote understanding of the intersections of individual and systemic biases and their impact on health outcomes for individuals and populations. The ideal approach then begins with identifying institutional exemplars that have embedded EDI into organizational values and practices. In addition to self-reflection using an EDI lens, best institutional practices to further a culture of equity include codesign of institutional policies, processes, and behavioral norms with broad representation from community members and leadership that strives to ensure that all voices are heard and valued.[85] In subsequent steps, such institutions can also serve as a source of effective curricular examples that have integrated content into these areas.

> **EXAMPLE**: *An Institution That Fosters Equity as an Organizational Value.* The University of California, San Francisco set a strategic goal of creating and maintaining a diverse, equitable, and inclusive environment. Efforts began with a mission statement to broadcast its goal of inclusivity; attention to recruitment of diverse faculty, residents, and students; broad representation of diversity on websites and social media; and addressing faculty equity in workload and compensation. The institutional effort also committed to teach and use a common language in diversity and inclusion to facilitate dialogue between students, faculty, and administration. Teaching cultural humility to faculty and students; enhancing collaboration, trust, and cohesion of the student body; and recognizing the impact of implicit bias in student assessment were also part of the initiative.[86,87]

Accreditation standards that include EDI, social responsibility, and advocacy as core professional values are powerful resources in this engagement. Instruction in population health and community needs, leadership, and advocacy for vulnerable populations is included in nearly all health professions accreditation standards and competency frameworks.[88–93] One example is the transformation of public health accreditation standards rooted in health equity that "is naturally aligned with the goal of improving population health which is defined by a shift from individual health behaviors and risk factors to examining the social and structural contexts that impact entire populations and lead to disparate distribution of outcomes."[94]

A systematic review of interventions to improve diversity in the health professions found several initiatives that can impact diversity in matriculants, including an admissions process that uses a points system, weighs nonacademic criteria versus academic criteria, includes holistic reviews, and offers application assistance.[95] (The AAMC Holistic Review tools and resources are available to medical schools and training programs on the AAMC website.) Enrichment and outreach programs have also had some impact.[95] Interestingly, a curricular program that values training in health disparities and preparation for working with vulnerable populations may be more attractive for URM applicants.[96]

> **EXAMPLE:** *Addressing Implicit Bias in the Admissions Process.* Recognizing that implicit racial bias may affect admissions decisions, all members of a medical school's admissions committee completed the Black-White Implicit Association Test (IAT) online.[31] The results indicated a strong white preference for

all groups, with the strongest preference in men and faculty members. A post-IAT survey indicated that 48% of committee members were conscious of the IAT results when interviewing applicants in the next cycle, and 21% thought it would impact admissions decisions in the next cycle. The next matriculating class was the most diverse in the school's history.[97]

While single initiatives have shown impact, most reviews conclude that the diversity efforts need to be multifaceted and need to address the continuum from pipelines into the matriculant pool, through student recruitment, faculty recruitment, support, and retention, to institutional culture.[59,95,98,99]

Completing the analysis of the ideal approach includes identifying best practices and common themes in published competencies, educational strategies, assessments, and evaluation approaches across the health professions education continuum. This is a rapidly evolving area in health professions education; suggested resources for this information include recent educational meeting abstracts, online collections such as MedEdPORTAL, and published literature.

EXAMPLE: *Published Learning Objectives and Competencies.* A Dutch medical school undertook a three-phase multimethod approach to create a more "diversity-responsive" curriculum. The educators began the work with a qualitative analysis of interviews with relevant stakeholders and a literature search to develop essential learning objectives. This analysis led to three overarching learning objectives: *medical knowledge* needed for physicians to approach diversity, patient-physician *communication* to effectively communicate with patients from diverse sociocultural backgrounds, and *reflexivity* (critical thinking that focuses on self-awareness).[100]

With respect to educational strategies, health professions education has shifted focus from teaching cross-cultural communication skills to educating learners about societal structural factors beyond the health care system that perpetuate health inequities.[33] The bridge from learning about SDOH to utilizing that knowledge in clinical encounters is termed *structural competency*. *Structural competency* allows health providers to recognize that clinical presentations can represent the downstream effects of societal factors, such as stress, food insecurity, environmental exposures, inadequate education, housing, and racism.[33] This holistic view of the clinical encounter reflects ST engendered by HSS, an awareness of a "web of interdependencies with multidirectional cause-effect relationships."[7,15,33]

EXAMPLE: *Tool to Build Structural Competency.* To address health disparities at the individual clinical encounter, a clinical tool, the *Structural Vulnerability Assessment Tool*, was developed to enhance the clinician's social history–taking beyond risk-taking behaviors. The tool informs the clinician of potential social services provisions and advocacy needs that enhance the clinical care provided to the individual and collects needed population-level data by the health system.[101]

Learner attitudes and biases may also be barriers to learning this content. As a first step, curricula will often incorporate exercises in implicit bias awareness in the cross-cultural communications training. Rather than stand-alone exercises, an integrated approach that combines clinical experiences with medically vulnerable populations, didactic and self-reflection across the curriculum is most likely to enhance student awareness and knowledge.[102,103] Learners educated in these environments are more likely to enter primary care fields and practice in underserved communities.[104]

EXAMPLE: *Residency Curriculum on Structural Competency.* An internal medical residency program developed a longitudinal curriculum focused on *structural competency, structural racism, implicit bias, microaggressions, and cultural humility*. The educators evaluated the curriculum using a previously validated instrument, the *Clinical Cultural Competency Questionnaire*, with additional questions developed from structural competency literature.[105,106]

To address the call for social accountability, there are many health professional schools that have a primary mission to educate a health care workforce that will meet the needs of vulnerable populations, both in the United States and abroad.[107,108] Established programs have developed dedicated tracks for learners with an interest in health equity and underserved populations. Typically, these curricula have *longitudinal curricular threads* and *community-based placements* that support the development of knowledge, attitudes, and skills for socially accountable practice.[107,109]

EXAMPLE: *An Integrated Curriculum Addressing Health Equity.* A. T. Still University School of Osteopathic Medicine expounds a stated mission to develop physicians and leaders who serve medically underserved populations. The school focuses on recruiting students from the communities served by the medical school and their partner community health centers. Once admitted, students learn through a health-equity-grounded curriculum and spend years 2 through 4 embedded in community placements. While living and working in the community longitudinally, students develop a deep understanding of the systems and structures impacting health and are trained as "community-minded healers."[110]

A General Needs Assessment in Health Equity Curricula

In summary, the general needs assessment for a health equity curriculum will provide important population-level data on health disparities and evidence for the structural causes of inequities that occur at the societal, institutional, community, patient, and practitioner levels. The educational gaps that need to be addressed in training future health care providers will be identified and may include the following: ensuring *knowledge of SDOH* and structural factors that contribute to health inequity; *ST approaches* to analyzing clinical presentation that includes the patient's context of illness (supporting structural competency); *awareness of one's own implicit biases* and behaviors; a *commitment to fostering health equity*; applying these skills as an effective *change agent*; and the *skills of patient-centered cross-cultural communications*.

STEP 2: TARGETED NEEDS ASSESSMENT

This step identifies and assesses both targeted learners and the learning environment, a critical step in developing a health equity curriculum. Attempting to deliver meaningful learning about health equity in a learning environment that is perceived as inequitable for students, patients, and communities can be disastrous. Unlike the traditional basic science or clinical science–focused curricula, a robust health equity curriculum requires work at three levels: (1) institutional composition (diversity of students, faculty, and staff), (2) inclusive organizational values and educational environment, and (3) comprehensive curricular attention to upstream and midstream determinants, such as *structural racism* and SDOH, respectively.[111] Multiple targeted needs assessments, as outlined in Chapter 3, are used in this step and may result in both qualitative and quantitative data. The following considerations should guide the approach to the targeted needs assessment for health equity curricula.

Since the institutional setting is so important to the effective delivery of a health equity curriculum, Step 2 should begin with the assessment of the institutional and school/program overarching missions and their alignments with the needs of society/community, as well as the commitment to EDI. Such assessments may require collaboration with other institutional departments and efforts to ensure a comprehensive analysis of all elements of the learning environment, including institutional policies, processes, and behavioral norms.[85]

EXAMPLE: *Institutional Assessment of Racism.* In 2019, the Boston University School of Medicine (BUSM) Medical Education Committee commissioned a vertical integration group (VIG), composed of students, faculty, and staff, to assess how systemic racism impacted the learning climate at BUSM. The VIG summary report highlighted strengths in the curriculum, such as presentation of racial health disparities with population data and personal narratives, and weaknesses, such as the use of race as a risk factor for pathology. Opportunities to strengthen the longitudinal presentation of an antiracism curriculum and recommendations with associated competencies emerged from this work.[112]

While not every school/program has committed to social accountability, an assessment of how well the program is meeting the criteria for social accountability indicates receptivity of the learning environment to a health equity curriculum. North American medical schools may use the AAMC Mission Management Tool, published annually since 2009.[113] The Tool, using multisourced data, benchmarks schools' performances in selected mission areas, including graduating a workforce that will address priority health needs of the nation, preparing a diverse physician workforce, and preparing physicians to fulfill the needs of the community.

Selecting Learners

Targeted learners may include undergraduate or graduate students, practitioners-in-training, faculty, staff, or community members. As noted in Chapter 3, they are "the group most likely, with further learning, to contribute to the solution of the problem." As noted above, selection of learners to the program or school may have a profound impact on the educational outcomes of a health equity curriculum. Step 2, then, should include an assessment of local institutional efforts and success in increasing health care workforce diversity.

Assessing Targeted Learners

Once targeted learners have been identified, it is important for curriculum developers to identify skills of ST and the lived experience of learners related to EDI. Due to a paucity of formal assessment tools for ST, educators may find themselves using admission personal statements or answers to interview questions to understand an applicant's ST skills. These narratives give educators a glimpse of how learners connect seemingly disparate events, take on a holistic approach when it comes to problem-solving, or appreciate complexity. For EDI, lived experiences are particularly important as URM learners have disproportionately experienced bias and discrimination, while majority counterparts may have varied understanding of these concepts. Even advanced learners can lack self-awareness or self-reflexive capacity or perceive themselves already knowledgeable.[114] Unlike most topics in a health professions curriculum, topics of racism, poverty, and inequity can be emotionally charged and/or triggering for learners, who may be reluctant to participate in surveys or even group discussions to share their lived experience. The methods used for this type of targeted assessment will require careful attention to psychological safety and cultural humility.

EXAMPLE: *Development and Validation of a Cultural Attitudes Survey for Medical Students.* A survey was developed to understand medical students' attitudes toward sociocultural issues they might encounter during medical school. The survey topics included examination of patients, intercultural interactions, discussions of race and ethnicity, interactions with individuals of diverse sexual orientation, interaction with institutional representatives, learning about alternative medicine, and identification of skin conditions in people of different skin color. The survey was administered to incoming medical students and psychometric properties were assessed. Meaningful differences were noted between white students' responses versus URM students.[115,116]

The vulnerability of learners may explain the paucity of published literature on health professionals' knowledge and attitudes regarding health equity, and the resulting paucity of validated measurement instruments. A few instruments have been used to assess learners' attitudes toward poverty, including the *Attitude toward Poverty Scale*, used in nursing education, the *Systems and Individual Responsibility for Poverty (SIRP) Scale*, and the *Inner City Attitudinal Assessment Tool (ICAAT)*, which has been validated across health care professions.[117–119] The validated *Medical Student Attitude toward the Medically Underserved (MSATU)* questionnaire has repeatedly shown that the attitudes of medical and dental students, but not pharmacy students, deteriorate from the first to the last year of professional school, showing a decreased commitment to care for vulnerable populations and a lack of efficacy in working with this population.[120–125]

Assessment of targeted learners should include methods that elucidate an understanding of the intersection of the current local curriculum (or lack thereof) and learner experience regarding systemic bias, EDI, ST and HSS.

Assessing the Targeted Learning Environment

The targeted learning environment includes the formal curriculum, informal curriculum, and the hidden curriculum. The AAMC has recommended the use of the Tool for Assessing Cultural Competency Training (TACCT) (https://www.aamc.org/media/20841/download) to understand the formal curriculum.[126] The tool surveys five domains: (1) rationale, definitions, and context; (2) key aspects of cultural competence; (3) impact of stereotyping on medical decision-making; (4) health disparities; and (5) cross-cultural clinical skills. Ideally, the TACCT is completed by faculty and students to identify content gaps in the formal curriculum. With the ideal approaches in mind, the developer for a health equity curriculum should assess not only whether these domains are represented but also how well they are integrated vertically and horizontally, and whether the curriculum fosters ST and advocacy as core professional values.

The formal curriculum may also need close inspection for evidence of *structural racism*, such as the presentation of race as biology. A review of 63 published virtual patient teaching cases found six common pitfalls in the presentation of race and culture including (1) presentation of race as a genetic risk factor rather than a social or structural risk factor, (2) lack of presentation of upstream factors, (3) reductionist and essentialist portrayals of non-Western culture and people of color, (4) providers who ignore or portray frustration in dealing with social and structural causes of disease or illness, (5) lack of critical reflection on health disparities and implicit bias in medicine, and (6) minority identities displayed in patients, physicians, and providers that do not reflect the US population.[68] The study authors proposed a guide for authors of teaching cases to address these pitfalls.

Understanding the informal and hidden curriculum can be more challenging. This involves clarifying issues as perceived by the targeted learners and considering the intersection of individual and systemic bias, as well as elements of EDI and their impact on the learning environment.

EXAMPLE: *Residents' Experience of the Learning Environment.* A qualitative study of the training experiences of 27 URM residents attending a national meeting found three themes: "a daily barrage of microaggressions and bias, minority residents tasked as race/ethnicity ambassadors, and challenges negotiating personal and professional identity while seen as 'other.'"[127]

EXAMPLE: *Medical Students' Experience of the Learning Environment.* An analysis of over 27,000 graduation questionnaires in 2016 and 2017 found that medical students who were female, multiracial, or sexual and gender minorities experienced higher rates of mistreatment than their peers. Mistreatment included public humiliation, being subjected to offensive remarks, being denied opportunities or receiving lower evaluations based on gender, sexual orientation, or race. URM females reported the highest prevalence of mistreatment and discrimination.[128]

At the conclusion of Step 2, the curriculum developer has examined the local institutional history and culture related to EDI, the commitment to recruitment and retention of a diverse educational community, the existing infrastructure for addressing bias, and processes to ensure an equitable learning environment. The curriculum developer has surveyed the learners, the curriculum, and the learning environment for receptivity and potential barriers to addressing the educational gaps identified in the general needs assessment.

STEP 3: GOALS, OBJECTIVES, AND COMPETENCIES

Health equity curricular goals and objectives need to align both with societal needs, as identified in Step 1, and relevant institutional missions, as identified in Step 2. As noted in several of the examples below, consensus is building around the broad domains needed to address health equity. These include

1. knowledge of SDOH and structural factors that contribute to health inequity,
2. awareness of one's own implicit biases and behaviors,
3. ST approaches to understanding the context of illness,
4. the skills of patient-centered cross-cultural communication, and
5. a commitment to fostering health equity.

It is challenging to write goals and examples in ways that respect learners' lived experience, minimize bias, and enhance change agency and self-efficacy in working with communities in need while also addressing the hidden curriculum.

EXAMPLE: *Writing Health Professional Education Goals to Address Societal Needs.* A task force of educators from the Society for General Internal Medicine used a review and consensus process to develop recommendations for teaching about racial and health disparities.[129] The task force condensed the recommendations to the broad goal of developing within one's professional role a commitment to eliminating health inequities. Three areas of learning were advised:

1. Identifying attitudes such as mistrust, bias, and stereotyping that practitioners and patients may bring to the clinical encounter.
2. Knowledge of the existence, extent, underlying causes, and potential solutions to health disparities.
3. Skills to communicate effectively across cultures, languages, and literacy.

This framework was subsequently used to create a national Train-the-Trainer course for faculty in health disparities education and a longitudinal health disparities curriculum for medical residents.[130,131]

EXAMPLE: *Learning Objectives for a Longitudinal Health Equity and Social Justice Curriculum for Medical Students.* Preclerkship learning objectives from a medical student longitudinal Health Equity and Social Justice course reflected these same areas of learning:

"1. Recognize and appropriately address biases in ourselves.
2. Describe the impact that gender, race/ethnicity, sexual orientation, culture, religion, socioeconomic status, disabilities, literacy level and health disparities have on health status.
3. Describe the social determinants of health and recognize the impact of health care policy and community partnerships on population health.
4. Develop skills to better understand the manner in which diverse cultures and belief systems perceive health and illness.
5. Demonstrate a commitment to life-long learning, social justice and community service."[132]

The example below illustrates assessing and aligning goals and objectives with learner lived experience identified in Step 2. Goals and objectives also need to align with competencies that enable learners to meet societal needs, such as minimizing bias and fostering change agency. Well-written objectives will direct the educational design in Step 4.

EXAMPLE: *Writing Equity-Grounded Goals and Objectives That Foster Change Agency while Minimizing Bias: Health Equity Rounds.* In developing a health equity curriculum for medical students, the faculty educators were mindful that faculty and resident team leaders needed this curriculum as well. The educational objectives were written respecting these various "learners" and their lived experiences:

"By the end of this activity, learners will be able to:

1. Identify and analyze the effects of implicit bias and structural racism in clinical scenarios.
2. Describe the historical context and present-day role of structural racism and its impact on the health care system.
3. Employ evidence-based tools to recognize and mitigate the effects of implicit biases.
4. Use newly learned strategies to combat structural racism at the institutional level and reduce the impact of implicit bias on patient care and interprofessional relationships."[133]

Learners were involved in the planning of the curricula in both above examples. The inclusion of learners in the planning process can be helpful to focus the curriculum, avoid redundancies, and ensure that the curriculum will address the learners' needs and expectations. In developing goals and objectives, it can also be helpful to seek multidisciplinary input. For example, patients, community leaders, and experts from the fields of sociology, social work, psychology, anthropology, public health, and law can help shape objectives that deepen understanding of the historical context of racism, bias, and structural determinants of health.

EXAMPLE: *Engagement of Nontraditional Stakeholders.* Curricular faculty designed a curriculum for medical students and residents that encouraged patient-centered, culturally sensitive care for transnational patients (i.e., living in the United States but with strong ties to their communities of origin). The faculty used one-on-one interviews and focus groups with transnational patients to develop teaching vignettes that reflect the challenges facing patients and their providers. Two goals for the curriculum that emerged from these interviews were (1) "enhance their (learners') awareness of transnational community context by examining quotations and narratives based on first-hand experiences," and (2) "elicit relevant migration history as well as patient's values and goals during the medical interview."[134]

Step 1 should yield key examples of *competencies* for health equity curricula, such as ST, change agency, and elements of equity-grounded health professions practice.

Existing public health and preventive medicine programs can serve as resources for creating the competency framework.[135] In Step 3, goals and objectives should align with the competencies and content that have been identified in the ideal approach (Step 1).

> **EXAMPLE:** *Interprofessional Competency Map for Teaching Population Health.* A medical school's Department of Community and Family Medicine, with a long history of community engagement, sought to improve the training of future health professionals in improving the health of local communities. A group of interprofessional faculty reviewed and synthesized published competencies and developed a population health competency map. The map details four competency domains—public health practice, community engagement, critical thinking, and team skills—with learning objectives written at three training levels (medical students, physician assistant students, and family medicine residents).[136]

Finally, goals and objectives need to align with external requirements. As an example, the AAMC, in its new and emerging competencies initiative, is currently engaged in the development of a diversity, equity, and inclusion (DEI) competency framework that will be tiered across the education continuum from students to residents to faculty.[137]

STEP 4: EDUCATIONAL STRATEGIES: ALIGNING AND INTEGRATING CONTENT AND CHOOSING METHODS

Critical Pedagogy in Health Equity Curricula

The content and methods used to achieve the identified goals and objectives are defined in Step 4. As outlined in Chapter 5, learning theory must be carefully considered and applied to the determination of content and identification of educational methods. Health equity curricula can be seen to build on Freire's critical pedagogy, which empowers learners to rethink social and political norms and become actively engaged in social change.[138] The foundation of critical pedagogy is dialogue within learning communities of individuals who bring prior experience and knowledge to the discussions. Building in learners' prior knowledge and/or lived experience is critical to the authenticity of a health equity curriculum. Because of the moral and ethical dimensions of the health equity construct, most educators strive for a *longitudinal integrated* curriculum that prompts learners to return repeatedly to the concepts and reflect on their meaning in clinical work and the impact on their professional identity formation. Embedded in these longitudinal curricula are educational methods that particularly promote targeted health equity competencies, as discussed in the sections that follow.

Cultural Competence, Cultural Humility, Cultural Safety, and Awareness of Bias

Cultural competence is the set of communication skills and practice behaviors that facilitate patient-centered care in multicultural encounters.[24] A systematic review of cultural competence training of health professions found a variety of methods were used to address the knowledge, attitudes, and skills objectives.[139] These included lectures, discussions, cases, cultural immersions, interviewing other cultures, and role-play. The length of interventions ranged from hours to several weeks. These training programs improved provider knowledge, attitudes, and skills, and several showed improved patient satisfaction. None have shown impact on patient outcomes.[139] Additionally, the focus of cultural competence training on the individual encounter may perpetuate stereotypes of "other" in the clinical encounter.[26,140] It has been suggested that these concepts be embedded in a larger framework of *cultural humility*, which includes a lifelong commitment to self-evaluation and self-critique, analysis and correction of the power dynamics in a patient-provider relationship, and the development of mutually beneficial partnerships with communities.[25]

Cultural safety is another example of ST and extends beyond cultural competence training to focus on the structural, social, and power inequities in patient-provider relationships, and it encourages providers to challenge those power dynamics.[26] Its outcomes are the sense of safety experienced by the patient and shared decision-making. A review of 44 international publications with a focus on Indigenous populations, found that cultural safety training and application to practice improved relationships, health outcomes, interest in working with Indigenous populations, and the number of Indigenous people entering health professional careers.[141] A literature review of 59 articles focused on cultural safety concluded that, to practice culturally safe care, health care practitioners, organizations, and systems must provide mechanisms for challenging power structures and overtly link culturally safe activities in the clinical setting to achieving health equity.[26]

As noted, many health equity curricula share attitudinal objectives that involve awareness of implicit bias and challenging one's assumptions about people different from oneself. Strategies to accomplish this have been taken from social-cognitive psychology as well as anthropology and include enhancing the internal motivation to reduce bias by learning the historical evidence of bias in health care; knowing one's own implicit bias through a tool such as the Implicit Association Test;[31] understanding the psychological basis of bias; and enhancing confidence in working with socially disadvantaged persons, usually with direct patient contact.[142]

Facilitating Systems Thinking Habits

Health equity courses frequently use longitudinal experiential learning that highlights lived experiences of patients and prompts discussions of structural and SDOH to demonstrate how historical policies or neighborhood structures impact health. Such curriculum design allows educators and learners to recognize the dynamic interplay of different aspects of the biopsychosocial health model. This complexity can be captured with clinical case discussions, with concept-mapping, or by using a systems thinking framework, encouraging learners to articulate how determinants of health are not limited to physiology alone. Many health care professionals employ ST but may not necessarily define it as such. Teaching methods such as reflection and concept-mapping allow this tacit thinking to come into focus as learners discuss and map out the relationship of the various parts to each other and to the larger whole.

Social and Structural Determinants of Health

Lower-level knowledge about health disparities, historical context, and SDOH can be presented with readings, multimedia formats, and lectures. For higher-order cognitive objectives, such as the ability to analyze the impact of SDOH and structural vulnerability in clinical encounters (i.e., the application of ST), programs often use case-based discussions with tools or frameworks that prompt the learner to challenge assumptions and consider alternative perspectives.

EXAMPLE: *Using a Tool for Understanding Patient Perspective.* A residency-based health disparities track seminar series includes a session on Language, Acculturation, and Immigrant Health. Residents are assigned a documentary, *Unnatural Causes: Becoming American* (unnaturalcauses.org), prior to the seminar. After a didactic on immigrant health, residents practice using the ETHNIC (explanation, treatment, healers, negotiate, intervention, collaboration) mnemonic to elicit and incorporate the patient's perspective.[131,143]

EXAMPLE: *Using a Tool to Challenge Assumptions.* Three interactive workshops for clinical year medical students were developed to extend the Health Equity and Social Justice curriculum into the clinical year. Educators built a framework, based on a previous lecture in unconscious bias, to describe efforts practitioners can use to address unconscious bias in clinical encounters, called CHARGE2. This framework opens with "C: Change your context: Is there another perspective possible?"[144]

Advocacy and Commitment to Foster Health Equity

Nearly every health equity curriculum recognizes the power of longitudinal authentic experiences with vulnerable populations to achieve health equity objectives, including a long-term commitment to address health care disparities. Working with disadvantaged populations provides learners authentic experiences that can foster empathy, trust, and cultural humility, while forging elements of partnership with vulnerable populations. Approaches include community-based service learning, continuity clinics, or longitudinal clerkships in clinics for underinsured, refugee/immigrant populations, or community-based advocacy work. Medical students who have clinical experience in vulnerable and/or rural areas are significantly more likely to eventually practice primary care and to practice in medically underserved areas.[145]

EXAMPLE: *Early Training and Use of Medical Interpreters.* In a patient navigator program, first- and second-year medical students are paired with newly arrived refugee families and begin utilizing medical interpreters both in person and by phone. Faculty model and directly teach the appropriate use of medically trained interpreter services, including maintaining eye contact and nonverbal communication with the patient, short direct verbal communication to allow for accurate verbal interpretation, and providing printed materials translated in the patient's preferred language.[146]

In the past, *service learning* occurred in one of three ways: health education in communities and schools, community clinic placements, or participating in social justice and philanthropic activities.[147] More recently, these activities purposely overlap. *Critical service learning* includes a social justice orientation to the community activity; students are often assigned the task of responding to a social injustice with advocacy or projects.[148] Critical service learning may be especially effective in helping students see themselves as agents of change.[148]

EXAMPLE: *Critical Service Learning in Nursing Education.* At the request of community members for more access to early cardiac screening, a nursing education program worked to establish a community cardiac screening clinic. Community nursing students, who had completed an enhanced curriculum in social justice and health, worked a minimum of 32 hours as members of an interdisciplinary team, conducting cardiac screenings and reporting cardiac risks to community members, followed by counseling regarding treatment and follow-up monitoring. Students subsequently engaged in structured discussions with faculty, peers, and community members. Community members provided local community knowledge and perspectives on root causes of health inequities. Students were required to submit examples of reflective journaling and to describe, in a formal presentation, the nursing service provided, the need for the service, inequities underlying the need, and lastly, the nurse's role in responding to the need.

Students' reflective writing showed growth in their understanding of clients, a reorientation of the power dynamic with their clients, and progress in building authentic relationships. Students also demonstrated a shift in their thinking about the nurse's role and responsibilities for social justice.[149]

The example above addresses the *advocacy* competency sought in many health equity curricula and exemplifies hallmarks of successful advocacy training programs: incorporation of *critical self-reflection, interdisciplinary work, collaborative teamwork, and experiential learning*.[150] As with other aspects of professional identity formation, advocacy is best acquired through socialization with role models/mentors and experiential learning.[151]

Many longitudinal curricula use a *personal learning portfolio* to build reflective practice, track commitment to health equity, and guide professional identity formation. This may include a requirement to formally create a personal statement of commitment to EDI.

Minimizing Bias in a Health Equity Curriculum

In a health equity curriculum, activities should emphasize the overarching concepts of ST and change agency while minimizing reinforcement of biases. This requires a careful balance of presentation of the problem with proposed *solutions*, such as examples of communities that have successfully addressed health disparities, balancing descriptions of risk factors with descriptions of *community strengths*, and highlighting *exemplars as leaders of social change*.[152]

As the educational design takes form, multiple layers of alignment for both content and methods are also necessary, to ensure congruence with learner lived experience identified in Step 2, as well as goals and objectives identified in Step 3.

STEP 5: IMPLEMENTATION

Barriers, Resources, Nontraditional Expertise

All elements of Step 5 (see Chapter 6) pertain to a health equity curriculum, with some additional considerations. Typical barriers of curricular time, competition with other curricular content, and resources exist for HSS and health equity curricula. HSS and health equity institutional expertise often extends across multiple institutional departments, so identifying the curriculum's administrative "home" will be important in sustaining its ongoing implementation. As noted above in Step 4, health equity is often presented as a longitudinal thread or course within a larger program, and the governance within the curriculum needs to be transparent, participatory, and equitable (see Chapter 10).

Resources for the curriculum, beginning with support of institutional leadership, should have been identified in Step 2. Institutions are turning more attention to EDI, and several have committed funding and effort to institutional transformation in this area. Health equity curricula are an important piece of this institutional cultural resetting, but multiple other areas also require effort, including admissions and faculty/staff recruitment and development, as well as student and faculty affairs. Resources need to be shared across these various centers; ideally, curricular faculty work collaboratively with other institutional leaders and initiatives to maximize available resources.

A unique aspect of HSS and health equity curricula is that they usually draw on expertise and resources that reside outside of the training program or school.[16] These curricula may use other professional school faculty, health system centers of excellence, government, or industry leaders to provide needed expertise. Students and community members have been instrumental in highlighting the need for curricula, implementing targeted needs assessments, and serving as faculty and mentors. The diversity of these participants enriches the curriculum but can be challenging to coordinate while ensuring that all voices are heard and respected.

Community-Engaged Medical Education

Community members enrich the needs assessment, provide key perspectives of the community regarding health and health care, serve as curriculum design consultants and as faculty in educational sessions, and identify community partners and preceptors who can assist in experiential learning. The alignment of community needs with learning objectives of the curriculum is termed *community-engaged medical education (CEME)*.[23] Unlike community-based education, in which the community was viewed as a destination or learning venue, CEME implies an interdependent and mutually beneficial relationship.[23] This need for the educational process to add value to the community has led to experiential models of patient navigation, health coaching, and critical service learning described under Step 4. To be successful, CEME should rest within a larger collaboration between the academic/health system institution and the community it serves—a collaboration that recognizes historical context and seeks initiatives to improve the health of the community.[153] True community engagement is a complex and challenging process of building trust and harnessing resources. The AAMC and the Centers for Disease Control and Prevention have developed resources for institutional community engagement.[22,154] At a minimum, curricular faculty must model cultural humility and reflective practices in their conversations with community partners and ensure that community members are acknowledged for their work.

Faculty Development for All

To address the targeted learning environment, faculty development should build the faculty member's skills to create an inclusive and equitable learning environment, *regardless of what is being taught.* As learner cohorts become increasingly diverse in health professions education, these skills are needed by all teaching faculty. Faculty development may do the following: foster critical reflection on one's own implicit bias and teaching behaviors, examine structural problems with grading and assessment, present successful strategies for teaching diverse student groups, and offer practice recognizing and addressing microaggressions in the learning environment.[155,156]

Piloting and Phasing In

Given the complexity of health equity curricula, it is often wise to develop a piloting and phasing-in approach to implementation. Volunteer students in a "selective" may have deeper motivations and/or more background in equity issues and be more receptive and adaptive to the first implementation of a curriculum.

EXAMPLE: *Recruiting Volunteers for Community Electives and Service Learning.* Following completion of year 1 community field experiences, medical students were offered a variety of community-based electives in different clinical settings. These included a student-run interprofessional free clinic, quality improvement teams in intensive care units, geriatric home care, veterans' outpatient practices, and refugee clinics. This led students to find other community experiences in juvenile justice systems and tutoring for high school students. These pilot programs paved the way for an HSS service learning requirement and built a foundation for early community engagement in the curriculum.

STEP 6: EVALUATION AND FEEDBACK

In the final step, both learners and the curriculum are assessed for achievement of curricular goals and learning objectives.

Maintaining congruence between goals and objectives, methods, and assessments is essential to the development of an effective learner assessment plan. The Kirkpatrick framework for program evaluation is a useful tool for health equity curricula, since it reminds the curriculum planners to include outcomes that impact local health systems and communities. The Kirkpatrick framework describes four levels of program evaluation: (1) learner satisfaction; (2) changes in knowledge, attitudes, and skills; (3) changes in practice behavior; and (4) program outcomes in context.[157]

Learner Satisfaction

Level 1 learner satisfaction is straightforward and easily measured through existing trainee evaluation systems, such as end-of-course, end-of-rotation, and end-of-clerkship evaluations. Health equity curricula, which are often novel, provocative, and unanticipated by learners, need to be nimble and responsive. To make prompt adjustments, curriculum leaders should also consider just-in-time learner feedback.

Measures of Change in Learners

Level 2 measures of change in learner attitudes, knowledge, and skills can use traditional methods of survey and attitudinal instruments (see Step 2, above), knowledge tests, and demonstration of skills with real or standardized patients (see Chapter 7).

EXAMPLE: *Measure of Student Structural Skills.* Faculty at Vanderbilt University developed a prehealth 36-credit undergraduate major, Medicine, Health and Society (MHS), which uses an interdisciplinary approach to develop structural competency, the ability to understand how structural factors affect health. A new survey, the Structural Foundations of Health Survey, was developed to assess students' analytic skills. The survey was administered to MHS majors, premed science majors, and first-year students; MHS majors identified structural factors and health outcomes at higher rates and in deeper ways and demonstrated higher awareness of *structural racism* and *health disparities* than the comparison students.[158]

EXAMPLE: *Concept-Mapping in Patient Navigation.* As part of a patient navigator program, early medical students are presented with complex case scenarios that they use to develop concept maps, identifying factors that led to the patient's presentation. Students work in teams as they craft a visual of all the causes for the current presentation from the system to the individual levels. This is followed by a facilitated ST debrief and reflection to present explicitly how the different factors are interconnected. To model ST, the maps are then assessed for interconnectedness and causal loops that illuminate layers of complexity and intersectionality.

There are several published instruments, with validity evidence, to assess ST, cultural competence, empathy/compassion, professionalism, and teamwork.[159,160] For cultural competence, there are more than 20 published self-administered, validated assessment instruments.[161] Several are grounded in self-efficacy theory and may translate into clinical practice behaviors.[162]

Assessing Practice Behavior

Level 3 practice behavior changes are often measured by practitioner self-report. A more rigorous approach, however, involves direct observation or audit of practice.

EXAMPLE: *Measuring Change in Practice Behaviors in Sexual History–Taking.* Sexual and gender minority (SGM) patients experience numerous health disparities and poorer outcomes in preventive care, mental health, cancer, substance use, and violence. Structural barriers as well as personal attitudes and behaviors of providers and patients during the clinical encounter contribute to health disparities, often by inhibiting disclosure.[163] A majority of surveyed physicians in one study reported that they did not have the skills to work with SGM patients.[164] An internal medicine residency program designed a brief intervention of three sessions on sexual history–taking. Chart audits of resident patients pre- and post-intervention showed improved documentation of sexual history (22% vs. 31%, respectively).[165]

Because health equity curricular goals often include instilling the habit of ST, and a professional identity that embraces advocacy for patients, communities, and populations, the evaluation plan will want to include insight into achievement of these learner competencies.

Assessing Reflective Capacity and Professional Identity Formation

Developing reflection and reflective practice is a goal of many curricula and embedded in the competencies of cultural humility, advocacy, and structural competence.[166,167] While reflective capacity has been assessed with self-report questionnaires,[156] reflective capacity is more often encouraged and tracked with *reflective writing*, *journaling*, or maintenance of personal *learning portfolios*[156,167–170] (see also Chapter 7). Rubrics and qualitative analysis support the validity of the learning portfolio assessment.[171–174]

EXAMPLE: *Reflective Writing in a Longitudinal Integrated Clerkship (LIC) Focused on Care of the Underserved.* Medical students participating in an 11-month LIC, with experiences in a public safety-net hospital and community health centers, were required to submit three reflective essays, responding to specific prompts, over the course of time in the clerkship. The essays were subsequently analyzed using an inductive analytic process. The six themes identified in the analysis of 45 essays were care for the underserved, therapeutic alliance, humility and gratitude, altruism, resilience, and aspirations. The authors concluded that professional identity construction in students was observed through the essays.[175]

Focus groups of learners, coupled with qualitative analysis, can provide rich information about the learner experience—what was learned and how learners perceived their own professional development in a health equity curriculum.[176]

Assessing the Curriculum's Added Value to the Community

Although Level 4 is often the most challenging level of program evaluation for curricula, this should be a natural product of a well-designed health equity curriculum. When community activities are designed with an intent to "add value" to the community, or the community partner's mission, the evaluation plan should easily accommodate collection of this information.[177] (Refer to the Example "Critical Service Learning" under Step 4, above.) Patient navigator programs can track completed appointments, adherence to treatment recommendations, and patient satisfaction. Student-run clinics have documented improved cancer screening rates and chronic disease metrics, as well as improved access to health insurance.[178–181] Student health coaches can monitor patient satisfaction and behavioral change.[182] Tracking, analyzing, and communicating these outcomes in the evaluation reinforce the community engagement in the curriculum.

Evaluation criteria for social accountability of schools are in development.[12,29,47,183] Schools and programs with a mission of social accountability can have difficulty in documenting population health outcomes, but they have successfully documented improved recruitment of underrepresented students into health professions, increased selection of primary care careers, and eventual practice of graduates in underserved areas.[145,176,184]

> **EXAMPLE**: *Career Choices of Graduates from an Integrated Curriculum Addressing Health Equity.* A medical school in Israel was founded with a mission of humanism and community-oriented primary care. Half of alumni were subsequently found to be involved with social medicine and working in areas of health inequities versus 30% of alumni of research-oriented medical schools.[107]

CONCLUSION

The next generation of health professionals must be equipped to care for both individuals and populations. Inherent in population health curricula is recognizing the differences in health among populations and communities that cannot be explained by biology alone. This requires an appreciation of the systemic and structural determinants of health to develop an understanding of health disparities and advocacy tools for health professionals. This tall order demands that learners possess both the content and process expertise to understand and transform the systems and structures that result in contemporary health inequities. The six-step approach outlined here provides health professions educators with a systematic methodology to develop innovative health equity curricula that prepare the next generation of health care change agents.

QUESTIONS

Assuming that you are developing a curriculum in health equity relevant to a local community in which your school/training program resides:

1. Describe your institution's history, mission, and commitment to health equity. Does your institution have a mission statement that addresses equity, diversity, and inclusion (EDI)? If so, what institutional activities are currently in place to promote this mission? Who is directing those activities?

2. Describe your institution's resources to support a health equity curriculum. Does your institution have external partnerships aimed at improving the health of the community? Are there other professional school faculty, government or health system leaders, or research centers that can serve as experts in development and implementation of a health equity curriculum? Can community members serve as experts in the development and implementation of this curriculum?

3. How do you define the community of focus? Is there a distinction between your local community and various populations served by the health professions school? What is known about the health outcomes of populations and local communities when examined by geography, race/ethnicity, socioeconomic status, and so on? Are there community health assessments/data (from public health, health care systems,

community-based organizations, or others) available that detail local/regional/state/territorial community health outcomes and the root causes or historical context of health disparities?

4. Describe your program's approach to preparing health professionals for practice and continuous improvement in modern health care systems. Is there an HSS curriculum? If not, what are the opportunities for integrating HSS into the current curriculum? How is the HSS curriculum integrated with the basic and clinical science curricula?

5. How do the learners experience the current curriculum and learning environment with respect to equity, diversity, and inclusion?

6. Are the social determinants of health currently taught in the curriculum? If so, how is this content integrated horizontally and vertically?

7. What emerging competencies in EDI are currently missing in your program for faculty and students? What knowledge, skills, attitudes, and behaviors will your curriculum address?

8. Will the current program/curriculum accommodate a longitudinal approach to teaching health equity? What educational methods will be congruent with achievement of these skills, attitudes, and behaviors?

9. Are there community-based engagement activities in the current school/program? If so, can they be structured as critical service learning opportunities for students or as longitudinal "added value" experiences for students with vulnerable populations?

10. What faculty development activities are currently in place to promote EDI? What new faculty skills will need development in your curriculum?

11. Could you identify learners who would be willing to pilot a new curriculum?

12. What curricular outcomes will you track? How do these outcomes align with the goals and objectives of the curriculum, and how do they support the achievement of competencies?

GENERAL REFERENCES

American Medical Association. "Organizational Strategic Plan to Embed Racial Justice and Advance Health Equity." Accessed October 7, 2021. https://www.ama-assn.org/about/leadership/ama-s-strategic-plan-embed-racial-justice-and-advance-health-equity.
    This plan was initiated by the AMA's Health Equity Task Force with the launch of the AMA Center for Health Equity. With multiple stakeholder voices both inside and outside the AMA, this plan provides an inclusive three-year map with five strategic approaches to advance a health equity agenda. In addition to helpful historical discussion, the plan provides specific actions and accountability for racial justice while discussing other forms of equity.

Dankwa-Mullan, Irene, Eliseo J. Perez-Stable, Kevin L. Gardner, Xinzhi Zhang, and Adelaida M. Rosario, eds. The Science of Health Disparities Research. Hoboken, NJ: Wiley Blackwell, 2021.
    A comprehensive text providing details on conducting clinical and translational health disparities studies. This 26-chapter textbook provides an all-inclusive view on the topic, ranging from basic definitions of health disparity science to conceptual frameworks for identifying disparities. The book

provides a practical guide for new areas of research, capacity-building strategies, and tools to advance health equity.

National Academies of Sciences, Engineering, and Medicine. *Communities in Action: Pathways to Health Equity*. Washington, DC: National Academies Press, 2017. https://doi.org/10.17226 /24624.
This report provides a review of the health disparities within the United States and discusses factors that cause such disparities, called determinants of health. It recognizes that community-wide problems, such as poverty, poor education, and inadequate housing, play a larger role in an individual's health than behavior. This report outlines these structural barriers to health equity coupled with solutions that guide a community as to what they can do to promote health for all.

National Collaborating Centre for Determinants of Health. "Let's Talk: Moving Upstream." Antigonish, NS: National Collaborating Centre for Determinants of Health, St. Francis Xavier University, 2014. Accessed October 7, 2021, https://nccdh.ca/resources/entry/lets-talk-moving-upstream.
The purpose of this publication is to use the classic public health parable to reframe the health inequities discussion into "upstream, midstream, and downstream" causes. This practical publication serves as a communication tool for public health teams and provides a guide for standard language. It helps teams to ask appropriate questions so they can identify the level of the root causes and respective strategies and resources that would be the most effective to address a given cause.

Plack, Margaret M., Ellen F. Goldman, Andrea R. Scott, and Shelley B. Brundage. *Systems Thinking in the Healthcare Professions: A Guide for Educators and Clinicians*. Washington, DC: George Washington University, 2019. Accessed October 7, 2021. https://hsrc.himmelfarb .gwu.edu/cgi/viewcontent.cgi?article=1000&context=educational_resources_teaching.
A thorough overview for health professional educators on how to integrate and assess systems thinking in their curriculum. This readable monograph uses a step wise approach from competency to assessment of systems thinking skills and provides instructional examples for course and clinical educators.

Skochelak, Susan E., Maya M. Hammoud, Kimberly D. Lomis, Jeffrey M. Borkan, Jed D. Gonzalo, Luan E. Lawson, and Stephanie R. Starr S, eds. *Health Systems Science*, Second Edition. St. Louis, MO: Elsevier, 2021.
A comprehensive textbook that reviews the emerging field of HSS and all the different domains of HSS that impact health care delivery at the patient and population level. The book offers challenges and solutions to a complicated health care system and practical exercises and learning strategies for the health care educator teaching HSS.

Waters Center for Systems Thinking. Accessed October 7, 2021. https://waterscenterst.org/.
An internationally recognized and practical website dedicated to dissemination of systems thinking knowledge and skills for all walks of life. The website provides resources to individuals and organizations on how to leverage systems thinking and apply it to their daily work. It also has important tools such as the 12 Habits of a Systems Thinker and practical exercises on how to teach and evaluate systems thinking.

REFERENCES CITED

1. National Collaborating Centre for Determinants of Health, "Let's Talk: Moving Upstream," (Antigonish, NS: National Collaborating Centre for Determinants of Health, St. Francis Xavier University, 2014), accessed October 7, 2021, https://nccdh.ca/resources/entry/lets-talk-moving-upstream.
2. Paula Braveman et al., "What Is Health Equity? And What Difference Does a Definition Make?" (Princeton, NJ: Robert Wood Johnson Foundation, 2017), accessed October 7, 2021, https:// nccdh.ca/resources/entry/what-is-health-equity-and-what-difference-does-a-definition-make.

3. National Academies of Sciences, Engineering, and Medicine, *Communities in Action: Pathways to Health Equity* (Washington, DC: National Academies Press, 2017), https://doi.org/10.17226/24624.

4. Brian C. Castrucci and John Auerbach, "Meeting Individual Social Needs Falls Short of Addressing Social Determinants of Health," Health Affairs Blog, 2019, accessed October 7, 2021, https://www.healthaffairs.org/do/10.1377/hblog20190115.234942.

5. Commission on Social Determinants of Health, *Closing the Gap in a Generation: Health Equity through Action on the Social Determinants of Health: Final Report of the Commission on Social Determinants of Health* (Geneva, World Health Organization, 2008), accessed October 7, 2021, https://www.who.int/publications/i/item/WHO-IER-CSDH-08.1.

6. Paula A. Braveman et al., "Health Disparities and Health Equity: The Issue Is Justice," *American Journal of Public Health* 101, no. Suppl 1 (2011): S149–55, https://doi.org/10.2105/ajph.2010.300062.

7. Peter S. Hovmand, *Community Based System Dynamics* (New York: Springer, 2014).

8. John A. Powell, *Structural Racism: Building upon the Insights of John Calmore*, 86 N.C. L. Rev. 791 (2008), accessed October 7, 2021, https://scholarship.law.unc.edu/nclr/vol86/iss3/8.

9. Margaret Whitehead, "The Concepts and Principles of Equity and Health," *International Journal of Health Services* 22, no. 3 (1992): 429–45, https://doi.org/10.2190/986L-LHQ6-2VTE-YRRN.

10. Julian T. Hart, "The Inverse Care Law," *The Lancet* 1, no. 7696 (1971): 405–12, https://doi.org/10.1016/s0140-6736(71)92410-x.

11. Paula A. Braveman et al., "Socioeconomic Disparities in Health in the United States: What the Patterns Tell Us," *American Journal of Public Health* 100, no. S1 (2010): S186–96, https://doi.org/10.2105/ajph.2009.166082.

12. Charles D. Boelen et al., "Accrediting Excellence for a Medical School's Impact on Population Health," *Education for Health (Abingdon)* 32, no. 1 (2019): 41–48, https://doi.org/10.4103/efh.EfH_204_19.

13. Donald M. Berwick and Jonathan A. Finkelstein, "Preparing Medical Students for the Continual Improvement of Health and Health Care: Abraham Flexner and the New 'Public Interest,'" *Academic Medicine* 85, no. 9 Suppl (2010): S56–65, https://doi.org/10.1097/ACM.0b013e3181ead779.

14. Hilary S. Daniel, Sue S. Bornstein, and Gregory C. Kane, "Addressing Social Determinants to Improve Patient Care and Promote Health Equity: An American College of Physicians Position Paper," *Annals of Internal Medicine* 168, no. 8 (2018): 577–78, https://doi.org/10.7326/M17-2441.

15. Susan E. Skochelak et. al., *Health Systems Science*, 2nd ed. (St. Louis, MO: Elsevier, 2021).

16. Mamta K. Singh, Heidi L. Gullett, and Patricia A. Thomas, "Using Kern's Six-Step Approach to Integrate Health Systems Science in Medical Education," *Academic Medicine* 96, no. 9 (2021), 1282–90, https://doi.org/10.1097/ACM.0000000000004141.

17. Peter M. Senge, *The Fifth Discipline: The Art and Practice of the Learning Organization* (New York: Doubleday/Currency, 2006).

18. Thelma P. Quince et al., "Undergraduate Medical Students' Empathy: Current Perspectives," *Advanced Medical Education Practice* 7 (2016): 443–55, https://doi.org/10.2147/amep.S76800.

19. Margaret M. Plack et al., "Systems Thinking and Systems-Based Practice across the Health Professions: An Inquiry into Definitions, Teaching Practices, and Assessment," *Teaching and Learning in Medicine* 30, no. 3 (2018): 242–54, https://doi.org/10.1080/10401334.2017.1398654.

20. "Habits of a Systems Thinker," Waters Center for Systems Thinking, accessed October 7, 2021, https://waterscenterst.org/.

21. Mark A. Earnest, Shale L. Wong, and Steven G. Federico, "Perspective: Physician Advocacy: What Is It and How Do We Do It?" *Academic Medicine* 85, no. 1 (2010): 63–67, https://doi.org/10.1097/ACM.0b013e3181c40d40.

22. Center for Disease Control and Prevention, *Principles of Community Engagement*. 2nd ed. (Atlanta: CDC/ATSR Committee on Community Engagement, 2011), accessed May 31, 2021, https://www.atsdr.cdc.gov/communityengagement/index.html.

23. Roger Strasser et al., "Putting Communities in the Driver's Seat: The Realities of Community-Engaged Medical Education," *Academic Medicine* 90, no. 11 (2015): 1466–70, https://doi.org/10.1097/ACM.0000000000000765.

24. Cayla R. Teal and Richard L. Street, "Critical Elements of Culturally Competent Communication in the Medical Encounter: A Review and Model," *Social Science & Medicine* 68, no. 3 (2009): 533–43, https://doi.org/10.1016/j.socscimed.2008.10.015.

25. Melanie Tervalon and Jann Murray-García, "Cultural Humility versus Cultural Competence: A Critical Distinction in Defining Physician Training Outcomes in Multicultural Education," *Journal of Health Care for the Poor and Underserved* 9, no. 2 (1998): 117–25, https://doi.org/10.1353/hpu.2010.0233.

26. Elana Curtis et al., "Why Cultural Safety Rather Than Cultural Competency Is Required to Achieve Health Equity: A Literature Review and Recommended Definition," *International Journal of Equity in Health* 18, no. 1 (2019): 174, https://doi.org/10.1186/s12939-019-1082-3.

27. "11 Terms You Should Know to Better Understand Structural Racism," Aspen Institute, accessed October 7, 2021, https://www.aspeninstitute.org/blog-posts/structural-racism-definition/.

28. "Health Inequities and Their Causes," World Health Organization, accessed October 7, 2021, https://www.who.int/features/factfiles/health_inequities/en/.

29. Institute of Medicine, *Unequal Treatment: Confronting Racial and Ethnic Disparities in Health Care* (Washington, DC: National Academies Press, 2003), https://doi.org/10.17226/10260.

30. "Healthy People 2020: Disparities," Office of Disease Prevention and Health Promotion, accessed October 7, 2021, https://www.healthypeople.gov/2020/about/foundation-health-measures/Disparities.

31. Project Implicit, accessed October 7, 2021, https://implicit.harvard.edu/implicit/takeatest.html.

32. "Diversity and Inclusion, Definitions of," in *The Sage Encyclopedia of Intercultural Competence*, ed. Janet M. Bennett (Thousand Oaks, CA: SAGE Publications, 2015), 267–69.

33. Jonathan M. Metzl and Helena Hansen, "Structural Competency: Theorizing a New Medical Engagement with Stigma and Inequality," *Social Science & Medicine* 103 (2014): 126–33, https://doi.org/10.1016/j.socscimed.2013.06.032.

34. Camara P. Jones, "Toward the Science and Practice of Anti-racism: Launching a National Campaign against Racism," *Ethnicity & Disease* 28, no. Suppl 1 (2018): 231–34, https://doi.org/10.18865/ed.28.S1.231.

35. "Underrepresented in Medicine Definition," Association of American Medical Colleges, accessed October 7, 2021, https://www.aamc.org/what-we-do/equity-diversity-inclusion/underrepresented-in-medicine.

36. Gopal K. Singh et al., "Social Determinants of Health in the United States: Addressing Major Health Inequality Trends for the Nation, 1935–2016," *International Journal of Maternal Child Health and AIDS* 6, no. 2 (2017): 139–64, https://doi.org/10.21106/ijma.236.

37. Jarvis T. Chen and Nancy Krieger, "Revealing the Unequal Burden of COVID-19 by Income, Race/Ethnicity and Household Crowding: US County versus Zip Code Analyses," *Journal of Public Health Management and Practice*, 27 Suppl 1 (2020): S43–56, https://doi.org/10.1097/PHH.0000000000001263.

38. Theresa Andrasfay and Noreen Goldman, "Reductions in 2020 US Life Expectancy Due to COVID-19 and the Disproportionate Impact on the Black and Latino Populations," *Proceedings of the National Academy of Sciences* 118, no. 5 (2021): e2014746118, https://doi.org/10.1073/pnas.2014746118.

39. Elizabeth Fee and Ana Rita Gonzalez, "The History of Health Equity: Concept and Vision," *Diversity & Equality in Health and Care* 14, no. 3 (2017): 148–52, https://diversityhealthcare.imedpub.com/the-history-of-health-equity-concept-and-vision.pdf.

40. "Healthy People 2010," Centers for Disease Control and Prevention, accessed October 7, 2021, https://www.cdc.gov/nchs/healthy_people/hp2010.htm.

41. Frederick J. Zimmerman and Nathaniel W. Anderson, "Trends in Health Equity in the United States by Race/Ethnicity, Sex, and Income, 1993–2017," *JAMA Network Open* 2, no. 6 (2019): e196386, https://doi.org/10.1001/jamanetworkopen.2019.6386.

42. Institute of Medicine, *Primary Care and Public Health: Exploring Integration to Improve Population Health* (Washington, DC: National Academies Press, 2012), https://doi.org/10.17226/13381.

43. Harvey V. Fineberg, "Public Health and Medicine: Where the Twain Shall Meet," *American Journal of Preventive Medicine* 41, no. 4 Suppl 3 (2011): S149–51, https://doi.org/10.1016/j.amepre.2011.07.013.

44. A. M. Brandt and M. Gardner, "Antagonism and Accommodation: Interpreting the Relationship between Public Health and Medicine in the United States During the 20th Century," *American Journal of Public Health* 90, no. 5 (2000): 707–15, https://doi.org/10.2105/ajph.90.5.707.

45. The Association of Faculties of Medicine in Canada, *The Future of Medical Education in Canada: A Collective Vision for MD Education,* (Ottawa: AFMC, 2010), accessed October 7, 2021, https://cou.ca/wp-content/uploads/2010/01/COU-Future-of-Medical-Education-in-Canada-A-Collective-Vision.pdf.

46. Robert F. Woollard, "Caring for a Common Future: Medical Schools' Social Accountability," *Medical Education* 40, no. 4 (2006): 301–13, https://doi.org/10.1111/j.1365-2929.2006.02416.x.

47. Charles Boelen, Jeffrey E. Heck, and the World Health Organization, Division of Development of Human Resources for Health, "Defining and Measuring the Social Accountability of Medical Schools," 1995, accessed October 7, 2021, https://apps.who.int/iris/handle/10665/59441.

48. James Rourke, "Social Accountability: A Framework for Medical Schools to Improve the Health of the Populations They Serve," *Academic Medicine* 93, no. 8 (2018): 1120–24, https://doi.org/10.1097/acm.0000000000002239.

49. "Community Health Assessment Toolkit," Association for Community Health Improvement, accessed October 7, 2021, https://www.healthycommunities.org/resources/community-health-assessment-toolkit.

50. "Mobilizing for Action through Planning and Partnerships (MAPP)," National Association of County and City Health Officials, accessed October 7, 2021, https://www.naccho.org/programs/public-health-infrastructure/performance-improvement/community-health-assessment/mapp.

51. Health Improvement Partnership–Cuyahoga, accessed October 7, 2021, https://hipcuyahoga.org.

52. "2018 National Healthcare Quality and Disparities Report," Agency for Healthcare Research and Quality, accessed October 7, 2021, https://www.ahrq.gov/research/findings/nhqrdr/nhqdr18/index.html.

53. "Cuyahoga Place Matters: History Matters Report," Kirwan Institute for the Study of Race and Ethnicity, accessed October 7, 2021, https://kirwaninstitute.osu.edu/research/cuyahoga-placematters-history-matters-report.

54. Anthony Nardone, Joey Chiang, and Jason Corburn, "Historic Redlining and Urban Health Today in U.S. Cities," *Environmental Justice* 13, no. 4 (2020): 109–19, https://doi.org/10.1089/env.2020.0011.

55. "Clark-Fulton MetroHealth EcoDistrict," MetroHealth, accessed October 7, 2021, https://www.metrohealth.org/transformation/transformation-blog/clark-fulton-metrohealth-ecodistrict.

56. East Baltimore Development, Inc., accessed October 7, 2021, www.ebdi.org.

57. "Care Process Model: Social Determinants of Health," Intermountain Healthcare, accessed October 7, 2021, https://intermountainhealthcare.org/ckr-ext/Dcmnt?ncid=529732182.

58. "Our Commitment to End Racism in Health Care," Froedtert and Medical College of Wisconsin, accessed October 7, 2021, https://www.froedtert.com/end-racism.

59. "American Hospital Association #123forEquity Campaign to Eliminate Health Care Disparities," AHA Institute for Diversity and Health Equity, accessed October 7, 2021, https://ifdhe.aha.org/123forequity.

60. Kevin A. Schulman et al., "The Effect of Race and Sex on Physicians' Recommendations for Cardiac Catheterization," *New England Journal of Medicine* 340, no. 8 (1999): 618–26, https://doi.org/10.1056/nejm199902253400806.

61. Robert C. Like, "Educating Clinicians about Cultural Competence and Disparities in Health and Health Care," *Journal of Continuing Education in the Health Professions* 31, no. 3 (2011): 196–206, https://doi.org/10.1002/chp.20127.

62. Lidia Horvat et al., "Cultural Competence Education for Health Professionals," *Cochrane Database of Systematic Reviews*, no. 5 (2014), https://doi.org/10.1002/14651858.CD009405.pub2.

63. Stephanie M. Shepherd, "Cultural Awareness Workshops: Limitations and Practical Consequences," *BMC Medical Education* 19, no. 1 (2019): 14, https://doi.org/10.1186/s12909-018-1450-5.

64. "Curriculum Reports: Social Determinants of Health by Academic Level," AAMC, accessed October 7, 2021, https://www.aamc.org/data-reports/curriculum-reports/interactive-data/social-determinants-health-academic-level.

65. Joy H. Lewis et al., "Addressing the Social Determinants of Health in Undergraduate Medical Education Curricula: A Survey Report," *Advances in Medical Education and Practice* 11 (2020): 369–77, https://doi.org/10.2147/amep.S243827.

66. George E. Thibault, "Reforming Health Professions Education Will Require Culture Change and Closer Ties between Classroom and Practice," *Health Affairs* 32, no. 11 (2013): 1928–32, https://doi.org/10.1377/hlthaff.2013.0827.

67. Christina Amutah et al., "Misrepresenting Race—the Role of Medical Schools in Propagating Physician Bias," *New England Journal of Medicine* 384 (2021): 872–78, https://doi.org/10.1056/NEJMms2025768.

68. Aparna Krishnan et al., "Addressing Race, Culture, and Structural Inequality in Medical Education: A Guide for Revising Teaching Cases," *Academic Medicine* 94, no. 4 (2019): 550–55, https://doi.org/10.1097/acm.0000000000002589.

69. Kimberly D. Acquaviva and Matthew Mintz, "Perspective: Are We Teaching Racial Profiling? The Dangers of Subjective Determinations of Race and Ethnicity in Case Presentations," *Academic Medicine* 85, no. 4 (2010): 702–5, https://doi.org/10.1097/ACM.0b013e3181d296c7.

70. Kelly M. Hoffman et al., "Racial Bias in Pain Assessment and Treatment Recommendations, and False Beliefs about Biological Differences between Blacks and Whites," *Proceedings of the National Academy of Sciences* 113, no. 16 (2016): 4296–301, https://doi.org/10.1073/pnas.1516047113.

71. Donna Cormack et al., "Ethnic Bias amongst Medical Students in Aotearoa/New Zealand: Findings from the Bias and Decision Making in Medicine (BDMM) Study," *PLOS One* 13, no. 8 (2018): e0201168, https://doi.org/10.1371/journal.pone.0201168.

72. Liaison Committee on Medical Education, *Functions and Structure of a Medical School: Standards for Accreditation of Medical Education Programs Leading to the MD Degree*, March 2021, accessed October 7, 2021, https://lcme.org/publications/.

73. Association of American Medical Colleges (AAMC), *Roadmap to Diversity and Educational Excellence: Key Legal and Educational Policy Foundations for Medical Schools*. 2nd ed. (Washington, DC: AAMC, 2014), accessed October 7, 2021, https://store.aamc.org/roadmap-to-diversity-and-educational-excellence-key-legal-and-educational-policy-foundations-for-medical-schools-pdf.html.

74. Doreen C. Parkhurst, Gerald Kayingo, and Shani Fleming, "Redesigning Physician Assistant Education to Promote Cognitive Diversity, Inclusion, and Health Care Equity," *Journal of Physician Assistant Education* 28 Suppl 1 (2017): S38–42, https://doi.org/10.1097/jpa.0000000000000128.

75. Ryan L. Crass and Frank Romanelli, "Curricular Reform in Pharmacy Education through the Lens of the Flexner Report of 1910," *American Journal of Pharmaceutical Education* 82, no. 7 (2018): 6804, https://doi.org/10.5688/ajpe6804.

76. Institute of Medicine (US) Committee on the Robert Wood Johnson Foundation Initiative on the Future of Nursing, "Transforming Education: The Need to Increase Diversity of the Nursing Workforce," in *The Future of Nursing: Leading Change, Advancing Health* (Washington, DC: National Academies Press, 2011), accessed October 7, 2021, https://www.ncbi.nlm.nih.gov/books/NBK209885/.

77. Committee on the Governance and Financing of Graduate Medical Education; Board on Health Care Services; Institute of Medicine; Jill Eden, Donald Berwick and Gail Wilensky, eds., *Graduate Medical Education That Meets the Nation's Health Needs* (Washington, DC: National Academies Press, 2014), accessed June 1, 2021, https://doi.org/10.17226/18754.

78. Samantha Saha et al., "Student Body Racial and Ethnic Composition and Diversity-Related Outcomes in US Medical Schools," *JAMA* 300, no. 10 (2008): 1135–45, https://doi.org/10.1001/jama.300.10.1135.

79. Brad N. Greenwood et al., "Physician-Patient Racial Concordance and Disparities in Birthing Mortality for Newborns," *Proceedings of the National Academy of Sciences* 117, no. 35 (2020): 21194–200, https://doi.org/10.1073/pnas.1913405117.

80. Louis W. Sullivan and Ilana Suez Mittman, "The State of Diversity in the Health Professions a Century after Flexner," *Academic Medicine* 85, no. 2 (2010): 246–53, https://doi.org/10.1097/ACM.0b013e3181c88145.

81. Gretchen Guiton, Mitchell J. Chang, and LuAnn Wilkerson, "Student Body Diversity: Relationship to Medical Students' Experiences and Attitudes," *Academic Medicine* 82, no. 10 (2007): S85–88, https://doi.org/10.1097/ACM.0b013e31813ffe1e.

82. Cyndy R. Snyder, Bianca K. Frogner, and Susan M. Skillman, "Facilitating Racial and Ethnic Diversity in the Health Workforce," *Journal of Allied Health* 47, no. 1 (2018): 58–65.

83. "Diversity in Medicine: Facts and Figures 2019," Association of American Medical Colleges, accessed October 7, 2021, https://www.aamc.org/data-reports/workforce/report/diversity-medicine-facts-and-figures-2019.

84. Association of American Medical Colleges (AAMC), *Altering the Course: Black Males in Medicine* (Washington, DC: AAMC, 2015), accessed October 7, 2021, https://store.aamc.org/altering-the-course-black-males-in-medicine.html.

85. Saleem Razack and Ingrid Philibert, "Inclusion in the Clinical Learning Environment: Building the Conditions for Diverse Human Flourishing," *Medical Teacher* 41, no. 4 (2019): 380–84, https://doi.org/10.1080/0142159X.2019.1566600.

86. Tomas Diaz, J. Renee Navarro, and Esther H. Chen, "An Institutional Approach to Fostering Inclusion and Addressing Racial Bias: Implications for Diversity in Academic Medicine," *Teaching and Learning in Medicine* 32, no. 1 (2020): 110–16, https://doi.org/10.1080/10401334.2019.1670665.

87. Arianne Teherani et al., "How Small Differences in Assessed Clinical Performance Amplify to Large Differences in Grades and Awards: A Cascade with Serious Consequences for Students Underrepresented in Medicine," *Academic Medicine* 93, no. 9 (2018): 1286–92, https://doi.org/10.1097/ACM.0000000000002323.

88. "Common Program Requirements (Residency)," Accreditation Council for Graduate Medical Education, 2020, accessed October 7, 2021, https://www.acgme.org/what-we-do/accreditation/common-program-requirements/.

89. "Diversity, Equity and Inclusion in Academic Nursing: AACN Position Statement," American Association of Colleges of Nursing, 2017, accessed October 7, 2021, https://www.aacnnursing.org/News-Information/Position-Statements-White-Papers/Diversity.

90. Jason R. Frank, Linda Snell, and Jonathan Sherbino, eds., *CanMEDS 2015 Physician Competency Framework* (Ottawa: Royal College of Physicians and Surgeons of Canada, 2015), accessed October 7, 2021, http://canmeds.royalcollege.ca/uploads/en/framework/CanMEDS%202015%20Framework_EN_Reduced.pdf.

91. General Medical Council, *Outcomes for Graduates 2018*, accessed October 7, 2021, https://www.gmc-uk.org/-/media/documents/dc11326-outcomes-for-graduates-2018_pdf-75040796.pdf.

92. "PharmD Program Accreditation," Accreditation Council for Pharmacy Education, accessed October 7, 2021, https://www.acpe-accredit.org/pharmd-program-accreditation/.

93. Interprofessional Education Collaborative, *Core Competencies for Interprofessional Collaborative Practice: 2016 Update* (Washington, DC: Interprofessional Education Collaborative, 2016), accessed October 8, 2021, https://www.ipecollaborative.org/ipec-core-competencies.

94. Public Health Accreditation Board, "Advancing Health Equity in Health Department's Public Health Practice," accessed October 7, 2021, https://www.phaboard.org/wp-content/uploads/HIP-Paper-Final.pdf.

95. Kristen Simone et al., "What Are the Features of Targeted or System-Wide Initiatives That Affect Diversity in Health Professions Trainees? A BEME Systematic Review: BEME Guide No. 50," *Medical Teacher* 40, no. 8 (2018): 762–80, https://doi.org/10.1080/0142159X.2018.1473562.

96. Monica B. Vela et al., "Improving Underrepresented Minority Medical Student Recruitment with Health Disparities Curriculum," *Journal of General Internal Medicine* 25, no. Suppl 2 (2010): S82–85, https://doi.org/10.1007/s11606-010-1270-8.

97. Quinn Capers IV et al., "Implicit Racial Bias in Medical School Admissions," *Academic Medicine* 92, no. 3 (2017): 365–69, https://doi.org/10.1097/acm.0000000000001388.

98. Alda Maria R. Gonzaga et al., "A Framework for Inclusive Graduate Medical Education Recruitment Strategies: Meeting the ACGME Standard for a Diverse and Inclusive Workforce," *Academic Medicine* 95, no. 5 (2019): 710–16, https://doi.org/10.1097/acm.0000000000003073.

99. Kelly E. Mahon, Mackenzie K. Henderson, and Darrell G. Kirch, "Selecting Tomorrow's Physicians: The Key to the Future Health Care Workforce," *Academic Medicine* 88, no. 12 (2013): 1806–11, https://doi.org/10.1097/acm.0000000000000023.

100. M. E. Muntinga et al., "Toward Diversity-Responsive Medical Education: Taking an Intersectionality-Based Approach to a Curriculum Evaluation," *Advances in Health Sciences Education* 21, no. 3 (2016): 541–59, https://doi.org/10.1007/s10459-015-9650-9.

101. Philippe Bourgois et al., "Structural Vulnerability: Operationalizing the Concept to Address Health Disparities in Clinical Care," *Academic Medicine* 92, no. 3 (2017): 299–307, https://doi.org/10.1097/ACM.0000000000001294.

102. Allison A. Vanderbilt et al., "Curricular Integration of Social Medicine: A Prospective for Medical Educators," *Medical Education Online* 21 (2016): 30586, https://doi.org/10.3402/meo.v21.30586.

103. Valarie B. Jernigan et al., "An Examination of Cultural Competence Training in US Medical Education Guided by the Tool for Assessing Cultural Competence Training," *Journal of Health Disparities Research and Practice* 9, no. 3 (2016): 150–67.

104. Lynn M. VanderWielen et al., "Health Disparities and Underserved Populations: A Potential Solution, Medical School Partnerships with Free Clinics to Improve Curriculum," *Medical Education Online* 20 (2015): 27535, https://doi.org/10.3402/meo.v20.27535.

105. Nicole Mareno, Patricia L. Hart, and Lewis VanBrackle, "Psychometric Validation of the Revised Clinical Cultural Competency Questionnaire," *Journal of Nursing Measurement* 21, no. 3 (2013): 426–36, https://doi.org/10.1891/1061-3749.21.3.426.

106. Erica V. Tate and Melanie Prestidge, "Evaluating the Effectiveness of a Structural Competency and Bias in Medicine Curriculum for Internal Medicine Residents," *Journal of General Internal Medicine* 35, no. 1 (2020): 725, https://doi.org/10.1007/s11606-020-05890-3.

107. Keren Dopelt et al., "Reducing Health Disparities: The Social Role of Medical Schools," *Medical Teacher* 36, no. 6 (2014): 511–17, https://doi.org/10.3109/0142159x.2014.891006.

108. World Summit on Social Accountability, *Tunis Declaration,* 2017, accessed October 7, 2021, http://thenetworktufh.org/wp-content/uploads/2017/06/Tunis-Declaration-FINAL-2.pdf.

109. Carole Reeve et al., "The Impact of Socially-Accountable Health Professional Education: A Systematic Review of the Literature," *Medical Teacher* 39, no. 1 (2017): 67–73, https://doi.org/10.1080/0142159x.2016.1231914.

110. Richard VanEck, Heidi L. Gullett, and Kimberly Lomis, "The Power of Interdependence: Linking Health Systems, Communities, and Health Professions Educational Programs to Better Meet the Needs of Patients and Populations," *Medical Teacher* 43, no. sup2 (2021): S32–38, https://doi.org/10.1080/0142159X.2021.1935834.

111. Sharon Parsons, "Addressing Racial Biases in Medicine: A Review of the Literature, Critique, and Recommendations," *International Journal of Health Services* 50, no. 4 (2020): 371–86, https://doi.org/10.1177/0020731420940961.

112. Kaye-Alese Green, Racism in Medicine Vertical Integration Group, "Is Race a Risk Factor? Creating Leadership and Education to Address Racism: An Analytical Review of Best Practices for BUSM Implementation," 2020, accessed October 7, 2021, https://www.bumc.bu.edu/busm/files/2021/06/Racism-in-Medicine-VIG-Final-Report-ExecSummary.pdf.

113. "Mission Matters: Trends in Graduates Practicing in Primary Care, Rural and Underserved Areas, and In State," 2020, Association of American Medical Colleges, accessed October 7, 2021, https://www.aamc.org/media/47636/download.

114. Rose Anne C. Illes et al., "Culturally Responsive Integrated Health Care: Key Issues for Medical Education," *The International Journal of Psychiatry in Medicine* 50, no. 1 (2015): 92–103, https://doi.org/10.1177/0091217415592368.

115. Juanyce Deanna Taylor, "Critical Synthesis Package: Cultural Attitudes Survey," MedEdPORTAL 9 (2013), https://doi.org/doi:10.15766/mep_2374-8265.9477.

116. L. S. Robins et al., "Development and Evaluation of an Instrument to Assess Medical Students' Cultural Attitudes," *Journal of American Medical Women's Association* 53, no. 3 Suppl (1998): 124–27.

117. Wendy L. Sword et al., "Baccalaureate Nursing Students' Attitudes toward Poverty: Implications for Nursing Curricula," *Journal of Nursing Education* 43, no. 1 (2004): 13–19, https://doi.org/10.3928/01484834-20040101-05.

118. Melissa Ehmke and Ericka Sanner-Stiehr, "Improving Attitudes toward Poverty among DNP Students: Implementing a Community Action Poverty Simulation©," *Journal of the American Association of Nurse Practitioners* 33, no. 2 (2020): 150–57, https://doi.org/10.1097/jxx.0000000000000361.

119. Rachel Shor, Jenna M. Calton, and Lauren B. Cattaneo, "The Development of the Systems and Individual Responsibility for Poverty (SIRP) Scale," *Journal of Community Psychology* 46, no. 8 (2018): 1010–25, https://doi.org/10.1002/jcop.22088.

120. Sonia J. S. Crandall, Robert J. Volk, and Vicki Loemker, "Medical Students' Attitudes toward Providing Care for the Underserved: Are We Training Socially Responsible Physicians?" *JAMA* 269, no. 19 (1993): 2519–23, https://doi.org/10.1001/jama.1993.03500190063036.

121. Delese Wear and Mark G. Kuczewski, "Perspective: Medical Students' Perceptions of the Poor: What Impact Can Medical Education Have?" *Academic Medicine* 83, no. 7 (2008): 639–45, https://doi.org/10.1097/ACM.0b013e3181782d67.

122. Sonia J. Crandall et al., "A Longitudinal Comparison of Pharmacy and Medical Students' Attitudes toward the Medically Underserved," *American Journal of Pharmaceutical Education* 72, no. 6 (2008): 148, https://doi.org/10.5688/aj7206148.

123. Mina Habibian, Hazem Seirawan, and Roseann Mulligan, "Dental Students' Attitudes toward Underserved Populations across Four Years of Dental School," *Journal of Dental Education* 75, no. 8 (2011): 1020–29.

124. Mark B. Stephens et al., "Medical Student Attitudes toward the Medically Underserved: The USU Perspective," *Military Medicine* 180, no. 4 Suppl (2015): 61–63, https://doi.org/10.7205/milmed-d-14-00558.

125. Sonia J. Crandall et al., "Medical Students' Attitudes toward Underserved Patients: A Longitudinal Comparison of Problem-Based and Traditional Medical Curricula," *Advances in Health Sciences Education* 12, no. 1 (2007): 71–86, https://doi.org/10.1007/s10459-005-2297-1.

126. Désirée A. Lie et al., "Revising the Tool for Assessing Cultural Competence Training (TACCT) for Curriculum Evaluation: Findings Derived from Seven US Schools and Expert Consensus," *Medical Education Online* 13 (2008): 1–11, https://doi.org/10.3885/meo.2008.Res00272.

127. Aba Osseo-Asare et al., "Minority Resident Physicians' Views on the Role of Race/Ethnicity in Their Training Experiences in the Workplace," *JAMA Network Open* 1, no. 5 (2018): e182723, https://doi.org/10.1001/jamanetworkopen.2018.2723.

128. Katherine A. Hill et al., "Assessment of the Prevalence of Medical Student Mistreatment by Sex, Race/Ethnicity, and Sexual Orientation," *JAMA Internal Medicine* 180, no. 5 (2020): 653–65, https://doi.org/10.1001/jamainternmed.2020.0030.

129. Wally R. Smith et al., "Recommendations for Teaching about Racial and Ethnic Disparities in Health and Health Care," *Annals of Internal Medicine* 147, no. 9 (2007): 654–65, https://doi.org/10.7326/0003-4819-147-9-200711060-00010.

130. Paula T. Ross et al., "A Strategy for Improving Health Disparities Education in Medicine," *Journal of General Internal Medicine* 25 Suppl 2 (2010): S160–63, https://doi.org/10.1007/s11606-010-1283-3.

131. Ashley H. Noriea et al., "Development of a Multifaceted Health Disparities Curriculum for Medical Residents," *Family Medicine* 49, no. 10 (2017): 796–802.

132. Michelle DallaPiazza, Manasa S. Ayyala, and Maria L. Soto-Greene, "Empowering Future Physicians to Advocate for Health Equity: A Blueprint for a Longitudinal Thread in Undergraduate Medical Education," *Medical Teacher* 42, no. 7 (2020): 806–12, https://doi.org/10.1080/0142159x.2020.1737322.

133. Joanna Perdomo et al., "Health Equity Rounds: An Interdisciplinary Case Conference to Address Implicit Bias and Structural Racism for Faculty and Trainees," MedEdPORTAL 15 (2019): 10858, https://doi.org/10.15766/mep_2374-8265.10858.

134. Triveni DeFries et al., "Health Communication and Action Planning with Immigrant Patients: Aligning Clinician and Community Perspectives," MedEdPORTAL 11 (2015), https://doi.org/doi:10.15766/mep_2374-8265.10050.

135. "The Preventive Medicine Milestone Project: Public Health and General Preventive Medicine," the Accreditation Council for Graduate Medical Education and the American Board of Preventive Medicine, July 2015, accessed October 7, 2021, https://www.acgme.org/Portals/0/PDFs/Milestones/PreventiveMedicineMilestones-PublicHealthandGeneralPreventiveMedicine.pdf.

136. Victoria S. Kaprielian et al., "Teaching Population Health: A Competency Map Approach to Education," *Academic Medicine* 88, no. 5 (2013): 626–37, https://doi.org/10.1097/ACM.0b013e31828acf27.

137. "Competencies Across the Learning Continuum Series: New and Emerging Areas in Medicine," Association of American Medical Colleges, accessed October 7, 2021, https://www.aamc.org/what-we-do/mission-areas/medical-education/cbme/competency.

138. Paul Freire, *Pedagogy of the Oppressed*, trans. M. B. Ramos (New York: Herder and Herder, 1970).

139. Mary Catherine Beach et al., "Cultural Competence: A Systematic Review of Health Care Provider Educational Interventions," *Medical Care* 43, no. 4 (2005): 356–73, https://doi.org/10.1097/01.mlr.0000156861.58905.96.

140. Zinzi D. Bailey et al., "Structural Racism and Health Inequities in the USA: Evidence and Interventions," *The Lancet* 389, no. 10077 (2017): 1453–63, https://doi.org/10.1016/s0140-6736(17)30569-x.

141. Donna L. M. Kurtz et al., "Health Sciences Cultural Safety Education in Australia, Canada, New Zealand, and the United States: A Literature Review," *International Journal of Medical Education* 9 (2018): 271–85, https://doi.org/10.5116/ijme.5bc7.21e2.

142. Diana M. Burgess et al., "Reducing Racial Bias among Health Care Providers: Lessons from Social-Cognitive Psychology," *Journal of General Internal Medicine* 22, no. 6 (2007): 882–87, https://doi.org/10.1007/s11606-007-0160-1.

143. Fred A. Kobylarz, John M. Heath, and Robert C. Like, "The ETHNIC(S) Mnemonic: A Clinical Tool for Ethnogeriatric Education," *Journal of the American Geriatrics Society* 50, no. 9 (2002): 1582–89, https://doi.org/10.1046/j.1532-5415.2002.50417.x.

144. Michelle DallaPiazza et al., "Exploring Racism and Health: An Intensive Interactive Session for Medical Students," MedEdPORTAL 14 (2018), https://doi.org/doi:10.15766/mep_2374 -8265.10783.

145. Ryan William Raymond Guilbault and Joseph Alexander Vinson, "Clinical Medical Education in Rural and Underserved Areas and Eventual Practice Outcomes: A Systematic Review and Meta-analysis," *Education for Health (Abingdon)* 30, no. 2 (2017): 146–55, https://doi .org/10.4103/efh.EfH_226_16.

146. Heidi L. Gullett, "Students as Patient Navigators: Case Western Reserve University School of Medicine," in *Value-Added Roles for Medical Students*, ed. Jed D. Gonzalo (Philadelphia: Elsevier, 2021).

147. Trae Stewart and Zane C. Wubbena, "A Systematic Review of Service-Learning in Medical Education: 1998–2012," *Teaching and Learning in Medicine* 27, no. 2 (2015): 115–22, https:// doi.org/10.1080/10401334.2015.1011647.

148. Tania D. Mitchell, "Traditional vs. Critical Service-Learning: Engaging the Literature to Differentiate Two Models," *Michigan Journal of Community Service Learning* 14, no. 2 (2008): 50–65, accessed October 7, 2021, https://files.eric.ed.gov/fulltext/EJ831374.pdf.

149. Angela Gillis and A. MacLellan Marian, "Critical Service Learning in Community Health Nursing: Enhancing Access to Cardiac Health Screening," *International Journal of Nursing Education Scholarship* 10, no. 1. (2013): 63, https://doi.org/10.1515/ijnes-2012-0031.

150. Martha E. Gaines et al., "Medical Professionalism from the Patient's Perspective: Is There an Advocate in the House?" in *Patient Care and Professionalism*, ed. Catherine D. DeAngelis (New York: Oxford University Press, 2013), 1–18.

151. Richard L. Cruess et al., "Reframing Medical Education to Support Professional Identity Formation," *Academic Medicine* 89, no. 11 (2014): 1446–51, https://doi.org/10.1097/acm .0000000000000427.

152. George Rust and Joedrecka S. Brown Speights, "Creating Health Equity Curricula," *Family Medicine* 50, no. 3 (2018): 242–43, https://doi.org/10.22454/FamMed.2018.397067.

153. Syed M. Ahmed et al., "Towards a Practical Model for Community Engagement: Advancing the Art and Science in Academic Health Centers," *Journal of Clinical and Translational Science* 1, no. 5 (2017): 310–15, https://doi.org/10.1017/cts.2017.304.

154. "Community Engagement Toolkits," Association of American Medical Colleges, accessed October 7, 2021, https://www.aamc.org/what-we-do/mission-areas/medical-research/health -equity/community-engagement/toolkits.

155. "Creating a Positive Classroom Climate for Diversity," UCLA Diversity & Faculty Development, accessed October 7, 2021, https://equity.ucla.edu/wp-content/uploads/2019/12/Cr eatingaPositiveClassroomClimateWeb-2.pdf.

156. Shane L. Rogers et al., "Applications of the Reflective Practice Questionnaire in Medical Education," *BMC Medical Education* 19, no. 1 (2019): 47, https://doi.org/10.1186/s12909 -019-1481-6.

157. James D. Kirkpatrick and Wendy Kayser Kirkpatrick, *Kirkpatrick's Four Levels of Training Evaluation* (Alexandria, VA: Association for Talent Development Press, 2016).

158. Jonathan M. Metzl, Juleigh Petty, and Oluwatunmise V. Olowojoba, "Using a Structural Competency Framework to Teach Structural Racism in Pre–Health Education," *Social Science & Medicine* 199 (2018): 189–201, https://doi.org/10.1016/j.socscimed.2017.06.029.

159. Patricia A. Carney et al., "Tools to Assess Behavioral and Social Science Competencies in Medical Education: A Systematic Review," *Academic Medicine* 91, no. 5 (2016): 730–42, https://doi.org/10.1097/ACM.0000000000001090.

160. Mary A. Dolansky et al., "Development and Validation of the Systems Thinking Scale," *Journal of General Internal Medicine* 35 (2020): 2314–20, https://doi.org/10.1007/s11606-020 -05830-1.
161. S. Osmancevic et al., "Psychometric Properties of Instruments Used to Measure the Cultural Competence of Nurses: A Systematic Review," *International Journal of Nursing Studies Advances* 113 (2021):103789, https://doi.org/10.1016/j.ijnurstu.2020.103789.
162. Zuwang Shen, "Cultural Competence Models and Cultural Competence Assessment Instruments in Nursing: A Literature Review," *Journal of Transcultural Nursing* 26, no. 3 (2015): 308–21, https://doi.org/10.1177/1043659614524790.
163. Adekemi O. Sekoni et al., "The Effects of Educational Curricula and Training on LGBT-Specific Health Issues for Healthcare Students and Professionals: A Mixed-Method Systematic Review," *Journal of the International AIDS Society* 20, no. 1 (2017): 21624, https://doi.org /10.7448/IAS.20.1.21624.
164. Robert Li Kitts, "Barriers to Optimal Care between Physicians and Lesbian, Gay, Bisexual, Transgender, and Questioning Adolescent Patients," *Journal of Homosexuality* 57, no. 6 (2010): 730–47, https://doi.org/10.1080/00918369.2010.485872.
165. Danielle F. Loeb et al., "Modest Impact of a Brief Curricular Intervention on Poor Documentation of Sexual History in University-Based Resident Internal Medicine Clinics," *Journal of Sexual Medicine* 7, no. 10 (2010): 3315–21, https://doi.org/10.1111/j.1743-6109.2010.01883.x.
166. Candice Chen and Andrea Anderson, "How Should Health Professionalism be Redefined to Address Health Equity?," *AMA Journal of Ethics* 23, no. 3 (2021): E265–70, https://doi.org /10.1001/amajethics.2021.265.
167. Karen Mann, Jill Gordon, and Anna MacLeod, "Reflection and Reflective Practice in Health Professions Education: A Systematic Review," *Advances in Health Sciences Education* 14, no. 4 (2009): 595–621, https://doi.org/10.1007/s10459-007-9090-2.
168. Hedy S. Wald et al., "Fostering and Evaluating Reflective Capacity in Medical Education: Developing the Reflect Rubric for Assessing Reflective Writing," *Academic Medicine* 87, no. 1 (2012): 41–50, https://doi.org/10.1097/ACM.0b013e31823b55fa.
169. Frances K. Wong et al., "Assessing the Level of Student Reflection from Reflective Journals," *Journal of Advanced Nursing* 22, no. 1 (1995): 48–57, https://doi.org/10.1046 /j.1365-2648.1995.22010048.x.
170. Tracy Moniz et al., "Considerations in the Use of Reflective Writing for Student Assessment: Issues of Reliability and Validity," *Medical Education* 49, no. 9 (2015): 901–8, https://doi.org /10.1111/medu.12771.
171. Jan Van Tartwijk and Erik W. Driessen, "Portfolios for Assessment and Learning: AMEE Guide No. 45," *Medical Teacher* 31, no. 9 (2009): 790–801, https://doi.org/10.1080/0142159 0903139201.
172. Carol Carraccio and Robert Englander, "Evaluating Competence Using a Portfolio: A Literature Review and Web-Based Application to the ACGME Competencies," *Teaching and Learning in Medicine* 16, no. 4 (2004): 381–87, https://doi.org/10.1207/s15328015tlm1604_13.
173. Jeremy H. Neal and Laura D. M. Neal, "Self-Directed Learning in Physician Assistant Education: Learning Portfolios in Physician Assistant Programs," *Journal of Physician Assistant Education* 27, no. 4 (2016): 162–69, https://doi.org/10.1097/jpa.0000000000000091.
174. Eric S. Holmboe, Stephen J. Durning, and Richard E. Hawkins, *Evaluation of Clinical Competence*, 2nd ed. (Philadelphia: Elsevier, 2018).
175. Jennifer Adams et al., "Reflective Writing as a Window on Medical Students' Professional Identity Development in a Longitudinal Integrated Clerkship," *Teaching and Learning in Medicine* 32, no. 2 (2020): 117–25, https://doi.org/10.1080/10401334.2019.1687303.
176. Karen Sokal-Gutierrez et al., "Evaluation of the Program in Medical Education for the Urban Underserved (PRIME-US) at the UC Berkeley–UCSF Joint Medical Program (JMP): The First 4 Years," *Teaching and Learning in Medicine* 27, no. 2 (2015): 189–96, https://doi.org /10.1080/10401334.2015.1011650.

177. Jed D. Gonzalo, ed., *Value-Added Roles for Medical Students* (Philadelphia: Elsevier, 2021).

178. Sabrina Khalil et al., "Addressing Breast Cancer Screening Disparities among Uninsured and Insured Patients: A Student-Run Free Clinic Initiative," *Journal of Community Health* 45, no. 3 (2020): 501–5, https://doi.org/10.1007/s10900-019-00767-x.

179. Corley Rachelle Price et al., "Enhancing Adherence to Cervical Cancer Screening Guidelines at a Student-Run Free Clinic," *Journal of Community Health* 45, no. 1 (2020): 128–32, https://doi.org/10.1007/s10900-019-00724-8.

180. Phillip Gorrindo et al., "Medical Students as Health Educators at a Student-Run Free Clinic: Improving the Clinical Outcomes of Diabetic Patients," *Academic Medicine* 89, no. 4 (2014): 625–31, https://doi.org/10.1097/acm.0000000000000164.

181. Sunny D. Smith et al., "Longitudinal Hypertension Outcomes at Four Student-Run Free Clinic Sites," *Family Medicine* 49, no. 1 (2017): 28–34.

182. Chalee Engelhard et al., "The Implementation and Evaluation of Health Professions Students as Health Coaches within a Diabetes Self-Management Education Program," *Currents in Pharmacy Teaching and Learning* 10, no. 12 (2018): 1600–608, https://doi.org/10.1016/j.cptl.2018.08.018.

183. Simone J. Ross et al., "The Training for Health Equity Network Evaluation Framework: A Pilot Study at Five Health Professional Schools," *Education for Health (Abingdon)* 27, no. 2 (2014): 116–26, https://doi.org/10.4103/1357-6283.143727.

184. Anneke M. Metz, "Medical School Outcomes, Primary Care Specialty Choice, and Practice in Medically Underserved Areas by Physician Alumni of MEDPREP, a Postbaccalaureate Premedical Program for Underrepresented and Disadvantaged Students," *Teaching and Learning in Medicine* 29, no. 3 (2017): 351–59. https://doi.org/10.1080/10401334.2016.1275970.

Example Curricula

This appendix provides three examples of curricula that have progressed through all six steps of curriculum development. The curricula were chosen to demonstrate differences in learner level and longevity. One focuses on medical students (Topics in Interdisciplinary Medicine: High-Value Health Care), one on residents (Neurology Graduate Training Program in Zambia), and one on faculty, which was subsequently adapted to interprofessional trainees (The Kennedy Krieger Curriculum: Equipping Frontline Clinicians to Improve Care for Children with Behavioral, Emotional, and Developmental Disorders). The curricula demonstrate a range of resources, funding, and time for curriculum development. The reader may want to review one or more of these examples to see how the various steps of the curriculum development process can relate to one another and be integrated into a whole.

TOPICS IN INTERDISCIPLINARY MEDICINE: HIGH-VALUE HEALTH CARE

Amit K. Pahwa, MD

In 2014, the American Association of Medical Colleges (AAMC) recommended that selecting cost-effective diagnostic tests should be included as a core entrustable professional activity (EPA) for medical students.[1] High-value care (HVC) is defined by the Institute of Medicine as the best care for the patient, with the optimal result for the circumstances, delivered at the right cost.[2] An Introduction to HVC curriculum was developed in 2015 as an optional intersession for students at the Johns Hopkins University School of Medicine (JHUSOM). This curriculum is presented as an example of how a preclinical curriculum can be developed and piloted in response to a nationally and locally identified need.

Step 1: Problem Identification and General Needs Assessment

The author conducted a literature search in preparing this step. Much of what was learned in that step has been subsequently summarized in the referenced publications by others which represent examples of scholarly contributions related to Step 1.

Problem Identification	Constantly rising health care costs cannot be sustained by society. Cost pressures have been attributed to technology, population factors, and fiscal constraints. Finance, health, and policy experts, as well as individual patients, have struggled to figure out how to contain overall spending while maintaining gains achieved in life expectancy and quality of life. While much of this is necessary, nearly 20% of spending on health care has been estimated to be unnecessary.[3,4] Physicians are responsible for ordering tests and treatments for their patients. This awareness has led to efforts to improve the education of physicians, residents, and patients about the importance of practicing HVC and reducing unnecessary tests and treatments.[5,6] Studies had shown that resident physicians who had trained in high utilizing regions would spend more than their peers who had trained in low utilizing regions.[7] Medical students in environments with higher health care intensity observed wasteful practices.[8] The AAMC recommended in 2014 that graduating medical students should be able to incorporate cost awareness and principles of cost-effectiveness in developing diagnostic plans.[1]
Current Approach	Based on the AAMC Curriculum Inventory in 2014, most medical schools had some required coursework on HVC, but the effect on clinical management was unclear.[9] Previously published curricula had targeted students during their clinical rotations.[10] Almost half of the internal medicine clerkship directors in the United States, however, felt HVC concepts should be introduced prior to clinical rotations.[11] Previously published curricula had not demonstrated an effective HVC curriculum for first-year or preclinical medical students.[10] While programs like Choosing Wisely STARS (Students

and Trainees Advocating for Resource Stewardship) are now empowering first-year medical students to begin integrating curriculum in HVC at their respective institutions, that initiative did not start until after the introduction of this course.[12]

Ideal Approach	The ideal approach should include effective knowledge transfer, reflective practice, and a supportive clinical environment.[13] Efforts were underway to change these environments through value-based quality improvement. However, since environmental change was expected to take time, a complementary ideal approach would be to prepare clinical students to recognize examples of low- and high-value care. For example, students on some internal medicine clerkships had already been tasked with educating the inpatient team when low-value care was occurring.[10] Thus, there was reason to believe that teaching these concepts preclinically could shape students' future behaviors during clinical rotations. For education to promote retention of material and ultimately change behaviors, it has to be implemented throughout training rather than at one time.[14] This is based on spaced learning, which has been shown to be one of the most efficacious ways to transmit knowledge.[15] Core knowledge can facilitate deliberate practice, which is required to achieve mastery.[16] HVC concepts incorporated into the preclinical curriculum could allow learners to have repeated practice with those concepts followed by feedback to prepare them to be a part of the changes in the clinical training environment.

Step 2: Needs Assessment of Targeted Learners

Targeted Learners	For this step, we assessed the adequacy of the HVC curriculum at our institution. One of the missions of JHUSOM was "to prepare clinicians to practice patient-centered medicine of the highest standard," and one of the school's objectives was for graduates to "exhibit the highest level of effective and efficient performance in data gathering, organization, interpretation, and clinical decision-making in the prevention, diagnosis, and management of disease." Both of these were therefore shared learning goals of enrolled students and both involved concepts of HVC. Prior to initiation of this course, only the core clerkship in internal medicine had a formal HVC curriculum. After the internal medicine clerkship, only 33% of our students felt their education in HVC was appropriate, and 68% agreed that additional HVC training should be added. Therefore, we sought to identify an opportunity to introduce HVC concepts to preclerkship students.
Targeted Environment	During the first year at this medical school, between major subject blocks, the students also take a three- or four-day intersession

course from a series titled "TIME: Topics in Interdisciplinary Medicine," which included topics such as health care disparities, nutrition, global health, disaster medicine, and pain. As students desired some choice in intersession topics, we seized this opportunity to ask about piloting an HVC intersession option as an elective, and the deans were quite open to that idea. Since first-year medical students (MS1) also participated in a longitudinal ambulatory clerkship (LAC) consisting of weekly precepted outpatient clinic sessions with real patients, they could witness low- or high-value care throughout the year and reflect upon real patient scenarios to apply to their classroom learning.

Facilities/Resources: We knew many local experts willing to share their knowledge through lectures, and we had a 100-person lecture hall with modern audiovisual equipment and multiple 15-person small-group discussion rooms.

.The first year, 20 students enrolled in the pilot. Subsequently, 60 (out of 120) students enrolled.

Step 3: Goals and Objectives

Goals	Given the existing clinical experiences in LAC, the communication and shared-decision-making skills taught in the Foundations in Clinical Medicine course, and the existing medicine clerkship HVC curriculum, the fundamental goals of the intersession curriculum were to

1. understand the financial burden of health care costs for patients and society,

2. improve student attitudes regarding health care providers' responsibility to decrease unnecessary testing, and

3. empower students to understand HVC and advocate for its practice on clinical rotations.

Specific Measurable Objectives	By the end of the HVC intersession course ("By When"), all first-year medical students who have taken this intersession course ("Who") will be able to do the following:

Objective 1

a. Differentiate between health and health care.

b. Interpret laboratory tests and imaging results based on prevalence and pretest probability of a condition.

c. Identify three common health care issues in the outpatient setting where overutilization of resources is a problem and formulate a method to decrease it.

Objective 2

a. Rate as high the physician's role in decreasing overutilization of health care resources.

b. Describe how the Centers for Medicare & Medicaid Services (CMS) Innovation Center is changing how government pays for health care.

c. Recognize causes for geographical variation in spending per Medicare beneficiary.

Objective 3

a. Describe how insurance companies and beneficiaries pay for health care.

b. Demonstrate the ability to decrease a patient's financial burden from pharmaceuticals.

Step 4: Educational Strategies

To achieve the largely higher-order cognitive learning objectives, the primary educational strategies used were lecture and small-group application exercises. During the first year, the course was allotted 16 contact hours. Approximately nine hours were lectures and seven were small group. Lectures were used to deliver foundational material, while the small groups help reinforce those concepts.

Educational Content   Lectures by content experts were used to achieve lower-order cognitive objectives 1a, 1b, 2a, 2b, 2c, and 3a.

- *Objective 1a:* A health economist from the Johns Hopkins School of Public Health discussed economic theory applied to health. This involved the Grossman Model, which included inputs other than health care into health. (1 hour)

- *Objective 1b:* A radiologist focused on overutilization of imaging, and a pathologist focused on laboratory overutilization, as well as diagnostic limitations of labs. (2 hours)

- *Objective 2a:* The executive vice president of the ABIM Foundation (the organization that started the Choosing Wisely campaign) lectured on how Choosing Wisely has promoted conversations of value by physicians. (1 hour)

- *Objective 2b:* The former director of the CMS Innovation Center summarized the different health care payment models the Innovation Center was testing to place more emphasis on value rather than volume. (1 hour)

- *Objective 2c:* A member from the Dartmouth Institute discussed the large regional differences in health care utilization in the United States despite similarities among populations in each region. (1 hour)

- *Objective 3a:* A former director of a health insurance company described how health care costs are distributed among the beneficiary and an insurance company. A pharmacist outlined the pharmaceutical cost impact on both the patient and health care industry. The information in these lectures provided the background necessary for students to proceed to the higher-order cognitive objective 3b. (3 hours)

Educational Methods	Interactive small groups sessions were used to achieve some of the higher-order cognitive learning objectives as well as reinforce the material taught by lecturers.
	- *Objective 1c:* Groups of 6–10 students, with the help of a faculty facilitator, recalled specific times when they had observed a health care provider order an "unnecessary" test or treatment. This could have occurred during their longitudinal ambulatory clerkship, previous shadowing experiences, or with a family member. As a group, they chose one test or treatment and created a way to help health care providers decrease unnecessary use. Each group then presented to a panel of facilitators who selected a "best project idea" based on feasibility and likelihood to have an impact. (3 hours)
	- *Objective 3b:* Students were asked to estimate a sample patient's annual health care expenditures and the insurance company's portion. Two patients were compared: one who was relatively healthy and one who had diabetes mellitus. We used the most commonly purchased bronze- and silver-level insurance plans from the insurance marketplace. As time permitted, students could also use the insurance plan offered by the Johns Hopkins School of Medicine to the medical students not on their parent's insurance. After lectures from the pharmacists, students were given a list of medications from a patient case. Students were then asked to recommend therapeutic interchanges to reduce the out-of-pocket costs for that patient. (4 hours)

While the educational strategies remained constant, certain elements of the curriculum were refined over the years in response to assessment data (see "Step 6: Evaluation and Assessment" and "Curriculum Maintenance and Enhancement," below).

Step 5: Implementation

Resources	Classrooms for small groups / large lecture hall
	16 contact hours over four days
	Content expert faculty for lectures (10)

	Faculty to facilitate small-group sessions (one faculty instructor for every six to eight students)
	Simulation center for objective structured clinical examination (OSCE)
Support	Salary support for course director (0.1 full-time equivalent)
	Budget for outside speakers ($2,500)
Administration	A single faculty member as director of the course
	Administrative staff from the Office of Curriculum for scheduling and communications
Barriers	There were only a few months to implement the course.
	The course was only 16 contact hours, so material and time with students was limited.
	Could not assess communication in the course since standardized patients were too expensive for the budget.
	Faculty availability was not guaranteed (the time for the intersession had already been set by the academic schedule).
	Much of the material had to be created as this had not been done before.
Introduction	The first offering of the course was considered a pilot.
	Targeted needs assessment served as pilot for the assessment tool as well as providing valuable insight for curriculum development.

The curriculum was initially implemented as an intersession in June 2015 at JHUSOM. First-year students could choose to take this course or an intersession course on pain. Since that year, it has been offered as an alternative to the global health intersession. Approximately 50% of each class chooses the HVC intersession course.

Step 6: Evaluation and Assessment

Users	Users of the evaluation include students, the course director, participating faculty, and the Office of Medical Student Curriculum.
Uses	<ul><li>Students—to assess personal achievement of learning objectives and offer feedback for course improvement</li><li>Course director—to assess student experience and attitudes toward the course</li><li>Faculty—to assess student experience and attitudes about individual sessions</li><li>Office of Medical Student Curriculum—to assess the success of the course in providing education to medical students</li></ul>

Resources	• The course director was granted institutional support that provided protected time for curriculum development and implementation.
	• Collation and analysis of the data was performed through the Office of Medical Student Curriculum.
	• Although we did not have resources for a new standardized patient assessment specifically for HVC, we were able to get some data relevant to HVC from another standardized patient assessment already planned for the LAC. During one standardized encounter, students interviewed a patient with acute low back strain due to heavy lifting. During the encounter, the patient asked the student if imaging was needed. Student responses in this scenario were collected by the longitudinal clerkship coordinator and shared with us. The standardized patient encounter and questions were developed prior to the first iteration of this course.
Evaluation Questions	1. How much did students who completed the intersession improve their scores on the knowledge quiz pre-/post-intersession?
	2. Did students who had completed the HVC intersession course incorporate HVC principles in their response to the standardized patient with back pain, compared with those who chose a different intersession course?
	3. Could students synthesize HVC lessons learned sufficiently to identify an instance of low-value care that they had witnessed and propose a way to teach others to provide higher value care?
	4. How did the quality of the HVC intersession compare to other intersession courses?
Evaluation Design	1. $O_1 - - - X - - - O_2$
	2. E X - - - O
	C - - - O
	3. X - - - O
	4. X - - - O
Measurement Methods	1. Quiz—A timed one-hour 20-question open-book quiz was administered prior to the course and after the course. Questions were written by lecturers or the course director.
	2. Standardized Patient—During the encounter, the standardized patient asked if imaging was needed. The response was categorized into one of five responses. Standardized patients did not give any feedback to the students.
	3. Shark Tank—Groups of 6–10 students were required to present a method to decrease an unnecessary test or treatment at the end of the course.

4. Overall Course Evaluations—Data was also collected from standardized end-of-course questions used for all intersessions:

- Received clear learning objectives?
- Performance assessed against those learning questions?
- Sufficient time to complete out-of-class assignments?
- Facilitated development of lifelong learning habits?
- Organization of the course?
- Quality of course?

Ethical Concerns	Access to assessment data was restricted to the course leaders, and all data were stored in password-protected devices. Learners were informed in advance of how their individual assessment data would be used in determining the effectiveness of the course. An institutional review board approved the research aspects of this program, as all data were de-identified and analyzed only in aggregate.
Data Collection	We collected assessment data as an end-of-course evaluation and pre-post quizzes. Participation in the end-of-course evaluation was required of 25% of the class per school policy. Participation in the pre-post quizzes and Shark Tank were mandatory for all students in the class. The standardized patient data was collected by the LAC coordinator, who obtained it from the school's online recording system.
Data Analysis	Psychometric analysis was performed on the quizzes. The responses of the standardized patients were analyzed using a chi-square test of independence.

Student evaluations of the curriculum through the years have been uniformly positive, with 90% rating the quality of the course as good or excellent. While there was no difference in the percentage of students who ordered imaging for the standardized patient with back pain, students who took the HVC intersession were more likely to reassure the patient it was simple back strain and less likely to ask their preceptor for help. The course was rated as either excellent or very good at developing lifelong learning habits in HVC practices by 89% of students.

Curriculum Maintenance and Enhancement

The fundamental goal of the curriculum was to empower students to understand HVC and be able to advocate for its practice on clinical rotations. Changes have been made each year in response to feedback to move closer to this goal.

In review of the evaluations from the first two years of the course, the lecture on regional variation in physician practices and lab ordering practices was not well received by students. This lecture was subsequently removed for future iterations. The lecture on lab ordering practices was redesigned based on feedback from students that the lecture was too focused on statistics and less clinically relevant. For future iterations, we invited an internal medicine physician educator, who provided more clinical relevance, and it has become one of the highest rated lectures. On further review, the content of the lecture on Choosing Wisely did not align with the learning objectives and also was given by a nonphysician. For subsequent years this lecture was realigned with the course objectives and given by a physician.

After the second year, the TIME course allotment was contracted from four half-days to three half-days, requiring moving some of the material to out-of-class assignments. Prior to the contraction there was time built into the in-person class to complete them. This change has not affected overall rating of the course, nor student ratings of the appropriateness of the amount of out-of-class work.

The timed, open-book quiz was meant to simulate just-in-time search and recall of knowledge related to HVC. Students did demonstrate improved scores, with an average pretest score of 46% and an average posttest score of 73% ($p < 0.001$). However, psychometrics showed the exam had poor reliability and poor discrimination, and students did not feel it had value as an open-book test. Therefore, the quiz was dropped as a summative assessment. Instead, the small-group activity worksheets, originally designed as formative assessments, contributed to the summative assessment.

From year 3 on, the major assessment of students has been the Shark Tank activity, thus requiring the development of a rubric. The rubric included five points for the following categories:

1. Background to the problem summarized well
2. Intervention was feasible and creative
3. Well delineated outcome
4. Clear presentation
5. All members spoke

Two faculty not involved as faculty facilitators graded each presentation. Removal of the quiz has also allowed students to focus on the group presentations, which overall have become richer each year.

The structure of the course has been maintained for the last three years and continues to receive among the highest ratings from the students.

Dissemination

Educational outcome data from this curriculum have been presented at national professional meetings, in both poster and oral forms. The data has also been published in *The Clinical Teacher*.[17] One faculty member modeled health system curricula at his institution based on this course. Another institution adopted the Shark Tank to assess their HVC course.

REFERENCES CITED

1. Drafting Panel for Core Entrustable Professional Activities for Entering Residency, *Core Entrustable Professional Activities for Entering Residency: Faculty and Learners' Guide*, accessed July 5, 2015, https://www.aamc.org/what-we-do/mission-areas/medical-education/cbme/core-epas/publications.

2. Institute of Medicine, *Best Care at Lower Cost: The Path to Continuously Learning Health Care in America* (Washington, DC: National Academies Press, 2013), https://doi.org/10.17226/13444.

3. OECD, *Fiscal Sustainability of Health Systems: Bridging Health and Finance Perspectives* (Paris: OECD Publishing, 2015), https://doi.org/10.1787/9789264233386-en.

4. OECD, *Tackling Wasteful Spending on Health* (Paris: OECD Publishing, 2017), https://doi.org/10.1787/9789264266414-en.

5. M. Behmann, I. Brandes, and U. Walter, "[Teaching Health Economics, Health-Care System and Public Health at German Medical Faculties]," [in German], *Gesundheitswesen* 74, no. 7 (2012): 435–41, https://doi.org/10.1055/s-0031-1280847.

6. Raymond Oppong, Hema Mistry, and Emma Frew, "Health Economics Education in Undergraduate Medical Training: Introducing the Health Economics Education (HEE) Website," *BMC Medical Education* 13 (2013): 126, https://doi.org/10.1186/1472-6920-13-126.

7. Candice S. Chen et al., "Spending Patterns in Region of Residency Training and Subsequent Expenditures for Care Provided by Practicing Physicians for Medicare Beneficiaries," *JAMA* 312, no. 22 (2014): 2385–93, https://doi.org/10.1001/jama.2014.15973.

8. Andrea N. Leep Hunderfund et al., "Role Modeling and Regional Health Care Intensity: U.S. Medical Student Attitudes toward and Experiences with Cost-Conscious Care," *Academic Medicine* 92, no. 5 (2017): 694–702, https://doi.org/10.1097/acm.0000000000001223.

9. "Curriculum Inventory," Association of American Medical Colleges, accessed September 10, 2014, https://www.aamc.org/what-we-do/mission-areas/medical-education/curriculum-inventory.

10. G. Dodd Denton et al., "Abstracts from the Proceedings of the 2014 Annual Meeting of the Clerkship Directors of Internal Medicine (CDIM)," *Teaching and Learning in Medicine* 27, no. 3 (2015): 346–50, https://doi.org/10.1080/10401334.2015.1044752.

11. Danelle Cayea et al., "Current and Optimal Training in High-Value Care in the Internal Medicine Clerkship: A National Curricular Needs Assessment," *Academic Medicine* 93, no. 10 (2018): 1511–16. https://doi.org/10.1097/acm.0000000000002192.

12. Karen B. Born et al., "Learners as Leaders: A Global Groundswell of Students Leading Choosing Wisely Initiatives in Medical Education," *Academic Medicine* 94, no. 11 (2019): 1699–703, https://doi.org/10.1097/acm.0000000000002868.

13. Lorette A. Stammen et al., "Training Physicians to Provide High-Value, Cost-Conscious Care: A Systematic Review," *JAMA* 314, no. 22 (2015): 2384–400, https://doi.org/10.1001/jama.2015.16353.

14. Prathibha Varkey et al., "A Review of Cost-Effectiveness, Cost-Containment and Economics Curricula in Graduate Medical Education," *Journal of Evaluation in Clinical Practice* 16, no. 6 (2010): 1055–62, https://doi.org/10.1111/j.1365-2753.2009.01249.x.

15. S. Barry Issenberg et al., "Features and Uses of High-Fidelity Medical Simulations That Lead to Effective Learning: A BEME Systematic Review," *Medical Teacher* 27, no. 1 (2005): 10–28, https://doi.org/10.1080/01421590500046924.

16. William C. McGaghie et al., "Medical Education Featuring Mastery Learning with Deliberate Practice Can Lead to Better Health for Individuals and Populations," *Academic Medicine* 86, no. 11 (2011): e8–9, https://doi.org/10.1097/ACM.0b013e3182308d37.

17. Christopher Steele et al., "Novel First-Year Curriculum in High-Value Care," *Clinical Teacher* 16, no. 5 (2019): 513–18 https://doi.org/10.1111/tct.12989.

NEUROLOGY GRADUATE TRAINING PROGRAM IN ZAMBIA

Deanna Saylor, MD, MHS

Introduction

The author began curriculum development in 2015 to create the first neurology graduate training program in Zambia at the request of the University of Zambia School of Medicine (UNZA-SOM). Development coincided with the Zambian Ministry of Health's initiative to begin training specialist physicians within Zambia. As part of this initiative, local public health, medical, and government officials recognized the significant burden of neurologic disease in the Zambian population and the lack of neurologists to care for these patients. When this neurology graduate training program began in 2018 at UNZA-SOM and the University Teaching Hospital (UTH) in Lusaka, Zambia, there were no Zambian neurologists, and care for neurologic disorders was provided by general practitioners and internal medicine physicians.

Step 1: Problem Identification and Needs Assessment

The author conducted a literature review and interviews of key university and government officials in completing this step.

Problem Identification	According to the Global Burden of Disease study, neurologic disorders (e.g., stroke, epilepsy, meningitis, neuropathy, dementia, Parkinson's disease) were the leading cause of disability-adjusted life years and second-leading cause of mortality globally.[1] The absolute burden of neurologic disease was sixfold higher in low- and middle-income countries (LMICs) compared to higher-income countries,[2] but LMICs had the least resources to care for these patients.[3] While high-income countries averaged five or more neurologists per 100,000 population, low-income and lower-middle-income countries averaged 0.03 and 0.13 neurologists per 100,000 population, respectively. The situation was particularly dire in Africa, which had the lowest neurologist per population ratio (0.04 per 100,000 population) of any world region.[3] Unfortunately, with very few neurology graduate training programs on the continent, this situation was unlikely to change soon.[4] The burden of neurologic disorders in Zambia specifically was significant, with stroke alone as the seventh-leading cause of death, while other leading causes of death, such as HIV/AIDS, tuberculosis, diabetes, and road traffic accidents, were frequently associated with neurologic complications.[5] Zambia had a population of 17 million people but no Zambian-born practicing neurologists; all specialist neurologic care was provided by three expatriate neurologists living in Zambia and others who intermittently visited for shorter durations. The majority of this care was provided in the outpatient setting, so specialty neurologic care was inaccessible for most patients requiring hospitalization.

Current Approach	In most countries in Africa, including Zambia, patients with neurologic disorders were cared for by nonphysician health care workers, general practitioners, and internal medicine physicians, who had largely been taught neurology by non-neurologists. If a physician wanted to obtain training in neurology, government sponsorship or personal funds were needed to travel to international sites. These international programs were usually in better-resourced settings, many of which had a different spectrum of neurologic diseases (e.g., more autoimmune neurologic disorders and less neuro-infectious diseases) than in the trainees' home countries. Training in an international setting also increased the chances that trainees would not return to their home countries to practice. In the few existing neurology training programs established in Africa, and in similar LMICs outside of Africa, most began after a critical mass of internationally trained neurologists returned to offer local graduate training.[6] These programs often received significant external support initially before becoming self-sustaining as local graduates became faculty.[7,8] In Zambia, government sponsorship for local and international training was unavailable.
Ideal Approach	In-country graduate training in neurology would allow trainees to gain experience diagnosing and managing the spectrum of neurologic disorders that are most common in the local population with resources available in that health care setting.[9] Local clinical training also would allow for an immediate impact on the treatment of neurologic disease. The ideal training program would use contemporary educational strategies in graduate medical education, including an emphasis on clinical reasoning and bedside teaching,[10–12] case-based learning,[13] and experiential learning,[14] and it would apply traditional (e.g., written and oral examinations) and newer forms of assessment (e.g., learning portfolios,[15] objective structured clinical examinations, or OSCEs,[16] and individualized learning goals and self-assessment[17]) against competency-[18] and milestones-based[19] frameworks. The curriculum would need to accomplish all of this while optimizing use of limited resources and complying with local regulations, such as those set by the UNZA Senate and Office of Post-Graduate Education and the Ministry of Education's Higher Education Authority. For example, graduate education in Zambia would need to be offered through master's degree programs that define particular courses that graduate trainees would complete each year and specify formal summative assessments for each course. Ideally, the program would eventually become locally sustainable and contribute to national neurology education, research, and policy-making capacity by orienting learners to population needs and helping participants develop teaching and scholarly capabilities. This ideal approach, as applied to Zambia, could serve as a model for other LMICs seeking to build capacity in neurology or other subspecialty areas of medicine.

Step 2: Targeted Needs Assessment

Targeted Learners	The targeted learners were trainees enrolled in the graduate neurology program offered through UNZA, namely the Master of Medicine in Neurology (MMED Neurology) program, which was first offered in 2018. Because neurology is considered a subspecialty of internal medicine in Zambia, the MMED Neurology program was structured in the same way as other established subspecialty training programs such that trainees first completed three years of postgraduate internal medicine training followed by two years of dedicated postgraduate training in neurology.
Targeted Environment	The clinical setting for all graduate medical training programs offered through the UNZA-SOM were the inpatient wards and outpatient clinics of UTH in Lusaka, Zambia. UTH was the national referral hospital and primary teaching hospital in Zambia. With 1,655 beds, 56 wards, and ~20,000 admissions per year, it was a large-volume high-acuity hospital that served individuals within the Lusaka area who were self-referred for care, as well as individuals transferred from primary health care centers, first-level hospitals, and second-level hospitals from across Zambia for more specialized care. The neurology case-mix was unknown, and there was no dedicated neurology service when the program started. As such, the launch of the training program also coincided with the creation of a neurology inpatient and consult service at UTH.
Needs Assessment /Targeted Learners	Informal polls of graduate trainees in internal medicine showed high levels of neurophobia, the fear of clinical neurology,[20] and dissatisfaction with their neurology training. These conversations also identified three internal medicine graduate trainees interested in transferring to the neurology training program if it were to gain approval.
Needs Assessment /Targeted Environment	The author met with, and obtained support from, clinical and medical education leaders in the Department of Medicine at UNZA-SOM and UTH, all of whom affirmed the lack of formal training opportunities in neurology and the unmet need for neurology specialists in Zambia.

There were no funds available to support educators for the program, but the Zambian Ministry of Health would support learners' salaries during training.

The author met with the program directors for the UNZA-SOM Master of Medicine in Infectious Diseases program, the first graduate training program that had been developed in Zambia. This program's curriculum documents offered a template for the format and content expected by the UNZA Senate, the accreditation body for UNZA's graduate medical training programs. This |

template was essential in facilitating strong early drafts of the program curricula and minimizing the number of revisions requested in subsequent discussions with administration officials.

Step 3: Goals and Objectives

Goals	The overall goals of the curriculum were to train neurologists who would

- competently assess, diagnose, and manage a broad range of neurologic disorders, including stroke, epilepsy, meningitis/encephalitis, neurological complications of other infections (e.g., tuberculosis, malaria, and HIV), movement disorders, headache, and neuropathy, across the lifespan;
- undertake a significant role in developing public health policy as it relates to neurologic disorders;
- carry out an independent research project and disseminate knowledge gained locally and, ideally, regionally and internationally; and
- educate medical students, graduate medical trainees, and primary care providers in the evaluation and treatment of the most common neurologic disorders in the Zambian population.

Objectives	By the end of the program, graduates would be able to do the following:

1. Describe the incidence and prevalence of common neurologic disease in Zambia, the most common risk factors for these diseases, and the populations at highest risk for developing them.

2. Demonstrate mastery of the neurological clinical evaluation, including the neurologic physical examination to localize a pathologic process within the nervous system.

3. Identify the appropriate use and limitations of common neurologic diagnostic procedures, including electroencephalogram (EEG), nerve conduction studies and electromyography (NCS/EMG), computed tomography (CT), magnetic resonance imaging (MRI), and lumbar puncture (LP), and be able to appropriately interpret their data in clinical context.

4. Describe the mechanism of action, appropriate indications, and common risks of medications used to treat neurologic disorders.

5. Demonstrate sufficient clinical expertise to practice independently as a neurologist in Zambia.

6. Describe how local epidemiological data could be used to advocate for public health policies to benefit the greatest number

of patients with neurologic disorders with limited local resources for neurologic care.

7. Complete a scholarly project on a neurologic topic of their choice and present the results in a regional or national meeting and/or publication in a medical journal.

8. Competently teach the epidemiology, diagnosis, and management of neurologic disorders to medical students, internal medicine trainees, other physicians, and other non-neurologist clinical providers.

Step 4: Educational Strategies

Guided by the educational principles identified in the ideal approach in Step 1, and conforming to local requirements, the final structure of the UNZA-SOM MMED Neurology program consisted of two years of training in neurology after three years of training in internal medicine as part of the UNZA-SOM Master of Medicine in Internal Medicine curriculum. The two-year UNZA-SOM MMED Neurology curriculum was subdivided into four courses.

One course, the Introduction to Neuroscience & Neuroanatomy course, ran during the first half of the first year and consisted of traditional didactic lectures with weekly case-based discussions. Three courses were clinically oriented: Introduction to Clinical Neurology ran for the first half of the first year, Introduction to Principles & Practice of Neurology ran for the second half of the first year, and Principles & Practice of Neurology ran during the second year. The three clinically oriented courses used multiple teaching methods:

Clinical Rounds	Daily clinical rounds with a neurology faculty member were the predominant educational method and included intentional bedside teaching and discussion of diagnosis and management of neurological disorders with an emphasis on clinical reasoning, public health approaches to resource utilization, and adapting clinical practice guidelines from high-income settings to the local setting. Residents also played a primary role in bedside teaching of medical students on rounds.
One-on-One Precepting	Faculty preceptors provided in-the-moment individualized feedback during weekly outpatient clinic.
Lectures	Lectures occurred in-person, and virtual platforms allowed international experts to provide expert teaching to neurology trainees.
Clinical Case Conferences	Five weekly case conferences focused on management of active clinical cases: (1) discussion of complex cases encountered that week on the inpatient wards or in outpatient clinic; (2) NCS/EMG review; (3) EEG review; (4) neuroradiology conference; and (5) pediatric neurology case conference. Conferences were resident-led with feedback from local and visiting faculty, both on the cases themselves and on residents' presentation and teaching skills.

Journal Clubs	Residents led weekly conferences to discuss a recent publication applicable to clinical neurology. These conferences focused on critical appraisal of the literature and were moderated by neurology faculty.
Research Methods Seminars and Dissertation Project	Weekly conferences consisted of a mini-lecture on a relevant clinical or public health research topic and works-in-progress presentations from neurology residents for their required MMED dissertation project. Residents were encouraged to choose dissertation projects that addressed a locally relevant public health issue in neurology.

Step 5: Implementation

The curriculum was approved by the UNZA Senate and the Zambia Ministry of Health in 2016 and enrolled its first trainees in a full implementation in 2018.

Support	The MMED Neurology program was highly supported by Department of Internal Medicine leadership at both UNZA-SOM and UTH, as well as by the Zambia Ministry of Health.
Administration	No administrative support was available for the program. The author handled all administrative duties. The UNZA-SOM Post-Graduate Office provided general support to all graduate medical education programs in registering grades and ensured all UNZA graduation requirements were met by trainees.
Barriers	The primary barrier to implementation was the high level of external personnel support required to develop, launch, and maintain the MMED Neurology program. With no local Zambian neurologists and no funding to support the effort of international teaching faculty, the program relied heavily on the author's efforts and efforts of volunteer visiting faculty to meet the teaching obligations and administrative requirements during the initial years. Other barriers included the following: - There was limited funding and administrative support. - High patient volumes required daily rounds to be efficient and left less time for clinical teaching. - There was limited preprogram neurology exposure. Initial groups of learners required extra teaching to develop foundational knowledge consistent with early-stage neurology trainees in other settings. However, this barrier was expected to lessen as undergraduate medical students at UNZA-SOM were concurrently gaining increased exposure to clinical neurology during their preclinical and clinical years through exposure to the MMED Neurology program.

| Introduction | The MMED Neurology curriculum began development in 2015 and was fully introduced in the 2018–2019 academic year with plans to continue indefinitely. |

Step 6: Evaluation

Users	- Neurology trainees
	- MMED Neurology program director and teaching faculty
	- Clinical leadership in the Department of Medicine at UNZA-SOM and UTH
	- Zambia Ministry of Health
Uses	- Formative information to enable neurology trainees to achieve learning objectives
	- Formative evaluation of the strengths and weaknesses of the program to guide improvement of the curriculum for program leadership and teaching faculty
	- Summative information for stakeholders, including officials at the Zambia Ministry of Health and departmental leadership at UNZA-SOM and UTH, on the program's effectiveness and impact on clinical care for Zambians with neurologic disorders
	- Summative information to demonstrate worthiness of continued support, aid applications for future grants and funding mechanisms, and enable dissemination
Resources	The author received mentorship in curriculum design, implementation, and evaluation through the Johns Hopkins University Faculty Development Program. In addition, undergraduate medical students and graduate neurology trainees with an interest in global neurology research volunteered their time to support program evaluation.
Evaluation Questions, Designs, and Measurement Methods	Please see Table A.1 for examples of the some of the most important evaluation questions and approaches to answering them.
Data Analysis	Quantitative data were analyzed using descriptive statistics. Qualitative data obtained from open-ended responses to survey questions and individual in-depth interviews were analyzed using thematic coding.
Reporting of Results	At the time of this writing, results were being collected and analyzed with plans for submission of several manuscripts to peer-reviewed journals.

Table A.1.   Curriculum Evaluation Plan

Evaluation Question	Evaluation Design	Evaluation Measurement	Data Collection
Do MMED Neurology program graduates demonstrate the knowledge and clinical skills necessary to provide appropriate and high-quality care to patients with neurological disorders within the resource constraints of the local setting?	X - - - O	- Written examinations - Oral examinations - Objective structured clinical examinations - Assessment of oral presentations and written clinical documentation - Competency-based individualized learning plans and portfolios - Monthly clinical evaluations - Self-assessment of knowledge - Milestone assessment	Anonymized score reports from all assessments completed as part of the MMED Neurology program
Are MMED Neurology program graduates satisfied with the quality of their education, clinical skills, and readiness for independent practice as a clinical neurologist?	X - - - O	Electronic surveys	Survey software
From the perspective of the MMED Neurology program faculty and graduates, which components of the curriculum content, delivery, and assessment methods are strongest? Which components offer opportunities for improvement?	X - - - O	Electronic surveys	Survey software
What are the career trajectories of program graduates, such as practice model (public vs. private vs. hybrid practice and outpatient vs. inpatient practice), further subspecialty training, and teaching roles?	X - - - O	Annual surveys of program graduates evaluating current employment, practice model, and teaching involvement	Survey software

Table A.1.   *(continued)*

Evaluation Question	Evaluation Design	Evaluation Measurement	Data Collection
Does the program emphasis on completing a scholarly activity and providing training in research methods result in graduates who continue to pursue research or other scholarly activity after graduation?	X - - - O	Annual surveys of program graduates evaluating current employment, practice model, and research/scholarly activity products (e.g., successful grants, published manuscripts, conference presentations)	Survey software
Is the MMED Neurology program expanding access to specialist care for patients with neurological disorders in Zambia?	X - - - O	Clinical logs	Review of neurology inpatient admission and outpatient clinical logs to determine the number of admissions and patient visits over a six-month period and how these compared to total medical admissions and outpatient visits at UTH
Is the overall performance of the MMED Neurology program satisfactory to key stakeholders and funders?	X - - - O	In-depth qualitative interviews and anonymous surveys	Qualitative interviews with key program participants, beneficiaries, and stakeholders; survey software

Curriculum Maintenance and Enhancement

In the first two years ($n = 7$ trainees), trainee evaluations were uniformly positive. Visiting faculty members were impressed with trainees' knowledge, clinical skills, and clinical decision-making, and clinical evaluations completed by visiting faculty ranked trainees as very good to excellent in all domains. All assessments (e.g., written examinations, oral examinations, OSCEs, and clinical evaluations; see Table A.1) administered had a 100% pass rate, and trainees expressed satisfaction with their training and personal growth in feedback meetings. In particular, trainees cited the emphasis on bedside teaching and clinical reasoning as strengths of the program. The addition of virtual lectures helped to meet a previously identified area of weakness—that there were several areas of neurology that had not been covered in didactic sessions because faculty with subspecialty expertise were unavailable locally. Furthermore, scholarly outputs were high with trainees presenting oral abstracts and poster presentations at national, regional, and international scientific conferences. Several scientific manuscripts with trainees as first-authors were submitted to international peer-reviewed journals.

Early evidence suggested that the MMED Neurology program was also meeting a significant clinical need with ~1,500 inpatient admissions making the new neurology services the second-busiest medical service at UTH. In addition, ~2,500 outpatient visits for neurologic issues were completed annually. Departmental and hospital leadership were pleased with the quality of training and clinical care and remained supportive of efforts to further refine and build on these gains. Several neurology residents transferred into the program from postgraduate training programs in internal medicine, suggesting that neurophobia may also be decreasing among medical student and medicine residents exposed to more neurology teaching.

In addition to adding virtual lectures during the second year of the program, other enhancements intended to address educational goals and objectives more robustly were the addition of mini-curricula on patient-physician communication and patient-centered care, physician wellness, and teaching skills. Trainees also received targeted training in the evaluation of patients using teleneurology platforms as part of a new teleneurology program.

The program also gained support from philanthropic donors, international nongovernmental organizations, such as the Encephalitis Society, and academic adult and pediatric neurology faculty who volunteered their time as teaching faculty through the American Academy of Neurology Global Health Section and the American Neurological Association International Outreach Committee.

Anticipated challenges to curriculum maintenance and enhancement centered around the lack of dedicated funding and administrative support for a program director and teaching faculty. Of note, because the program was based in a public hospital where care was provided largely free of charge, clinical volume did not translate into program revenue. Thus, lack of funding for teaching activities and program leadership was likely to continue to be a threat to maintaining a high level of program quality. As local graduates were expected to enter the teaching faculty and take on greater leadership responsibilities, the program could become self-sustaining independent of external support. Continued mentoring and faculty development programs by external faculty were expected to incentivize graduates to remain actively involved in the MMED Neurology program.

Dissemination

The rationale and overall concept for this curriculum were presented at the Neurological Association of South Africa Annual Congress and as virtual abstracts for the 2020 American Academy of Neurology Annual Meeting and American Neurological Association Annual Meeting. At the time this was written, the author had published one manuscript[21] and was developing several others to highlight curricular innovations and modifications made to adapt pedagogical and assessment methods established in high-resourced settings to the local context in Zambia with its associated resource constraints. The aim with disseminating the structure of the curriculum as early as possible was to allow similar resource-limited settings lacking postgraduate training in neurology to review whether this format might be applicable to their own settings. Much of the quantitative and qualitative data on trainee performance and satisfaction, as well as stakeholder satisfaction, were still being collected as the first class of graduates had only recently graduated. Once data on a larger number of program graduates have been collected, the author plans to pursue additional dissemination opportunities in peer-reviewed medical education and neurology-focused journals.

REFERENCES CITED

1. Valery L. Feigin et al., "Global, Regional, and National Burden of Neurological Disorders, 1990–2016: A Systematic Analysis for the Global Burden of Disease Study 2016," *The Lancet Neurology* 18, no. 5 (2019): 459–80, https://doi.org/10.1016/S1474-4422(18)30499-X.
2. Jerome H. Chin and Nirali Vora, "The Global Burden of Neurologic Diseases," *Neurology* 83, no. 4 (2014): 349–51, https://doi.org/10.1212/WNL.0000000000000610.
3. World Health Organization, *Atlas: Country Resources for Neurological Disorders*, 2nd ed. (Geneva: World Health Organization, 2017).
4. Farrah J. Mateen et al., "Neurology Training in Sub-Saharan Africa: A Survey of People in Training from 19 Countries," *Annals of Neurology* 79, no. 6 (2016): 871–81, https://doi.org/10.1002/ana.24649.
5. Martin Nyahoda et al., "Mortality and Cause of Death Profile for Deaths from the Civil Registration System: 2017 Facts and Figures," *Health Press Zambia Bulletin* 2, no. 9 (2018): 17–25.
6. Marco T. Medina et al., "Developing a Neurology Training Program in Honduras: A Joint Project of Neurologists in Honduras and the World Federation of Neurology," *Journal of the Neurological Sciences* 253, no. 1–2 (2007): 7–17, https://doi.org/10.1016/j.jns.2006.07.005.
7. Mehila Zebenigus, Guta Zenebe, and James H. Bower, "Neurology Training in Africa: The Ethiopian Experience," *Nature Clinical Practice Neurology* 3, no. 7 (2007): 412–13, https://doi.org/10.1038/ncpneuro0531.
8. Kerling Israel et al., "Development of a Neurology Training Program in Haiti," *Neurology* 92, no. 8 (2019): 391–94, https://doi.org/10.1212/WNL.0000000000006960.
9. Deanna Saylor, "Developing a System of Neurological Care in Zambia," American Academy of Neurology without Borders, December 13, 2018, http://www.neurology.org/without_borders.
10. Meredith E. Young et al., "How Different Theories of Clinical Reasoning Influence Teaching and Assessment," *Academic Medicine* 93, no. 9 (2018): 1415, https://doi.org/10.1097/ACM.0000000000002303.
11. Brendan M. Reilly, "Inconvenient Truths about Effective Clinical Teaching," *The Lancet* 370, no. 9588 (2007): 705–11, https://doi.org/10.1016/S0140-6736(07)61347-6.
12. Judith L. Bowen, "Educational Strategies to Promote Clinical Diagnostic Reasoning," *New England Journal of Medicine* 355, no. 21 (2006): 2217–25, https://doi.org/10.1056/NEJMra054782.
13. Susan F. McLean, "Case-Based Learning and Its Application in Medical and Health-Care Fields: A Review of Worldwide Literature," *Journal of Medical Education and Curricular Development* 3 (2016): JMECD-S20377, https://doi.org/10.4137/JMECD.S20377.
14. David A. Kolb, *Experiential Learning: Experience as the Source of Learning and Development* (Englewood Cliffs, NJ: Prentice-Hall, 1984).
15. Claire Tochel et al., "The Effectiveness of Portfolios for Post-graduate Assessment and Education: BEME Guide No 12." *Medical Teacher* 31, no. 4 (2009): 299–318, https://doi.org/10.1080/01421590902883056.
16. David A. Sloan et al., "The Use of the Objective Structured Clinical Examination (OSCE) for Evaluation and Instruction in Graduate Medical Education," *Journal of Surgical Research* 63, no. 1 (1996): 225–30, https://doi.org/10.1006/jsre.1996.0252.
17. Su-Ting T. Li et al., "Resident Self-Assessment and Learning Goal Development: Evaluation of Resident-Reported Competence and Future Goals," *Academic Pediatrics* 15, no. 4 (2015): 367–73, https://doi.org/10.1016/j.acap.2015.01.001.

18. Accreditation Council for Graduate Medical Education, *ACGME Common Program Requirements (Residency)* (Chicago: Accreditation Council for Graduate Medical Education, 2018).

19. Accreditation Council for Graduate Medical Education, *The Neurology Milestone Project: Neurology Milestones* (Chicago: Accreditation Council for Graduate Medical Education, 2015).

20. Ralph F. Jozefowicz, "Neurophobia: The Fear of Neurology among Medical Students," *Archives of Neurology* 51, no. 4 (1994): 328–29, https://doi.org/10.1001/archneur.1994.00540160018003.

21. Rebecca Marie DiBiase et al., "Training in Neurology: Implementation and Evaluation of an Objective Structured Clinical Examination Tool for Neurology Post-graduate Trainees in Lusaka, Zambia," *Neurology* 97, no. 7 (2021): e750–54, https://doi.org/10.1212/WNL.0000000000012134.

THE KENNEDY KRIEGER CURRICULUM: EQUIPPING FRONTLINE CLINICIANS TO IMPROVE CARE FOR CHILDREN WITH BEHAVIORAL, EMOTIONAL, AND DEVELOPMENTAL DISORDERS

Mary L. O'Connor Leppert, MB BCh

This curriculum was designed to share the expertise of pediatric specialists at the Kennedy Krieger Institute (KKI) with rural and school-based health center pediatric primary clinicians (PPCs) caring for children with behavioral, emotional, and developmental disorders. Its components are also being used within KKI to standardize the learning of our many trainees who will be addressing the growing crisis of mental health/behavioral disorders in childhood in the United States. It illustrates use of technology and educational principles to transfer specialized knowledge to interprofessional clinicians and overcome geographic barriers to address health inequities in vulnerable populations.

Step 1: Problem Identification and General Needs Assessment

Problem Identification	• 17% of US children have a disability[1] and 10% to 20% have a disorder of behavior or mental health.[2] The top five chronic conditions of childhood are included within these two categories.[3]
	• This problem is compounded by a workforce shortage of neurodevelopmental, developmental, and behavioral[4] or child and adolescent psychiatry subspecialists. There is one board-certified subspecialist for every 11,000 children with a disability in the United States,[5] and these subspecialists are concentrated in urban areas around academic centers, leaving large rural areas of the country without access to their expertise.
	• The underpreparedness of the general pediatric workforce to meet the developmental and mental health care needs of this vulnerable population also contributes to the problem. In a survey of practicing pediatricians, only 31% felt comfortable caring for children with developmental disorders without the help of a subspecialist, and only 7% reported they were comfortable providing care for mental health disorders without a subspecialist.[6]

The general needs assessment combined literature on the crisis in developmental and behavioral/mental health care in children within the United States and the practical experience of our cohort of dedicated clinical educators at our organization, which has six decades of experience with clinical teaching in this field.

Current Approach	• Since 1997, the American Board of Pediatrics (ABP) has required that 1 out of 36 months of pediatrics residency be dedicated to Developmental and Behavioral Pediatrics (DBP).[7,8] However, the developmental and behavioral rotations vary tremendously in breadth and depth across residency programs.[9]

- The ABP also offers subspecialty certification for Neurodevelopmental Disabilities (since 2001), and Developmental and Behavioral Pediatrics (since 2002), but the number of graduates from these programs is insufficient to match the anticipated number of retiring subspecialists in the same programs.[4]

- Practicing pediatricians could choose to improve their own training in disorders of development, behavior, and mental health through continuing medical education (CME) activities such as regional or national conferences, special interest groups sessions, and webinars or learning collaboratives on topics such as autism, developmental disorders, and adverse childhood experiences. The difficulty with these limited learning venues is that they provide instruction regarding specific disorders, but the management of these conditions is nuanced by the frequency of co-occurring developmental and mental health disorders. Longitudinal learning allows for the nuanced context of the treatment of developmental disorders.

Ideal Approach	• Given the identified gap in clinical services to patients, an ideal approach would include blended learning that integrates access to a comprehensive, updated curriculum with actual provision of clinical care to patients. The Extension for Community Healthcare Outcomes (ECHO) format provides a structure for such professional development.[10]
	• Materials developed for CME could also improve developmental and behavioral pediatrics training in residency to better prepare pediatric residents for future practice and teaching.
	• Fellows in subspecialties that encounter higher volumes of children with disabilities, such as neurology, physical medicine and rehabilitation, and neonatology, are also likely to benefit from the materials developed for CME directly as well as in their training of other learners.
	• Materials could also be used to extend training to allied health professional learners and frontline clinicians, such as physical, occupational, speech and language, and behavioral therapists. This training extension to allied health professionals may be of particular value to those practicing in rural or underserved areas.

Step 2: Targeted Needs Assessment

The targeted learners described for this example were PPCs, which included not only pediatricians but also advanced practice providers, licensed social workers, and psychologists. These were recruited from rural areas where children with these disorders have very limited access to subspecialists. As mentioned in the Step 1 "Ideal

Approach," a second group of targeted learners for the larger grant-supported project was KKI "trainees," which represented the next generation of PPCs and subspecialists.

Targeted Learners	• PPC educational needs and priorities were assessed by electronic survey and semi-structured interviews. The survey listed specific developmental, behavioral, and mental health conditions and required participants to prioritize their learning needs on a Likert scale from greatest to least. PPC surveys also assessed the participants' knowledge of and confidence in their identification and management of children with developmental and behavioral disorders and their referral patterns for their patients with these disorders.
	• The top topics of interest to rural PPCs were anxiety disorders, psychotropic medication in preschoolers, adverse childhood experiences, autism, developmental delay, ADHD, and disruptive behavior. These topics correlated with the most frequent concerns prompting preschool referrals to KKI from across the state, supporting the generalizability of educational materials on these topics.
	• Content recommendations followed specifications of the certifying boards of our largest learner groups: general pediatrics, pediatric neurology, neonatology, and neurodevelopmental disabilities.
Targeted Learning Environment	• Longitudinal continuing medical education on development and behavior would allow PPCs to build on current skills while managing children with these disorders, and their co-morbidities, within the local community. The rise of telehealth specialty consultations meant that infrastructure was in place for distance learning for PPCs to address barriers of travel and time away from their practices.
	• Assessment of the experiences of KKI trainees revealed that learners of varied graduate and postgraduate experience and subspecialty backgrounds typically presented simultaneously for educational clinical experiences because the venues for supervised clinical exposure to patients with developmental disabilities were limited. Meeting the needs of such a diverse learning group has been a challenge to clinical educators.[11] There was no standardized curriculum available for teaching the multitude of KKI trainees. Since clinical training experiences were opportunistic, trainees were exposed to only a small subset of live clinical scenarios. It was impossible for program directors to know what had been learned by each trainee during their rotation. Therefore, there was interest in and support for simultaneously developing standardized instructional modules as part of the curriculum for KKI trainees.

Step 3: Goals and Objectives

Goal	The overarching goal is to provide a versatile, graduated learning program to amplify the workforce's capacity by arming PPCs, and the next generation of PPCs and subspecialists, with the requisite knowledge and confidence to diagnose and manage children's developmental, behavioral, and emotional health needs. The health outcome goal is to increase the number of children who receive appropriate care in their medical home[12] and timely access to needed subspecialists.
Specific Measurable Objectives	Some examples of learner objectives for PPCs ("Who") by the end of the 38-week longitudinal ECHO program ("By When") are listed below, organized by type of objective.

Cognitive

- Define diagnostic criteria for at least three developmental and three behavioral disorders.

- Describe at least four examples of co-occurring developmental and behavioral disorders.

- Identify when behavioral disorders are masking underlying developmental diagnoses.

- Identify local resources for the treatment of specific disorders.

Affective

- Express increased confidence in caring for children with developmental and behavioral disorders.

Skills

- Employ screening tests appropriate for specific disorders of behavior and development.

- Interpret school assessments and student plans.

- Recommend appropriate evaluations and services for individual children within the school program.

- Treat common disorders of behavior and development.

Behavior

- Reduce referrals to specialists for patients with common developmental and behavioral disorders, such as ADHD, anxiety, disruptive behavior, or developmental delay, by managing them in the medical home.

- Identify for referral patients with complicated developmental and behavioral disorders who would be best served by subspecialists, such as those with underlying genetic disorders or complex autism or those who have suffered significant emotional trauma.

.   Serve as practice or local experts in development and behavior and provide consultation to colleagues regarding communications with school programs, psychotropic medication use, screening tool use, and local resources.

Step 4: Educational Strategies

The curriculum design has the flexibility to be implemented as a stand-alone learning experience, as a model of just-in-time learning, and as a blended learning experience.

Educational Content	. We developed a modular system for organizing evidence-based, state-of-the-art information on developmental and behavioral topics. Each module includes a presentation with embedded pre-exposure test questions and posttest questions to assess learning. Each module has no more than 20 content slides and contains a final summary of content "pearls" to reinforce the most important teaching points.
	. The modules are grouped in topical chapters (e.g., autism, ADHD, anxiety disorders, developmental delay, language impairments). Within each chapter, the modules are organized into levels, which are semistandardized, as shown in Figure A.1.
	. In the year-long tele-education curriculum for the rural PPCs, the first semester didactics consist of mostly level 1 and 2 modules on the six priority topics: autism, ADHD, anxiety, developmental delay, speech language impairments, and behavioral disorders in early childhood. The second semester consists of level 3 and 4 modules on the same six topics. A one-month summer "mini-mester" allows for completion of up to four modules (e.g., a series on psychopharmacology in early childhood).
Educational Methods	. Following the ECHO model, rural PPCs participating in the weekly videoconference sessions take turns presenting cases relevant to common developmental and behavioral disorders of early childhood in a standardized format. The weekly case is discussed by participants and experts in an "all teach, all learn" approach. Experts summarize the diagnostic impressions and recommendations for the case and then present didactics.
	. During the didactic portion of the weekly videoconference, experts present module content from the designated topic chapter and level. The module pretest questions are embedded in the presentation as a live poll. Posttest questions are presented as a poll at the start of the next didactic session.

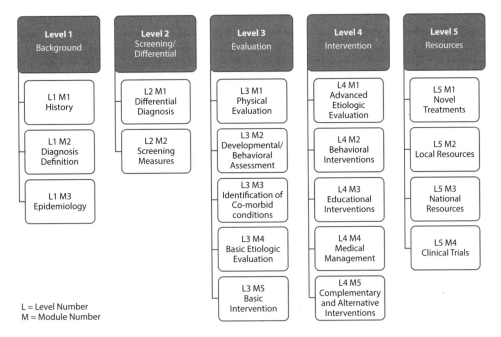

Figure A.1.   Organization of Modules by Level within Each Topical Chapter

- At the conclusion of the session, each participant is emailed a summary of the case, including recommendations, and local or national resources germane to the case. A copy of the didactic pearls is also sent to participants to serve as a review/reference for similar cases in their future practice.

- Modules are also stored on a KKI shared drive so that other faculty can assign modules to trainees relevant to their learning needs and anticipated clinical experiences, and successful completion of such modules can be documented.

Step 5: Implementation

The development and implementation of this curriculum to expand the clinical workforce in rural areas was supported by a four-year grant from the Health Resources and Services Administration (HRSA). Because this involved research as well as teaching, funding supported not only expert faculty and program leadership but also a research coordinator and IT support.

Resources	Personnel

- Principal Investigator: Write and maintain institutional review board (IRB) protocols, manage grant budget, write progress reports for funding agency, author modules, facilitate in person and remote learning sessions, and oversee data collection and analysis.

- Program Director: Determine syllabi for remote learning sessions, coordinate remote participant attendance and case presentation, author modules, facilitate in person and remote learning sessions, and oversee CME accreditation.

- Program Coordinator: Write syllabus, edit all learning modules, enter pre- and post-participation surveys, schedule learning sessions, track learners, distribute surveys, and track CME credit.

- Research Coordinator: Track and enter all data points, including pre- and post-participation responses, cumulative test responses, and survey responses.

- Expert Faculty: Seven to eight authors and editors for module content and delivery; three to four experts of varied backgrounds for each case discussion (e.g., pediatrician, psychiatrist, psychologist, and social worker).

Facilities/Equipment/Supplies

- KKI provided a large telehealth suite, properly fitted with television screens, and appropriate audiovisual equipment for large group videoconferencing.

- Project ECHO provided videoconferencing software.

Support	HRSA grant helped gain in-kind KKI support and protect faculty time. Research questions generated data to support applications for funding for future years.
Administration	See administrative responsibilities shared by personnel listed above.
Barriers	Recruitment of practicing pediatric clinicians was the first barrier. This was initially addressed by visiting rural primary care practices to garner interest in the program. Once the program was implemented, additional participants joined the program by "word of mouth" report of the value of the program.
Introduction of the Curriculum	The pilot program launched in March 2017 and included eight pediatric primary care clinicians in rural Maryland and in school-based health centers. This pilot met weekly by remote videoconferencing for 14 weeks.
	At the completion of week 14, participant feedback recommended that the longitudinal course be designed to encompass a full academic year of weekly meetings. Subsequent programs lasted an average of 38 weeks.

Step 6: Evaluation and Assessment

Users and Uses	• Learners (to monitor own growth)
	• Faculty (to plan future sessions)
	• Curriculum developers (to refine module content for relevance and accuracy)
	• Grant funders (to evaluate return on investment)
	• KKI administration (to base decisions about future funding support)
Resources	• HRSA funding
	• Institutional faculty support for research endeavors (e.g., statistical analysis resources)
Evaluation Questions and Evaluation Design	1. What are the learning priorities of the participants?
	2. Does the curriculum improve the participant's knowledge on topics of development, behavior, and mental health in early childhood?
	3. Are weekly learning objectives being met to the learners' satisfaction?
	4. Does the weekly longitudinal remote CME program improve the participants' confidence in caring for young children with developmental, behavioral, or mental health disorders?
	5. Does participation in the weekly longitudinal remote CME program change the practice of participants regarding the frequency with which they manage children with developmental, behavioral, or mental health disorder without the assistance of a subspecialist?
Evaluation Design	1. $O\text{-} \text{-} \text{-} \text{-} \text{-} \text{-} \text{-} \text{-} \text{-} \text{-} \text{-} X$
	2. $O_1 \text{-} \text{-} \text{-} X_1 \text{-} \text{-} \text{-} O_2$
	3. $\quad\quad X_1 \text{-} \text{-} \text{-} O$
	4. $O_1 \text{-} \text{-} \text{-} X_1 \text{-} \text{-} \text{-} O_2$
	5. $O_1 \text{-} \text{-} \text{-} \text{-} \text{-} \text{-} \text{-} \text{-} \text{-} \text{-} \text{-} X \text{-} \text{-} \text{-} \text{-} \text{-} \text{-} O_2$
Measurement Methods	1. Pre-participation surveys provide feedback about the participants' knowledge and confidence in caring for specific developmental, behavioral, and mental health disorders in early childhood. Embedded polls and open-ended questions provide ongoing formative information about participant learning goals and needs.

2. Precontent exposure multiple-choice questions were embedded in the didactic presentations. Individual and aggregate poll results were collected through Poll Everywhere. Postcontent exposure question results were also collected for individuals and in aggregate through polling.

3. At the completion of each session, the learning objectives are displayed on the final slide, and participants respond via poll to the question "How well were the learning objectives met?" using a five-point Likert scale ranging from "poorly" to "excellent."

4. Post-participation surveys (which included retro pre-participation assessments) assessed the participants' ratings of knowledge and confidence in caring for young children with developmental, behavioral, and mental health disorders using four-point Likert scales ranging from "no knowledge" to "a great deal of knowledge" and "not at all confident" to "very confident."

5. Post-participation satisfaction was an open text box response to the question "How has participating in this program impacted you and your work?"

Ethical Concerns	• As this was conducted as a research study, IRB approval was obtained prior to any data collection.
	• Each videoconferencing session offers participants AMA Category 1 credit, so individual participation needs to be tracked.
	• Individual and aggregate pre- and post-exposure performance are collected using polling software and are recorded by the research coordinator in a separate, secure evaluation database.
	• Results are presented in aggregate and in ways that protect individual participant's confidentiality.
Data Collection	• Pre- and post-participation survey data is collected electronically and recorded in the secure evaluation database by the research coordinator.
Data Analysis	1. Comparison analysis is done in aggregate for each longitudinal cohort.
	2. A paired t-test was used to determine statistical significance of knowledge gains by topic and topic group (developmental, behavioral, or mental health).
	3. Pre-post knowledge and confidence and practice patterns were analyzed using descriptive statistics.
	4. A paired Wilcoxon Signed Rank test was used to assess statistical significance of changes in confidence.
Reporting of Results	1. In addition to confirming interest in and need for instruction on the topics previously prepared, open-ended feedback identified additional topics which were added to subsequent courses

(see "Curriculum Maintenance and Enhancement," below, for examples).

2. Results of the longitudinal pre-/post-question results showed a statistically significant ($p < 0.001$) gain in knowledge measured by the percent of questions answered correctly.

3. When asked to rank on a five-point Likert scale whether the modules met the stated objectives, 95% of respondents answered "very well or excellent."

4. On a three-point Likert scale, there was a statistically significant increase in the PPCs level of confidence, from 1.82 pre-participation to 2.52 at the end of the program ($p < 0.001$). Prior to participation, for developmental disorders, 18.8% of PPCs reported deferring to specialists, and 17.5% reported managing them independently. Following participation, only 1.7% of PPCs deferred developmental concerns to subspecialists, and 38.3% reported managing them independently. For mental health conditions, prior to participation, 16.8% of PPCs deferred children to subspecialists, and 39.3% managed these conditions independently. Following participation in the longitudinal program, only 2.9% of PPCs continued to defer mental health concerns, and 53.33% reported managing them independently.

5. Responses to the open text box response to the question "How has participating in this program impacted you and your work?" were qualitatively analyzed, and the positive responses encouraged us to continue the program.

Curriculum Maintenance and Enhancement

Understanding the Curriculum	• In addition to being implemented with the rural PPCs, the curricular elements were also used to enhance didactic instruction for a wider variety of trainees, specifically future PPCs and subspecialists being trained at KKI.
	• Some trainees traversed the modules longitudinally in sequence from level 1 to level 5, working up to the level appropriate for their desired level of expertise. Other trainees sent to KKI for a targeted cross-sectional experience were assigned specific modules to cover in preparation for their planned clinical experience.
	• Assessment questions built into the structure of the modules provided data across different learners. These could then be combined with assessments of clinical skills development and application in the clinical environment for trainees.

- Such information helped to improve the module content and questions used in the CME program for subsequent cycles.

Management of Change	- *2017–2018*: Implementation over a full academic year: Fall semester covered levels 1 and 2 modules on screening, assessment, and early identification of developmental and behavioral disorders. Spring semester included level 3 and 4 modules as PPCs advanced to assessing co-morbidities and treatment of those disorders. At participant request, we added a four-week "mini-mester" on psychopharmacology in early childhood during the summer.

- *2018–2019:* The fall semester began with a new five-week mini-series on the epidemiology, epigenetics, and developmental and behavioral consequences of intrauterine substance exposure in early childhood, then continued with general developmental and behavioral topics. Modules followed the same curriculum design and levels 1–3 were covered. Two new groups of learners were recruited: PPCs from West Virginia via outreach through the American Academy of Pediatrics and health profession students placed in Maryland Area Health Education Centers (AHEC) as part of an educational program. The AHEC Scholars were not registered participants in the ECHO, as they were training in the primary care setting but not yet practicing. At the conclusion of each weekly session, the faculty offered to continue the videoconference for the AHEC Scholars to ask questions about cases or learning material.

- *2019–2020:* PPCs and AHEC Scholars continued in the same curriculum design, with levels 1 and 2 didactic modules in the first semester and levels 3 and 4 content at the start of the second semester. In mid-March 2020, the ECHO sessions continued through the COVID-19 pandemic but prompted changes in educational content for the second semester.

- Having the relationships, teleconferencing infrastructure, and module/level organizational structure in place facilitated an agile response to the pandemic and quick dissemination of newly desired expert knowledge effectively to frontline practice.

Networking Innovation and Scholarly Activity	- In mid-March 2020, the COVID-19 pandemic required our PPC participants to incorporate telemedicine into their regular practices. The PPCs continued attending the ECHO program and utilized those networking relationships. The time typically spent on didactics was replaced during the first two weeks of the pandemic with discussions of telehealth service delivery.

- It became immediately evident that the cases presented early after the start of the pandemic were related to the developmental and behavioral consequences of abrupt school closure; difficulties with online learning; interruption of behavioral and educational services; isolation from teachers, friends, and extended family; and the anxiety of the pandemic.

- New modules were written to address the behavioral and emotional implications of the pandemic in childhood, as well the educational rights of children with disabilities during the pandemic.

Dissemination

The core faculty involved in the Kennedy Krieger Curriculum have

- presented lectures and workshops on the curriculum design nationally and internationally, and
- authored one publication on the implementation of parts of this curriculum for learners of varied levels and disciplines.[11]

This tele-education model can reach additional pediatricians and others whose previous training did not fully equip them for managing developmental, behavioral, and mental health disorders in practice, particularly those in workforce shortage areas, such as rural areas of the United States.

The module resources can also be made accessible to program directors in general pediatrics and in pediatric subspecialty programs whose trainees' future practices will require an understanding of developmental disabilities and behavioral and mental health disorders.

REFERENCES CITED

1. Benjamin Zablotsky et al., "Prevalence and Trends of Developmental Disabilities among Children in the United States: 2009–2017," *Pediatrics* 144, no. 4 (2019), https://doi.org/10.1542/peds.2019-0811.
2. Carol Weitzman and Lynn Wegner, "Promoting Optimal Development: Screening for Behavioral and Emotional Problems," *Pediatrics* 135, no. 2 (2015): 384–95, https://doi.org/10.1542/peds.2014-3716.
3. Amy J. Houtrow et al., "Changing Trends of Childhood Disability, 2001–2011," *Pediatrics* 134, no. 3 (2014): 530–38, https://doi.org/10.1542/peds.2014-0594.
4. Carolyn Bridgemohan et al., "A Workforce Survey on Developmental-Behavioral Pediatrics," *Pediatrics* 141, no. 3 (2018), https://doi.org/10.1542/peds.2017-2164.
5. American Board of Medical Subspecialties, "ABMS Subspecialty Board Certification Report," accessed June 7, 2021, https://www.abms.org/wp-content/uploads/2020/11/ABMS-Board-Certification-Report-2019-2020.pdf.
6. Gary L. Freed et al., "Recently Trained General Pediatricians: Perspectives on Residency Training and Scope of Practice," *Pediatrics* 123 Suppl 1 (2009): S38–43, https://doi.org/10.1542/peds.2008-1578J.
7. "The Future of Pediatric Education II: Organizing Pediatric Education to Meet the Needs of Infants, Children, Adolescents, and Young Adults in the 21st Century. A Collaborative Project of the Pediatric Community. Task Force on the Future of Pediatric Education," *Pediatrics* 105, no. 1 Pt 2 (2000): 157–212.

8. Robert L. Johnson et al., "Final Report of the FOPE II Education of the Pediatrician Work-group," *Pediatrics* 106, no. 5 (2000): 1175–98.

9. Sarah M. Horwitz et al., "Is Developmental and Behavioral Pediatrics Training Related to Perceived Responsibility for Treating Mental Health Problems?" *Academic Pediatrics* 10, no. 4 (2010): 252–59, https://doi.org/10.1016/j.acap.2010.03.003.

10. Carrol Zhou et al., "The Impact of Project ECHO on Participant and Patient Outcomes: A Systematic Review," *Academic Medicine* 91, no. 10 (2016): 1439–61, https://doi.org/10.1097/acm.0000000000001328.

11. Mary L. O'Connor Leppert et al., "Teaching to Varied Disciplines and Educational Levels Simultaneously: An Innovative Approach in a Neonatal Follow-Up Clinic," *Medical Teacher* 40, no. 4 (2018): 400–406, https://doi.org/10.1080/0142159x.2017.1408898.

12. Medical Home Initiatives for Children with Special Needs Project Advisory Committee, American Academy of Pediatrics, "The Medical Home," *Pediatrics* 110 (2002): 184–86, https://doi.org/10.1542/peds.110.1.184.

Curricular, Faculty Development, and Funding Resources

Patricia A. Thomas, MD, and David E. Kern, MD, MPH

Lists of cited references and annotated general references appear at the end of each chapter. These lists provide the reader with access to predominantly published resources on curriculum development and evaluation. Recognizing that most people begin searches for information by looking at *online resources*, this appendix provides a selected list of online information resources for curriculum development, including content, faculty development, and funding resources. Since online information is frequently in flux, we chose in this edition to provide a few examples of each category here. In the experience of the editors, these examples are the most useful and stable over time. The list prioritizes open-source materials, although some organizations and websites require membership or registration. The appendix is directed to physician education, but many resources can be used across the health professions.

CURRICULAR RESOURCES

When searching for additional resources related to medical education curricula, we recommend the following approach:

a. Review websites and publications of the major accrediting bodies for standards that might apply to the curriculum once implemented and for other resources.

b. Review resources and organizations devoted to particular topics or fields.

c. Review general educational resources within the relevant health profession.

d. Review general educational resources beyond health professions education.

Many of these organizations sponsor meetings and peer-reviewed publications, a potential resource for the dissemination of the curriculum or its evaluation.

Oversight, Credentialing, and Accreditation Organizations

- *Accreditation Commission for Education in Nursing (ACEN):* Recognized as the accrediting body for all types of nursing education, from practical to doctorate level, in the United States
- *Accreditation Council for Continuing Medical Education (ACCME):* A voluntary accreditation body for activities related to continuing medical education; it sets the standards for qualifying educational programs
- *Accreditation Council for Graduate Medical Education (ACGME):* Accredits clinical residency training programs in the United States
- *Accreditation Council for Pharmacy Education (ACPE):* Recognized by US Department of Education for accreditation of professional pharmacy degrees
- *Accreditation Review Commission on Education for the Physician Assistant, Inc. (ARC-PA):* Sets standards and evaluates programs in physician assistant education in the territorial United States
- *American Medical Association (AMA):* Largest professional organization of physicians in the United States; AMA Council on Medical Education formulates educational policy and makes recommendations to the AMA; AMA launched the Accelerating Change in Medical Education Initiative in 2013 (created a consortium of grant-funded medical schools and residency programs to transform physician education)
- *American Osteopathic Association (AOA):* Charged with accreditation of predoctoral doctor of osteopathy (DO) degrees in the United States
- *Association of American Medical Colleges (AAMC):* Represents 172 US and Canadian medical schools and hundreds of teaching hospitals and health systems, as well as professional societies
- *Educational Commission for Foreign Medical Graduates (ECFMG):* Assesses readiness (through its program of certification) of international medical graduates to enter residency or fellowship programs in the United States that are accredited by the ACGME
- *General Medical Council (GMC):* Registers and provides oversight for all practicing physicians in the United Kingdom and sets the standards for undergraduate and postgraduate training in the United Kingdom
- *Health Professions Accreditors Collaborative (HPAC):* Brought multiple health professions accrediting bodies together (when founded in 2014) to address the IPEC Core Competencies (see below)
- *Joint Accreditation for Continuing Education:* Accredits organizations who meet criteria for *interprofessional and teamwork* education as providers of continuous professional development (CPD) programs for dentistry, medicine, nursing, optometry, physician assistant, and social work
- *Liaison Committee on Medical Education (LCME):* Joint committee of the AMA and the AAMC (above) recognized by US Department of Education as official accreditation body for MD degree

- *Society for Simulation in Healthcare (SSIH):* Provides accreditation for simulation centers and credentialing for simulation professionals
- *World Federation for Medical Education (WFME):* Publishes global standards for medical education; maintains *World Directory of Medical Schools*

Topic-Related Resources and Organizations

Basic Science

- *American Association for Anatomy:* International society of anatomy educators across the health professions
- *International Association of Medical Science Educators (IAMSE):* An international organization concerned with basic science medical education

Bioethics and Humanities

- *American Society of Bioethics and Humanities (ASBH):* Includes multidisciplinary and interdisciplinary professionals in academic and clinical bioethics and medical humanities
- *Arnold P. Gold Foundation:* Supports the integration of humanism in health care
- *Public Responsibility in Medicine and Research (PRIM&R):* A community of research administration and oversight individuals, with a goal of advancing ethical standards in conduct of biomedical, behavioral, and social science research

Clinical Sciences

- *Alliance for Clinical Education:* An umbrella organization for seven specialty medical student clerkship organizations
- *Consortium of Longitudinal Integrated Clerkships (CLIC):* An international organization of educators dedicated to implementation and research on the longitudinal integrated clerkship for medical students

Curriculum developers working in a particular clerkship or subspecialty discipline should review that specialty's website (see "Clinical Specialties," below) for developed core curricula that have been nationally peer-reviewed.

Communication and Clinical Skills

- *Academy of Communication in Healthcare (ACH) and International Association for Communication in Healthcare (EACH):* Organizations dedicated to improving communication and relationships in health care; they offer numerous resources in these areas
- *Clinical Skills Evaluation Collaboration (CSEC):* Jointly sponsored by the ECFMG and the National Board of Medical Examiners (NBME) to further the development and implementation of clinical skills assessments
- *Directors of Clinical Skills Course (DOCS):* Founded to promote scholarship in teaching clinical skills across the continuum
- *Society of Bedside Medicine:* Dedicated to the goal of fostering a culture of bedside medicine; links closely with humanistic aspects of bedside medicine
- *Society of Ultrasound in Medical Education (SUSME):* Founded to promote the use of ultrasound in medical education

Clinical Specialties (Selected List)

Curriculum developers should contact *professional societies in their relevant specialty/subspecialty* that are not listed below, because these societies may maintain curricular guidelines, curricular materials, or other resources helpful in developing specific curricula.

- *Academic Pediatric Association (APA)*
- *Alliance for Academic Internal Medicine (AAIM):* Consortium of five academically focused specialty organizations representing departments of internal medicine at medical schools and teaching hospitals in the United States and Canada
- *American College of Emergency Physicians (ACEP)*
- *American College of Physicians (ACP):* The largest professional organization for internists in the United States
- *Association for Surgical Education (ASE)*
- *Association of Professors of Gynecology and Obstetrics (APGO)*
- *Center to Advance Palliative Care (CAPC)*
- *Consortium of Neurology Clerkship Directors / The American Academy of Neurology*
- *Council on Medical Student Education in Pediatrics (COMSEP)*
- *Palliative Care Network of Wisconsin:* Site includes content from the *End of Life / Palliative Care Resource Center*, including core competencies, learning resources, learning assessments, and survey instruments (*American Academy of Hospice and Palliative Medicine (AAHPM)* and *National Hospice and Palliative Care Organization (NHPCO)* also provide educational resources in this content)
- *Portal of Geriatric Online Education (POGOe):* Online clearinghouse for educators
- *Society of General Internal Medicine (SGIM)*
- *Society of Teachers in Family Medicine (STFM)*

Preventive Medicine and Public Health

- *American Public Health Association (APHA)*
- *Association for Prevention Teaching and Research (APTR)*
- *Centers for Disease Control and Prevention (CDC)*
- *World Health Organization (WHO)*

General Education Resources within Health Professions

- *Association for Medical Education in Europe (AMEE):* International organization; publishes *Medical Teacher*, the e-journal *MedEdPublish*, and AMEE guides
- *Association for the Study of Medical Education (ASME)*
- *Association of Standardized Patient Educators (ASPE):* International organization of simulation educators promoting the advancement of standardized patient methodology for teaching, assessment, and research
- *Best Evidence Medical Education (BEME):* Provides systematic reviews
- *MedEdPORTAL:* Provides online access to peer-reviewed medical education curricular resources across the continuum of medical education
- *National Board of Medical Examiners (NBME):* Administers the US Medical Licensing Examination (USMLE), provides resources to build customized assessments
- *Society for Academic Continuing Medical Education (SACME):* North American organization that promotes research, scholarship, and evaluation and development

of continuing medical education (CME) and continuous professional development (CPD)

Educational and Information Technology

With the rapid diffusion of technology-enhanced learning in health professions education, there are numerous hardware and software applications potentially available to curriculum developers. When considering incorporation of technology into a curricular effort, we recommend that educators begin by consulting their institutional office of information technology. These offices often include instructional designers who can partner with the content experts and recommend best use of technology, not only from cost and feasibility perspectives but also from a regulatory issues standpoint, such as learner privacy (often an issue with software logins) and accessibility. Many educational organizations listed in this appendix have interest groups or sections committed to educational technology and can also be a source of expertise and faculty development. A few suggestions follow:

- *AAMC Group on Information Resources, Education Technology Work Group*
- *AMEE Technology Enhanced Learning (TEL) Committee*
- *American Medical Informatics Association (AMIA)*
- *EDUCAUSE:* Nonprofit association in the United States whose mission is to advance higher education through the use of information technology
- *MedBiquitous (www.medbiq.org):* International community of technology experts and innovators that has developed open technology standards for health care and health professions education

Interprofessional Education

- *Centre for Interprofessional Education:* A UK-based nonprofit community dedicated to improving health care through collaborative practice
- *Interprofessional Education Collaborative (IPEC):* Developed and publishes the *Core Competencies for Interprofessional Collaborative Practice*
- *National Center for Interprofessional Practice and Education:* Public-private organization dedicated to improving health care delivery through education

General Educational Resources beyond Health Professions

- *American Education Research Association (AERA)*
- *Carnegie Foundation for the Advancement of Teaching*
- *Educational Resource Information Center (ERIC):* Sponsored by the Institute of Education Research, the research arm of the US Department of Education, provides online access to a bibliography of educational research
- *Team-Based Learning Collaborative (TBLC):* International collaborative of educators devoted to advancing the use of team-based learning (TBL) method at all levels of education

FACULTY DEVELOPMENT RESOURCES

Listed below are selected programs, courses, and written resources that address the development of clinician-educators in general and educators for specific content areas. As medical education has become increasingly professionalized, many educators are seeking advanced degrees in education, and example degree programs are also noted. Individuals should also contact *professional societies* in their field, which frequently offer workshops, courses, certificates, and fellowships, and *health professional or educational schools* in their area, which may offer faculty development programs or courses.

Other potential resources are local offices of faculty development and academies of medical educators, which have become increasingly common.[1] In a 2013 report, 53 out of 136 schools hosted faculty academies.[2] The academy structures vary, but most support educators with faculty development programs (often with fellowships and/or innovation grants for junior faculty), enable research and scholarship among members, and mentoring. Several include interprofessional faculty.

Faculty Development Programs/Courses

In addition to the organizations listed above, many of which sponsor faculty development courses, workshops, and fellowships, curriculum developers may want to explore the following programs:

- *Center for Ambulatory Teaching Excellence (CATE)*
- *Essential Skills in Medical Education (ESME) and Masterclasses (AMEE)*
- *Foundation for Advancement of International Medical Education & Research (FAIMER) Institute and fellowships*
- *Harvard Macy Institute*
- *Johns Hopkins University Faculty Development Program*
- *McMaster University Faculty in Health Sciences Program for Faculty Development*
- *Medical Education Fellowship (IAMSE; see under "Basic Science," above)*
- *Medical Education Research Certificate (MERC) Program (AAMC)*
- *Stanford University Faculty Development Program*
- *Teaching for Quality (Te4Q):* AAMC-sponsored certificate program designed to provide clinical faculty the skills in teaching and learner assessment of *patient safety and quality improvement*

Degree Programs

The number of degree programs in health professions education have increased dramatically in recent decades.[3] Listed below are some of the American programs. In addition to the FAIMER-Keele distance degree, the FAIMER website lists a directory of international degree programs (both master's and PhD level). Interested readers are encouraged to do additional research looking for both Master of Education and Master of Science degrees.

- *FAIMER-Keele Master's in Health Professions Education*
- *Harvard Medical School:* Master's in Medical Education Program
- *Johns Hopkins University*: Master of Education in the Health Professions

- *Loma Linda University School of Allied Health Professions:* Graduate certificate or Master of Science in Health Professions Education
- *New York University School of Medicine and the NYU Steinhardt School of Education:* Master of Science in Health Professions Education
- *University of Cincinnati College of Education and the Division of Community and General Pediatrics at Cincinnati Children's Hospital:* Certificate in Medical Education or Master of Medical Education (MEd)
- *University of Illinois College of Medicine at Chicago*: Master of Health Professions Education (MHPE)
- *University of Michigan School of Education and the Medical School of the University of Michigan:* Master of Education with a Concentration in Medical and Professional Education
- *University of Pittsburgh, Institute for Clinical Research Education:* Master of Science in Medical Education
- *University of Southern California, Keck School of Medicine in collaboration with the schools of dentistry and pharmacy*: Master of Academic Medicine and Certificate in Academic Medicine

FUNDING RESOURCES

Funds for most medical education programs are provided through the sponsoring institution from tuition, clinical, or other revenues or government support of the educational mission of the institution. When asked to take on curriculum development, maintenance, or evaluation activities, it is advisable, before accepting, to elicit the requestor's goals, to think through what educational and evaluation strategies will be required (Chapters 5 and 7) to achieve and assess attainment of those or further refined goals (Chapter 4) and the resources that will be required for successful implementation (Chapter 6) and maintenance (Chapter 8), and to speak to others with experience and perspective for advice. One can then negotiate more effectively with one's institution for the support that will be required to do the job well.[4,5] Institutional funding, however, is usually limited. It is often desirable to obtain additional funding to protect faculty time, hire support staff, and enhance the quality of the educational intervention and evaluation. Unfortunately, the funding provided by external sources for direct support of the development, maintenance, and evaluation of specific educational programs is small when compared with sources that provide grant support for clinical and basic research. Some government and private entities that do provide direct support for health professional education, usually in targeted areas, are listed below. Additional funding can not only increase the quality of the educational intervention but also enhance the quality of related educational research,[6] increase the likelihood of publication,[7] and add to the academic portfolio of the curriculum developer.

General Information

Being familiar with one or two directories, and setting up regular notification of opportunities in your area(s) of interest, can facilitate the acquisition of funding. Librarians/informationists at your institution can also assist in locating funding and instruct you in resources to which your library subscribes. Below are a few directories subscribed to by many institutions.

- *The Foundation Directory Online:* Guide to foundations; lists funding opportunities from US foundations, corporate giving programs, public charities, and a growing number of international sources
- *Grant Forward:* Large US-focused database of funding opportunities from foundations, federal and state agencies, and universities; currently only institutional memberships
- *Pivot:* Database that provides a comprehensive global source of funding opportunities and scholarly profiles to match researchers with financial partners and collaborators (to create an account, you must be affiliated with an institution that subscribes to Pivot)

US Government Resources

Government grants, at least in the United States, provide generous funding. Applying for government grants in the United States is, however, a very competitive process. Having a mentor who has served on a review board or been funded by the type of grant being applied for is strongly recommended (see "Recommendations for Preparing a Grant Application," below). It is advisable for individuals from other countries to acquaint themselves with the government funding resources within their countries.

- *Agency for Healthcare Research and Quality (AHRQ):* Mission is to produce evidence to make health care safer, higher quality, more accessible, equitable, and affordable, and to make sure that the evidence is understood and used; sometimes research on promotion of improvements in clinical practice and dissemination activities can be framed in curriculum development terms
- *Federal Grants Wire:* Free resource that provides a directory for federal grants; includes a search function
- *Fogarty International Center:* Part of the *National Institutes of Health* (the mission of which is to support global health); Center supports research and research training focused on low- to middle-income nations; curriculum developers with a focus on international health should look at this organization's website
- *Fund for the Improvement of Postsecondary Education (FIPSE):* Nonmedical focus on precollege-, college-, and graduate-level curricula and faculty development to improve quality of and access to education; premedical or medical curricula that fit the criteria for specific programs could conceivably be funded
- *Grants.gov:* Guide to US government grants
- *Health Resources and Services Administration (HRSA), Bureau of Health Professions (BHPr):* Provides funding for training programs in primary care medicine, nursing, public health, oral health, behavioral health, geriatrics, and programs that support a diverse health workforce by providing education and training opportunities to individuals from disadvantaged backgrounds
- *National Institutes of Health (NIH):* Most funding is directed toward clinical, basic science, or disease-oriented research and awarded through disease-oriented institutes; sometimes educational research and development can be targeted toward specific disease processes and fall within the purview of one of the institutes; NIH's interest in translating research into practice may create opportunities for educators to incorporate educational initiatives into grant proposals; R25 (Education Projects), K07 (Academic/Teacher Award), and K30 (Clinical Research Curriculum Awards)

awards provide opportunity for curriculum development; website has a search function

- *National Science Foundation (NSF):* Funds research and education in science and engineering through grants, contracts, and cooperative agreements; might be a source for basic science curricula; ADVANCE program focuses on increasing participation and advancement of women in academic science and engineering careers
- *Veterans Administration (VA):* Faculty at VA hospitals in the United States should explore VA career development awards, as well as funding opportunities for individual projects

Private Foundations

Although generally smaller in amount, searching for funding from private foundations (see "General Information," above) is more likely to locate opportunities aligned with the curriculum developer's goals. Applying for funds from nongovernmental foundations, while usually less competitive than applying for government grants, is still quite competitive. It behooves applicants to discuss their ideas with a person at the foundation of interest, talk to individuals who have successfully competed for funding from it, review previously funded projects, and seek a mentor familiar with the foundation (see "Recommendations for Preparing a Grant Application," below.) Below are selected foundations that may fund curricular efforts in health professional education. Foundations that focus upon specific geographic locations or regions within the United States are not listed. Curriculum developers should also search for foundations/funding opportunities specific to their geographic area.

- *Arnold P. Gold Foundation:* In the past has supported projects related to humanism, ethics, and compassion
- *Arthur Vining Davis Foundations:* Current areas of focus include private higher education, public educational media, and palliative care (grant proposals are considered only from designated partners)
- *Cambia Health Foundation:* Has a Sojourns Scholar Leadership Program Award to support development of leaders in palliative care; includes professional development and project plan
- *Commonwealth Fund:* Aims to promote a high-performing health care system that achieves better access, improved quality, and greater efficiency, particularly for society's most vulnerable; predominantly supports health services research, but some needs assessment, educational intervention studies, and conferences might be supported
- *Hearst Foundations:* Funds programs in the areas of culture, education, health, and social service; funds programs designed to enhance skills and increase the number of practitioners and educators across roles in healthcare and to increase access for low-income populations; includes faculty development
- *John A. Hartford Foundation:* In the past has funded numerous programs related to geriatrics and health services; normally makes grants to organizations in the United States that have tax-exempt status and to state colleges and universities, not to individuals
- *Josiah Macy Jr. Foundation:* Focus on medical education; priorities change over time; two grant programs: Board Grants (one to three years of funding, starts with letter of inquiry) and discretionary President's Grants (one year or less in duration) in priority

areas; also has Macy Faculty Scholar program in medicine and nursing to implement an educational change project in one's institution

- *McDonnell Foundation:* Reviews proposals submitted in response to foundation-initiated programs and calls for proposals; a focus area has been "Understanding Human Cognition"; recent program area was "Teachers as Learners"
- *National Board of Medical Examiners (NBME) / Stemmler Fund:* NBME accepts proposals from LCME or AOA accredited medical schools; goal of Stemmler Fund is to support research or development of innovative assessment/evaluation methods
- *Retirement Research Foundation (RRF):* Mission is to improve quality of life for US elders; one funding area is professional education and training projects with regional or national impact for older Americans

Other Funding Resources

- *Fees/tuition:* For curricula serving multiple institutions, a user or subscriber fee can be charged.[8–10] Charging tuition may be an option for some programs (faculty may have tuition benefits).[11] Continuing education credits can be offered for curricula that qualify.
- *Institutional grant programs:* Educational institutions often have small grant programs available internally, which are usually less competitive than those from external sources. You should learn about grants offered by your own institution.
- *Professional organizations:* For specialty-oriented curricula, the curriculum developer should contact the relevant specialty organization. Below are a few examples of professional organizations offering education-related grants.
    - *The American College of Rheumatology's Rheumatology Research Foundation* offers a Clinician Scholar Educator Award.
    - *The American Medical Association Accelerating Change in Medical Education Initiative* was launched with undergraduate medical education in 2013 with a competitive grants program. Following two additional cycles, the number of consortium schools has increased to 37. The initiative continues to offer small annual grants to member schools as well as additional innovation awards. In 2019, the initiative was expanded to graduate medical education with the *Reimagining Residency* grant program.
    - *The American Medical Association Joan F. Giambalvo Fund for the Advancement of Women* provides small scholarships to support research related to women in the medical profession.
    - *The Association for Surgical Education (ASE) Foundation* of the Association for Surgical Education (ASE) funds *Center for Excellence in Surgical Education, Research and Training (CESERT)* one- to two-year grants.
    - *The Association of Professors of Gynecology and Obstetrics (APGO)* has a Medical Education Endowment Fund Grant Program that is able to fund curricular projects.
    - *The Radiologic Society of North America* has (1) an *Education Scholar Grant* that provides funding for educators whose focus is advancing radiologic education with an international scope, and (2) an *Education Research Development Grant* that encourages improvement of radiology education by funding all areas of education research, including the development of new education programs and teaching method pilot studies.

- *The Society for Academic Continuing Medical Education (SACME)* offers, every other year, a two-year *Phil R. Manning Research Award* for original research related to physician lifelong learning and physician change.
- *The Society for Academic Emergency Medicine Foundation (SAEMF)* has funded projects in curriculum development.
- *Pharmaceutical Corporations:* These corporations sometimes have foundations that will fund curricular projects.

Recommendations for Preparing a Grant Application

Based upon our experience, we offer the following recommendations:

- Identify focused goals that are based on your own passionate interests and could help you achieve your broader goals.
- Identify potential funding sources and opportunities (see above).
  - Chances are usually better if a funding agency has called for applications in a specific area than if you present an unsolicited idea to a funding agency. However, it does not hurt to ask an agency/program officer if they would consider a proposal on a topic of importance to you. Foundations may invite a short letter of inquiry before inviting a full application. This is time saving for both the applicant and the foundation.
  - Faculty development awards generally provide both partial salary support and some funding for research expenses. There is usually considerable flexibility in terms of the research project(s) the applicants may propose (i.e., unsolicited ideas for research are usually part of the process, although the award may specify a general area of focus).
- Get additional information, instructions, and application materials. Review the instructions in detail. Assess the complexity of the application process.
- Decide whether the focus of the grant award is appropriate and the potential financial award is worth the effort. A small grant may take nearly as much effort as a large one, so don't be afraid to think big.
- Identify and discuss the opportunity and the application process with a mentor or colleague who has received funding from this source previously or served in a role for the funding agency/foundation.
- If previous successful proposals are available, review them.
- Identify the most appropriate leader for the application, taking into consideration the skills, experience, and time needed to lead the project, as well as the funding agency's expectations for the leader. (Sometimes, because of curriculum development expertise, you may be asked to play a role in, and/or write part of, a grant for which someone else is principal investigator. For such a role, you are generally written in for partial salary support, which can provide protected time to accomplish the work to which you commit.)
- Assemble a team that has the appropriate combination of expertise. Look for opportunities to connect with colleagues who have been successful in obtaining peer-reviewed funding. Consider including colleagues from outside your own institution as advisors, if not as co-investigators. Aim for a balance between junior and senior team members, keeping in mind that junior colleagues are likely to have more time to spend on a project.

- Develop a list of components for the application and a timetable. Leave plenty of time to complete the process. Allow time for review of the proposal by all team members.
- Determine whether institutional review board (IRB) approval is required, begin the process early, and leave time for IRB review.
- Determine whether letters of support are required or desirable. Contact individuals early, and give them sample letters that they can revise.
- Delegate components of the application process / grant writing to colleagues when appropriate. Assign due dates and follow up. You are responsible for revising and consolidating individual contributions into a persuasive, coherent whole.
- Follow instructions precisely.
- Leave time for approval by your institution's Grants Administration Office (usually about two weeks).
- Grants are usually quite competitive. Put your best effort into the process, and get help/feedback/reviews from others. It is particularly helpful to obtain feedback from someone who was not involved in drafting the proposal.
- Be realistic in predicting needed time commitments, and budget appropriate salary support, whenever possible, to cover this time. Reviewers are likely to be critical of budgets that are unrealistically small or large.
- Be prepared to submit a proposal more than once to get it funded. For most funding agencies, only 20% to 30% (or less) of proposals are funded. Be persistent!
- Look for opportunities to learn more about grant writing (e.g., serve on a study section for a funding agency or take a course on grant writing).

REFERENCES CITED

1. Nancy S. Searle et al., "The Prevalence and Practice of Academies of Medical Educators: A Survey of U.S. Medical Schools," *Academic Medicine* 85, no. 1 (2010): 48–56, https://doi.org/10.1097/ACM.0b013e3181c4846b.
2. "Curriculum Reports: Faculty Academies at U.S. Medical Schools," AAMC, accessed October 5, 2021, https://www.aamc.org/data-reports/curriculum-reports/interactive-data/faculty-academies-us-medical-schools.
3. Ara Tekian and Ilene Harris, "Preparing Health Professions Education Leaders Worldwide: A Description of Masters-Level Programs," *Medical Teacher* 34, no. 1 (2012): 52–58, https://doi.org/10.3109/0142159x.2011.599895.
4. Kenneth W. Thomas, *Introduction to Conflict Management: Improving Performance Using the TKI* (Mountain View, CA: CPP, 2002).
5. Roger Fisher, William L. Ury, and Bruce Patton, *Getting to Yes: Negotiating Agreement without Giving In* (New York: Penguin Books, 2011).
6. Darcy A. Reed et al., "Association between Funding and Quality of Published Medical Education Research," *JAMA* 298, no. 9 (2007): 1002–9, https://doi.org/10.1001/jama.298.9.1002.
7. Darcy A. Reed et al., "Predictive Validity Evidence for Medical Education Research Study Quality Instrument Scores: Quality of Submissions to JGIM's Medical Education Special Issue," *Journal of General Internal Medicine* 23, no. 7 (2008): 903–7, https://doi.org/10.1007/s11606-008-0664-3.
8. Stephen D. Sisson et al., "Internal Medicine Residency Training on Topics in Ambulatory Care: A Status Report," *American Journal of Medicine* 124, no. 1 (2011): 86–90, https://doi.org/10.1016/j.amjmed.2010.09.007.

9. Ultrasound School of North American Rheumatologists (USSONAR), accessed October 5, 2021, https://ussonar.org/.

10. "Med Ed Curriculum Development," Johns Hopkins School of Medicine, accessed October 5, 2021, https://learn.hopkinsmedicine.org/learn/course/external/view/elearning/9/curriculum -development-for-medical-education.

11. "Programs in Curriculum Development," Johns Hopkins Medicine, accessed October 5, 2021, https://www.hopkinsmedicine.org/johns_hopkins_bayview/education_training/continuing _education/faculty_development_program/programs_curriculum_development.html.

Index